Autism
and Pervasive
Developmental
Disorders
SOURCEBOOK

Fourth Edition

Fourth Edition

Autism
and Pervasive
Developmental
Disorders
SOURCEBOOK

*Basic Consumer Health Information about Autism
Spectrum Disorder, and Pervasive Developmental Disorders
such as Asperger Syndrome and Rett Syndrome*

*Along with Facts about Causes, Symptoms, Assessment,
Interventions, Treatments, and Education, Tips for Family
Members and Teachers on the Transition to Adulthood,
a Glossary of Related Terms, and a Directory of
Resources for More Information*

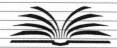

OMNIGRAPHICS

615 Griswold, Ste. 901, Detroit, MI 48226

Bibliographic Note
Because this page cannot legibly accommodate all the copyright notices, the Bibliographic
Note portion of the Preface constitutes an extension of the copyright notice.

* * *

OMNIGRAPHICS
Angela L. Williams, *Managing Editor*
* * *

Library of Congress Cataloging-in-Publication Data

Names: Omnigraphics, Inc., issuing body.

Title: Autism and pervasive developmental disorders sourcebook : basic consumer
health information about autism spectrum disorder, and pervasive developmental
disorders such as asperger syndrome and rett syndrome, along with facts about
causes, symptoms, assessment, interventions, treatments, and education. tips for
family members and teachers on the transition to adulthood, a glossary of related
terms, and a directory of resources for more information.

Description: 4th edition. | Detroit, MI : Omnigraphics, Inc., [2018] | Series:
Health reference series

Identifiers: LCCN 2018042235 (print) | LCCN 2018043142 (ebook) | ISBN
9780780816572 (ebook) | ISBN 9780780816565 (hard cover : alk. paper)

Subjects: LCSH: Autism in children--Popular works. | Developmental disabilities-
-Popular works.

Classification: LCC RJ506.A9 (ebook) | LCC RJ506.A9 A8929 2018 (print) | DDC
618.92/85882--dc23

LC record available at https://lccn.loc.gov/2018042235

Table of Contents

Part III: Identifying and Diagnosing Autism Spectrum Disorders

Part IV: Conditions That May Accompany Autism Spectrum Disorders

Part V: Interventions and Treatments for Autism Spectrum Disorders

Part VI: Education and Autism Spectrum Disorder

Part VII: Living with Autism Spectrum Disorder and Transitioning to Adulthood

Part VIII: Additional Help and Information

Preface

About This Book

The Centers for Disease Control and Prevention (CDC) reports that 1 in 59 children were identified with autism spectrum disorder (ASD). ASD includes autistic disorder, Asperger syndrome, Rett syndrome, childhood disintegrative disorder, and pervasive developmental disorder not otherwise specified. Studies indicate that the prevalence of these neurodevelopmental disabilities, which cause significant problems with social interaction and communication, is increasing. Researchers believe genes, brain dysfunction, and environmental factors play a role in causing ASD. Although there is no cure, early diagnosis and evidence-based interventions currently provide the best long-term outcomes.

Autism and Pervasive Developmental Disorders Sourcebook, Fourth Edition provides updated information about the specific types of ASDs. It explains symptoms, assessment, and diagnosis of ASD and describes the importance of early interventions. Evidence-based behavior, communication, and biomedical interventions are presented, along with educational guidelines for teachers and parents of children with ASD. Support, safety, transition, mental health, and employment information for families and individuals affected by ASD is also provided. The book concludes with a glossary of related terms and a directory of resources offer additional help and information.

How to Use This Book

This book is divided into parts and chapters. Parts focus on broad areas of interest. Chapters are devoted to single topics within a part.

Part One: Overview of Autism Spectrum Disorder describes autistic disorder, Asperger syndrome, Rett syndrome, and pervasive developmental disorder not otherwise specified. A separate chapter reviews the increasing prevalence and the diagnoses made for autism spectrum disorders in the United States.

Part Two: Causes and Risk Factors Associated with Autism Spectrum Disorder reviews causes and risk factors for autism, prenatal inflammation and autism risk, and presents current research about the many genes linked to ASD. Risk factors for ASD—including diseases, vaccines, premature birth, and early brain development risk factors for autism spectrum disorder are discussed.

Part Three: Identifying and Diagnosing Autism Spectrum Disorders describes the range of symptoms and developmental milestones and delays that indicate a need for further assessment of autism spectrum disorders. Developmental screening, medical and genetic tests, and other assessments are explained. The part also talks about speech and language development in children, diagnostic criterias, and measuring autistic intelligence.

Part Four: Conditions That May Accompany Autism Spectrum Disorders provides information about communication difficulties, nonverbal learning disability, seizures, and epilepsy. Genetic disorders that co-occur with ASD—such as Angelman syndrome, fragile X syndrome, Landau-Kleffner syndrome, and Prader-Willi syndrome—are also explained. The part also talks about conditions that may occur with autism spectrum disorder such as thin bones and high growth hormone in boys.

Part Five: Interventions and Treatments for Autism Spectrum Disorder gives detailed information about practices that are often effective for individuals with ASD. Topics include early intervention for children with developmental delays. Communication and behavior therapies such as applied behavior analysis, behavioral management therapy, cognitive behavior therapy, and joint attention therapy are described. Medical treatments, research study participation, communication therapies, and ASD medications are also discussed.

Part Six: Education and Autism Spectrum Disorder describes the special education process and promote social interaction. Separate chapters address secondary school experiences, preparing ASD students for postsecondary education, and teaching lifetime goals.

Part Seven: Living with Autism Spectrum Disorder and Transitioning to Adulthood provides practical information about safety and support for autism spectrum disorders adults focusing on specific concerns such as feeding and toilet training. The part also offers facts about oral care, transition plans, housing, career planning, and job accommodations for adults in the autism spectrum.

Part Eight: Additional Help and Information provides a glossary of terms related to ASDs. A directory of organizations with additional information about autism spectrum disorders is also included.

Bibliographic Note

This volume contains documents and excerpts from publications issued by the following U.S. government agencies: Administration for Children and Families (ACF); Centers for Disease Control and Prevention (CDC); Child Welfare Information Gateway; Effective Health Care Program; *Eunice Kennedy Shriver* National Institute of Child Health and Human Development (NICHD); Genetics Home Reference (GHR); Institute of Education Sciences (IES); National Aeronautics and Space Administration (NASA); National Council on Disability (NCD); National Human Genome Research Institute (NHGRI); National Institute of Dental and Craniofacial Research (NIDCR); National Institute of Environmental Health Sciences (NIEHS); National Institute of Mental Health (NIMH); National Institute of Neurological Disorders and Stroke (NINDS); National Institute of Standards and Technology (NIST); National Institute on Deafness and Other Communication Disorders (NIDCD); National Institutes of Health (NIH); Office of Minority Health (OMH); Office of the Assistant Secretary for Planning and Evaluation (ASPE); U.S. Bureau of Labor Statistics (BLS); U.S. Department of Education (ED); U.S. Department of Health and Human Services (HHS); U.S. Department of Labor (DOL); U.S. Environmental Protection Agency (EPA); U.S. Food and Drug Administration (FDA); and U.S. Office of Personnel Management (OPM).

It may also contain original material produced by Omnigraphics and reviewed by medical documents.

About the Health Reference Series

The *Health Reference Series* is designed to provide basic medical information for patients, families, caregivers, and the general public.

Each volume takes a particular topic and provides comprehensive coverage. This is especially important for people who may be dealing with a newly diagnosed disease or a chronic disorder in themselves or in a family member. People looking for preventive guidance, information about disease warning signs, medical statistics, and risk factors for health problems will also find answers to their questions in the *Health Reference Series*. The *Series*, however, is not intended to serve as a tool for diagnosing illness, in prescribing treatments, or as a substitute for the physician/patient relationship. All people concerned about medical symptoms or the possibility of disease are encouraged to seek professional care from an appropriate healthcare provider.

A Note about Spelling and Style

Health Reference Series editors use *Stedman's Medical Dictionary* as an authority for questions related to the spelling of medical terms and the *Chicago Manual of Style* for questions related to grammatical structures, punctuation, and other editorial concerns. Consistent adherence is not always possible, however, because the individual volumes within the *Series* include many documents from a wide variety of different producers, and the editor's primary goal is to present material from each source as accurately as is possible. This sometimes means that information in different chapters or sections may follow other guidelines and alternate spelling authorities. For example, occasionally a copyright holder may require that eponymous terms be shown in possessive forms (Crohn's disease vs. Crohn disease) or that British spelling norms be retained (leukaemia vs. leukemia).

Medical Review

Omnigraphics contracts with a team of qualified, senior medical professionals who serve as medical consultants for the *Health Reference Series*. As necessary, medical consultants review reprinted and originally written material for currency and accuracy. Citations including the phrase "Reviewed (month, year)" indicate material reviewed by this team. Medical consultation services are provided to the *Health Reference Series* editors by:

Dr. Vijayalakshmi, MBBS, DGO, MD
Dr. Senthil Selvan, MBBS, DCH, MD
Dr. K. Sivanandham, MBBS, DCH, MS (Research), PhD

Our Advisory Board

We would like to thank the following board members for providing initial guidance on the development of this series:

Health Reference Series *Update Policy*

The inaugural book in the *Health Reference Series* was the first edition of *Cancer Sourcebook* published in 1989. Since then, the *Series* has been enthusiastically received by librarians and in the medical community. In order to maintain the standard of providing high-quality health information for the layperson the editorial staff at Omnigraphics felt it was necessary to implement a policy of updating volumes when warranted.

Medical researchers have been making tremendous strides, and it is the purpose of the *Health Reference Series* to stay current with the most recent advances. Each decision to update a volume is made on an individual basis. Some of the considerations include how much new information is available and the feedback we receive from people who use the books. If there is a topic you would like to see added to the update list, or an area of medical concern you feel has not been adequately addressed, please write to:

Managing Editor
Health Reference Series
Omnigraphics
615 Griswold, Ste. 901
Detroit, MI 48226

Part One

Overview of Autism Spectrum Disorder

Chapter 1

What Are Autism Spectrum Disorder and Autistic Disorder?

What Is Autism Spectrum Disorder?

Autism spectrum disorder (ASD) refers to a group of complex neurodevelopment disorders characterized by repetitive and characteristic patterns of behavior and difficulties with social communication and interaction. The symptoms are present from early childhood and affect daily functioning.

The term "spectrum" refers to the wide range of symptoms, skills, and levels of disability in functioning that can occur in people with ASD. Some children and adults with ASD are fully able to perform all activities of daily living while others require substantial support to perform basic activities. The *Diagnostic and Statistical Manual of Mental Disorders (DSM-5)* includes Asperger syndrome (AS), childhood disintegrative disorder (CDD), and pervasive developmental disorders not otherwise specified (PDD-NOS) as part of ASD rather than as separate disorders. A diagnosis of ASD includes an assessment of intellectual disability and language impairment.

This chapter includes text excerpted from "Autism Spectrum Disorder Fact Sheet," National Institute of Neurological Disorders and Stroke (NINDS), October 10, 2018.

ASD occurs in every racial and ethnic group, and across all socio-economic levels. However, boys are significantly more likely to develop ASD than girls. An analysis from the Centers for Disease Control and Prevention (CDC) estimates that 1 in 68 children has ASD.

What Are Some Common Signs of Autism Spectrum Disorder?

Even as infants, children with ASD may seem different, especially when compared to other children their own age. They may become overly focused on certain objects, rarely make eye contact, and fail to engage in typical babbling with their parents. In other cases, children may develop normally until the second or even third year of life, but then start to withdraw and become indifferent to social engagement.

The severity of ASD can vary greatly and is based on the degree to which social communication, insistence of sameness of activities and surroundings, and repetitive patterns of behavior affect the daily functioning of the individual.

Social Impairment and Communication Difficulties

Many people with ASD find social interactions difficult. The mutual give-and-take nature of typical communication and interaction is often particularly challenging. Children with ASD may fail to respond to their names, avoid eye contact with other people, and only interact with others to achieve specific goals. Often children with ASD do not understand how to play or engage with other children and may prefer to be alone. People with ASD may find it difficult to understand other people's feelings or talk about their own feelings.

People with ASD may have very different verbal abilities ranging from no speech at all to speech that is fluent, but awkward and inappropriate. Some children with ASD may have delayed speech and language skills, may repeat phrases, and give unrelated answers to questions. In addition, people with ASD can have a hard time using and understanding nonverbal cues such as gestures, body language, or tone of voice. For example, young children with ASD might not understand what it means to wave goodbye. People with ASD may also speak in flat, robot-like or a sing-song voice about a narrow range of favorite topics, with little regard for the interests of the person to whom they are speaking.

Repetitive and Characteristic Behaviors

Many children with ASD engage in repetitive movements or unusual behaviors such as flapping their arms, rocking from side to side, or twirling. They may become preoccupied with parts of objects like the wheels on a toy truck. Children may also become obsessively interested in a particular topic such as airplanes or memorizing train schedules. Many people with ASD seem to thrive so much on routine that changes to the daily patterns of life—like an unexpected stop on the way home from school—can be very challenging. Some children may even get angry or have emotional outbursts, especially when placed in a new or overly stimulating environment.

What Disorders Are Related to Autism Spectrum Disorder?

Certain known genetic disorders are associated with an increased risk for autism, including fragile X syndrome (FXS) (which causes intellectual disability) and tuberous sclerosis (which causes benign tumors to grow in the brain and other vital organs)—each of which results from a mutation in a single, but different, gene. Researchers have discovered other genetic mutations in children diagnosed with autism, including some that have not yet been designated as named syndromes. While each of these disorders is rare, in aggregate, they may account for 20 percent or more of all autism cases.

People with ASD also have a higher than average risk of having epilepsy. Children whose language skills regress early in life—before age three—appear to have a risk of developing epilepsy or seizure-like brain activity. About 20–30 percent of children with ASD develop epilepsy by the time they reach adulthood. Additionally, people with both ASD and intellectual disability have the greatest risk of developing seizure disorder.

How Is Autism Spectrum Disorder Diagnosed?

ASD symptoms can vary greatly from person to person depending on the severity of the disorder. Symptoms may even go unrecognized for young children who have mild ASD or less debilitating handicaps.

Autism spectrum disorder is diagnosed by clinicians based on symptoms, signs, and testing according to the *Diagnostic and Statistical Manual of Mental Disorders-V*, a guide created by the American

Psychiatric Association (APA) used to diagnose mental disorders. Children should be screened for developmental delays during periodic checkups and specifically for autism at 18- and 24-month well-child visits.

Very early indicators that require evaluation by an expert include:

- No babbling or pointing by age 1
- No single words by age 16 months or two-word phrases by age 2
- No response to name
- Loss of language or social skills previously acquired
- Poor eye contact
- Excessive lining up of toys or objects
- No smiling or social responsiveness

Later indicators include:

- Impaired ability to make friends with peers
- Impaired ability to initiate or sustain a conversation with others
- Absence or impairment of imaginative and social play
- Repetitive or unusual use of language
- Abnormally intense or focused interest
- Preoccupation with certain objects or subjects
- Inflexible adherence to specific routines or rituals

If screening instruments indicate the possibility of ASD, a more comprehensive evaluation is usually indicated. A comprehensive evaluation requires a multidisciplinary team, including a psychologist, neurologist, psychiatrist, speech therapist, and other professionals who diagnose and treat children with ASD. The team members will conduct a thorough neurological assessment and in-depth cognitive and language testing. Because hearing problems can cause behaviors that could be mistaken for ASD, children with delayed speech development should also have their hearing tested.

What Causes Autism Spectrum Disorder?

Scientists believe that both genetics and environment likely play a role in ASD. There is great concern that rates of autism have been increasing in recent decades without full explanation as to why. Researchers have identified a number of genes associated with the disorder. Imaging studies of people with ASD have found differences in the development of several regions of the brain. Studies suggest that ASD could be a result of disruptions in normal brain growth very early in development. These disruptions may be the result of defects in genes that control brain development and regulate how brain cells communicate with each other. Autism is more common in children born prematurely. Environmental factors may also play a role in gene function and development, but no specific environmental causes have yet been identified. The theory that parental practices are responsible for ASD has long been disproved. Multiple studies have shown that vaccination to prevent childhood infectious diseases does not increase the risk of autism in the population.

What Role Do Genes Play?

Twin and family studies strongly suggest that some people have a genetic predisposition to autism. Identical twin studies show that if one twin is affected, then the other will be affected between 36–95 percent of the time. There are a number of studies in progress to determine the specific genetic factors associated with the development of ASD. In families with one child with ASD, the risk of having a second child with the disorder also increases. Many of the genes found to be associated with autism are involved in the function of the chemical connections between brain neurons (synapses). Researchers are look- ing for clues about which genes contribute to increased susceptibility. In some cases, parents and other relatives of a child with ASD show mild impairments in social communication skills or engage in repetitive behaviors. Evidence also suggests that emotional disorders such as bipolar disorder and schizophrenia occur more frequently than average in the families of people with ASD.

In addition to genetic variations that are inherited and are present in nearly all of a person's cells, a research has also shown that *de novo*, or spontaneous, gene mutations can influence the risk of developing autism spectrum disorder. *De novo* mutations are changes in sequences of deoxyribonucleic acid or DNA, the hereditary material in humans, which can occur spontaneously in a parent's sperm or egg cell or during fertilization. The mutation then occurs in each cell as the fertilized egg divides. These mutations may affect single genes or they may be changes called copy number variations, in which stretches of DNA containing multiple genes are deleted or duplicated. Studies have shown that people with ASD tend to have more copy number *de novo* gene mutations than those without the disorder, suggesting that for some the risk of developing ASD is not the result of mutations in individual genes but rather spontaneous coding mutations across many genes. *De novo* mutations may explain genetic disorders in which an affected child has the mutation in each cell but the parents do not and there is no family pattern to the disorder. Autism risk also increases in children born to older parents. There is still much research to be done to determine the potential role of environmental factors on spontaneous mutations and how that influences ASD risk.

Do Symptoms of Autism Change over Time?

For many children, symptoms improve with age and behavioral treatment. During adolescence, some children with ASD may become depressed or experience behavioral problems, and their treatment may need some modification as they transition to adulthood. People with ASD usually continue to need services and supports as they get older, but depending on severity of the disorder, people with ASD may be able to work successfully and live independently or within a supportive environment.

How Is Autism Treated?

There is no cure for ASD. Therapies and behavioral interventions are designed to remedy specific symptoms and can substantially improve those symptoms. The ideal treatment plan coordinates therapies and interventions that meet the specific needs of the individual. Most healthcare professionals agree that the earlier the intervention, the better.

Educational/behavioral interventions: Early behavioral/educational interventions have been very successful in many children with ASD. In these interventions, therapists use highly structured and intensive skill-oriented training sessions to help children develop social and language skills, such as applied behavioral analysis, which encourages positive behaviors and discourages negative ones. In addition, family counseling for the parents and siblings of children with ASD often helps families cope with the particular challenges of living with a child with ASD.

Medications: While medication can't cure ASD or even treat its main symptoms, there are some that can help with related symptoms such as anxiety, depression, and obsessive-compulsive disorder (OCD).

Antipsychotic medications are used to treat severe behavioral problems. Seizures can be treated with one or more anticonvulsant drugs. Medication used to treat people with attention deficit disorder can be used effectively to help decrease impulsivity and hyperactivity in people with ASD. Parents, caregivers, and people with autism should use caution before adopting any unproven treatments.

Chapter 2

Asperger Syndrome (High-Functioning Autism)

Asperger syndrome (AS) is a developmental disorder. It is an autism spectrum disorder (ASD), one of a distinct group of neurological conditions characterized by a greater or lesser degree of impairment in language and communication skills, as well as repetitive or restrictive patterns of thought and behavior.

Other ASDs include: classic autism, Rett syndrome (RTT), childhood disintegrative disorder (CDD), and pervasive developmental disorder not otherwise specified (usually referred to as PDD-NOS). Unlike children with autism, children with AS retain their early language skills.

Symptoms

The most distinguishing symptom of AS is a child's obsessive interest in a single object or topic to the exclusion of any other. Children with AS want to know everything about their topic of interest and their conversations with others will be about little else. Their expertise, high level of vocabulary, and formal speech patterns make them seem like little professors.

Other characteristics of AS include repetitive routines or rituals; peculiarities in speech and language; socially and emotionally inappropriate behavior and the inability to interact successfully with peers;

This chapter includes text excerpted from "Asperger Syndrome Information Page," National Institute of Neurological Disorders and Stroke (NINDS), June 20, 2018.

problems with nonverbal communication; and clumsy and uncoordinated motor movements.

Children with AS are isolated because of their poor social skills and narrow interests. They may approach other people, but make normal conversation impossible by inappropriate or eccentric behavior, or by wanting only to talk about their singular interest. Children with AS usually have a history of developmental delays in motor skills such as pedaling a bike, catching a ball, or climbing outdoor play equipment. They are often awkward and poorly coordinated with a walk that can appear either stilted or bouncy.

Treatment

The ideal treatment for AS coordinates therapies that address the three core symptoms of the disorder: poor communication skills, obsessive or repetitive routines, and physical clumsiness. There is no single best treatment package for all children with AS, but most professionals agree that the earlier the intervention, the better.

An effective treatment program builds on the child's interests, offers a predictable schedule, teaches tasks as a series of simple steps, actively engages the child's attention in highly structured activities, and provides regular reinforcement of behavior. It may include social skills training, cognitive behavioral therapy (CBT), medication for coexisting conditions, and other measures.

Prognosis

With effective treatment, children with AS can learn to cope with their disabilities, but they may still find social situations and personal relationships challenging. Many adults with AS are able to work successfully in mainstream jobs, although they may continue to need encouragement and moral support to maintain an independent life.

Chapter 3

Rett Syndrome

What Is Rett Syndrome?

Rett syndrome (RTT) is a neurodevelopmental disorder that affects girls almost exclusively. It is characterized by normal early growth and development followed by a slowing of development, loss of purposeful use of the hands, distinctive hand movements, slowed brain and head growth, problems with walking, seizures, and intellectual disability.

The disorder was identified by Dr. Andreas Rett, an Austrian physician who first described it in a journal article in 1966. It was not until after a second article about the disorder, published in 1983 by Swedish researcher Dr. Bengt Hagberg, that the disorder was generally recognized.

The course of Rett syndrome, including the age of onset and the severity of symptoms, varies from child to child. Before the symptoms begin, however, the child generally appears to grow and develop normally, although there are often subtle abnormalities even in early infancy, such as loss of muscle tone (hypotonia), difficulty feeding, and jerkiness in limb movements. Then, gradually, mental and physical symptoms appear. As the syndrome progresses, the child loses purposeful use of her hands and the ability to speak. Other early symptoms may include problems crawling or walking and diminished eye contact. The loss of functional use of the hands is followed by compulsive hand

This chapter includes text excerpted from "Rett Syndrome Fact Sheet," National Institute of Neurological Disorders and Stroke (NINDS), August 15, 2018.

movements such as wringing and washing. The onset of this period of regression is sometimes sudden.

Apraxia—the inability to perform motor functions—is perhaps the most severely disabling feature of Rett syndrome, interfering with every body movement, including eye gaze and speech.

Children with Rett syndrome often exhibit autistic-like behaviors in the early stages. Other symptoms may include walking on the toes, sleep problems, a wide-based gait, teeth grinding and difficulty chewing, slowed growth, seizures, cognitive disabilities, and breathing difficulties while awake such as hyperventilation, apnea (breath holding), and air swallowing.

What Are the Stages of the Disorder?

Scientists generally describe four stages of Rett syndrome. Stage I, called early onset, typically begins between 6 and 18 months of age. This stage is often overlooked because symptoms of the disorder may be somewhat vague, and parents and doctors may not notice the subtle slowing of development at first. The infant may begin to show less eye contact and have reduced interest in toys. There may be delays in gross motor skills such as sitting or crawling. Hand-wringing and decreasing head growth may occur, but not enough to draw attention. This stage usually lasts for a few months but can continue for more than a year.

Stage II, or the rapid destructive stage, usually begins between ages one and four and may last for weeks or months. Its onset may be rapid or gradual as the child loses purposeful hand skills and spoken language. Characteristic hand movements such as wringing, washing, clapping, or tapping, as well as repeatedly moving the hands to the mouth often begin during this stage. The child may hold the hands clasped behind the back or held at the sides, with random touching, grasping, and releasing. The movements continue while the child is awake but disappear during sleep. Breathing irregularities such as episodes of apnea and hyperventilation may occur, although breathing usually improves during sleep. Some girls also display autistic-like symptoms such as loss of social interaction and communication. Walking may be unsteady and initiating motor movements can be difficult. Slowed head growth is usually noticed during this stage.

Stage III, or the plateau or pseudo-stationary stage, usually begins between ages 2 and 10 and can last for years. Apraxia, motor problems, and seizures are prominent during this stage. However, there may be improvement in behavior, with less irritability, crying, and autistic-like features. A girl in stage III may show more interest in her surroundings and her alertness, attention span, and communication skills may improve. Many girls remain in this stage for most of their lives.

Stage IV, or the late motor deterioration stage, can last for years or decades. Prominent features include reduced mobility, curvature of the spine (scoliosis) and muscle weakness, rigidity, spasticity, and increased muscle tone with abnormal posturing of an arm, leg, or top part of the body. Girls who were previously able to walk may stop walking. Cognition, communication, or hand skills generally do not decline in stage IV. Repetitive hand movements may decrease and eye gaze usually improves.

What Causes Rett Syndrome

Nearly all cases of Rett syndrome are caused by a mutation in the methyl CpG binding protein 2, or *MECP2* gene. Scientists identified the gene—which is believed to control the functions of many other genes—in 1999. The *MECP2* gene contains instructions for the synthesis of a protein called methyl cytosine binding protein 2 (*MeCP2*), which is needed for brain development and acts as one of the many biochemical switches that can either increase gene expression or tell other genes when to turn off and stop producing their own unique proteins. Because the *MECP2* gene does not function properly in individuals with Rett syndrome, insufficient amounts or structurally abnormal forms of the protein are produced and can cause other genes to be abnormally expressed.

Not everyone who has a *MECP2* mutation has Rett syndrome. Scientists have identified mutations in the *CDKL5* and *FOXG1* genes in individuals who have atypical or congenital Rett syndrome, but they are still learning how those mutations cause the disorder. Scientists believe the remaining cases may be caused by partial gene deletions, mutations in other parts of the *MECP2* gene, or additional genes that have not yet been identified, and they continue to look for other causes.

Is Rett Syndrome Inherited?

Although Rett syndrome is a genetic disorder, less than one percent of recorded cases are inherited or passed from one generation to the next. Most cases are spontaneous, which means the mutation occurs randomly. However, in some families of individuals affected by Rett syndrome, there are other female family members who have a mutation of their *MECP2* gene but do not show clinical symptoms. These females are known as "asymptomatic female carriers."

Who Gets Rett Syndrome

Rett syndrome is estimated to affect one in every 10,000–15,000 live female births and in all racial and ethnic groups worldwide. Prenatal testing is available for families with an affected daughter who has an identified *MECP2* mutation. Since the disorder occurs spontaneously in most affected individuals, however, the risk of a family having a second child with the disorder is less than one percent.

Genetic testing is also available for sisters of girls with Rett syndrome who have an identified *MECP2* mutation to determine if they are asymptomatic carriers of the disorder, which is an extremely rare possibility.

The *MECP2* gene is found on a person's X chromosome, one of the two sex chromosomes. Girls have two X chromosomes, but only one is active in any given cell. This means that in a girl with Rett syndrome only a portion of the cells in the nervous system will use the defective gene. Some of the child's brain cells use the healthy gene and express normal amounts of the protein.

The severity of Rett syndrome in girls is in part a function of the percentage of their cells that express a normal copy of the *MECP2* gene. If the active X chromosome that is carrying the defective gene is turned off in a large proportion of cells, the symptoms will be mild, but if a larger percentage of cells have the X chromosome with the normal *MECP2* gene turned off, onset of the disorder may occur earlier and the symptoms may be more severe.

The story is different for boys who have a *MECP2* mutation known to cause Rett syndrome in girls. Because boys have only one X chromosome (and one Y chromosome) they lack a backup copy that could compensate for the defective one, and they have no protection from the harmful effects of the disorder. Boys with such a defect frequently do not show clinical features of Rett syndrome, but experience severe problems when they are first born and die shortly after birth. A very small number of boys may have a different mutation in the *MECP2* gene or a sporadic mutation after conception that can cause some degree of intellectual disability and developmental problems.

How Is Rett Syndrome Diagnosed?

Doctors clinically diagnose Rett syndrome by observing signs and symptoms during the child's early growth and development, and conducting ongoing evaluations of the child's physical and neurological status. Scientists have developed a genetic test to complement the clinical diagnosis, which involves searching for the *MECP2* mutation on the child's X chromosome.

A pediatric neurologist, clinical geneticist, or developmental pediatrician should be consulted to confirm the clinical diagnosis of Rett syndrome. The physician will use a highly specific set of guidelines that are divided into three types of clinical criteria: main, supportive, and exclusion. The presence of any of the exclusion criteria negates a diagnosis of classic Rett syndrome.

Examples of main diagnostic criteria or symptoms include partial or complete loss of acquired purposeful hand skills, partial or complete loss of acquired spoken language, repetitive hand movements (such as hand-wringing or squeezing, clapping or rubbing), and gait abnormalities, including toe-walking or an unsteady, wide-based, stiff-legged walk.

Supportive criteria are not required for a diagnosis of Rett syndrome but may occur in some individuals. In addition, these symptoms—which vary in severity from child to child—may not be observed in very young girls but may develop with age. A child with supportive criteria but none of the essential criteria does not have Rett syndrome. Supportive criteria include scoliosis. teeth-grinding, small cold hands, and feet in relation to height, abnormal sleep patterns, abnormal muscle tone, inappropriate laughing or screaming, intense eye communication, and diminished response to pain.

In addition to the main diagnostic criteria, a number of specific conditions enable physicians to rule out a diagnosis of Rett syndrome. These are referred to as exclusion criteria. Children with any one of the following criteria do not have Rett syndrome: brain injury secondary to trauma, neurometabolic disease, severe infection that causes neurological problems; and grossly abnormal psychomotor development in the first six months of life.

Is Treatment Available?

There is no cure for Rett syndrome. Treatment for the disorder is symptomatic—focusing on the management of symptoms—and supportive, requiring a multidisciplinary approach. Medication may be needed for breathing irregularities and motor difficulties, and anticonvulsant drugs may be used to control seizures. There should be regular monitoring for scoliosis and possible heart abnormalities. Occupational therapy can help children develop skills needed for performing self-directed activities (such as dressing, feeding, and practicing arts and crafts), while physical therapy and hydrotherapy may prolong mobility.

Some children may require special equipment and aids such as braces to arrest scoliosis, splints to modify hand movements, and nutritional programs to help them maintain adequate weight. Special academic, social, vocational, and support services may be required in some cases.

What Is the Outlook for Those with Rett Syndrome?

Despite the difficulties with symptoms, many individuals with Rett syndrome continue to live well into middle age and beyond. Because the disorder is rare, very little is known about long-term prognosis and life expectancy. While there are women in their forties and fifties with the disorder, currently it is not possible to make reliable estimates about life expectancy beyond the age of forty.

Chapter 4

Pervasive Developmental Disorder

The diagnostic category of pervasive developmental disorders (PDD) refers to a group of disorders characterized by delays in the development of socialization and communication skills. Parents may note symptoms as early as infancy, although the typical age of onset is before three years of age.

Symptoms

Symptoms may include problems with using and understanding language; difficulty relating to people, objects, and events; unusual play with toys and other objects; difficulty with changes in routine or familiar surroundings, and repetitive body movements or behavior patterns.

Types

Autism (a developmental brain disorder characterized by impaired social interaction and communication skills, and a limited range of activities and interests) is the most characteristic and best studied PDD. Other types of PDD include Asperger syndrome (AS), childhood disintegrative disorder (CDD), and Rett syndrome (RTT). Children

This chapter includes text excerpted from "Pervasive Developmental Disorders Information Page," National Institute of Neurological Disorders and Stroke (NINDS), July 2, 2018.

with PDD vary widely in abilities, intelligence, and behaviors. Some children do not speak at all, others speak in limited phrases or conversations, and some have relatively normal language development. Repetitive play skills and limited social skills are generally evident. Unusual responses to sensory information, such as loud noises and lights, are also common.

Treatment

There is no known cure for PDD. Medications are used to address specific behavioral problems; therapy for children with PDD should be specialized according to need. Some children with PDD benefit from specialized classrooms in which the class size is small and instruction is given on a one-to-one basis. Others function well in standard special education classes or regular classes with additional support.

Prognosis

Early intervention including appropriate and specialized educational programs and support services plays a critical role in improving the outcome of individuals with PDD. PDD is not fatal and does not affect normal life expectancy.

Chapter 5

Statistics on Autism Spectrum Disorder in the United States

About 1 in 59 children has been identified with autism spectrum disorder (ASD) according to estimates from the Centers for Disease Control and Prevention's (CDC) Autism and Developmental Disabilities Monitoring (ADDM) Network.

- ASD is reported to occur in all racial, ethnic, and socioeconomic groups.

- ASD is about four times more common among boys than among girls.

- Studies in Asia, Europe, and North America have identified individuals with ASD with an average prevalence of between one percent and two percent.

- About one in six children in the United States had a developmental disability in 2006–2008, ranging from mild disabilities such as speech and language impairments to serious developmental disabilities, such as intellectual disabilities, cerebral palsy (CP), and autism.

This chapter includes text excerpted from "Autism Spectrum Disorder (ASD)— Data and Statistics," Centers for Disease Control and Prevention (CDC), April 26, 2018.

Table 5.1. Identified Prevalence of Autism Spectrum Disorder

Surveillance Year	Birth Year	Number of ADDM Sites Reporting	Prevalence per 1,000 Children (Range)	This Is about 1 in X Children...
2000	1992	6	6.7 (4.5–9.9)	1 in 150
2002	1994	14	6.6 (3.3–10.6)	1 in 150
2004	1996	8	8.0 (4.6–9.8)	1 in 125
2006	1998	11	9.0 (4.2–12.1)	1 in 110
2008	2000	14	11.3 (4.8–21.2)	1 in 88
2010	2002	11	14.7 (5.7–21.9)	1 in 68
2012	2004	11	14.6 (8.2–24.6)	1 in 68
2014	2006	11	16.8 (13.1–29.3)	1 in 59

Risk Factors and Characteristics

- Studies have shown that among identical twins, if one child has ASD, then the other will be affected about 36–95 percent of the time. In nonidentical twins, if one child has ASD, then the other is affected about 0–31 percent of the time.

- Parents who have a child with ASD have a 2–18 percent chance of having a second child who is also affected.

- ASD tends to occur more often in people who have certain genetic or chromosomal conditions. About 10 percent of children with autism are also identified as having Down syndrome (DS), fragile X syndrome (FXS), tuberous sclerosis (TSC), or other genetic and chromosomal disorders.

- Almost half (44%) of children identified with ASD has average to above-average intellectual ability.

- Children born to older parents are at a higher risk for having ASD.

- A small percentage of children who are born prematurely or with low birth weight are at greater risk for having ASD.

- ASD commonly co-occurs with other developmental, psychiatric, neurologic, chromosomal, and genetic diagnoses. The co-occurrence of one or more non-ASD developmental diagnoses is 83 percent. The co-occurrence of one or more psychiatric diagnoses is 10 percent.

Diagnosis

- Research has shown that a diagnosis of autism at age two can be reliable, valid, and stable.

- Even though ASD can be diagnosed as early as age two years, most children are not diagnosed with ASD until after age four years. The median age of first diagnosis by subtype is as follows:

  - Autistic disorder: 3 years, 10 months

  - ASD/pervasive developmental disorder (PDD): 4 years, 8 months

  - Asperger disorder: 5 years, 7 months

- Studies have shown that parents of children with ASD notice a developmental problem before their child's first birthday. Concerns about vision and hearing were more often reported in the first year, and differences in social, communication, and fine motor skills were evident from six months of age.

Economic Costs

- The total costs per year for children with ASD in the United States were estimated to be between $11.5 billion to $60.9 billion (2011 U.S. dollars). This significant economic burden represents a variety of direct and indirect costs, from medical care to special education to lost parental productivity.

- Children and adolescents with ASD had average medical expenditures that exceeded those without ASD by $4,110 to $6,200 per year. On average, medical expenditures for children and adolescents with ASD were 4.1–6.2 times greater than for those without ASD. Differences in median expenditures ranged from $2,240 to $3,360 per year with median expenditures 8.4–9.5 times greater.

- In 2005, the average annual medical costs for Medicaid-enrolled children with ASD were $10,709 per child, which was about six times higher than costs for children without ASD ($1,812).

- In addition to medical costs, intensive behavioral interventions (IBI) for children with ASD cost $40,000 to $60,000 per child per year.

Part Two

Causes and Risk Factors Associated with Autism Spectrum Disorder

Chapter 6

Causes and Risk Factors for Autism

While scientists don't know the exact causes of autism spectrum disorder (ASD), research suggests that genes can act together with influences from the environment to affect development in ways that lead to ASD. Although scientists are still trying to understand why some people develop ASD and others don't, some risk factors include:

- Having a sibling with ASD

- Having older parents

- Having certain genetic conditions—people with conditions such as Down syndrome, fragile X syndrome (FXS), and Rett syndrome (RTT) are more likely than others to have ASD

- Very low birth weight

This chapter contains text excerpted from the following sources: Text in this chapter begins with excerpts from "Autism Spectrum Disorder," National Institute of Mental Health (NIMH), March 2018; Text under the heading "What Causes Autism?" is excerpted from "What Causes Autism?" *Eunice Kennedy Shriver National Institute of Child Health and Human Development* (NICHD), January 31, 2017; Text under the heading "What Are the Risk Factors for Autism?" is excerpted from "Neurodevelopmental Disorders," U.S. Environmental Protection Agency (EPA), October 2015. Reviewed October 2018.

What Causes Autism?

Autism was first described in the 1940s, but very little was known about it until the last few decades. Even today, there is a great deal that we don't know about autism. Because the disorder is so complex and no two people with autism are exactly alike, there are probably many causes for autism. It is also likely that there is not a single cause for autism, but rather that it results from a combination of causes

Scientists are studying some of the following as possible causes of or contributors to ASD.

Genes and ASD

A great deal of evidence supports the idea that genes are one of the main causes of or a major contributor to ASD. More than 100 genes on different chromosomes may be involved in causing ASD, to different degrees.

Many people with autism have slight changes, called mutations, in many of these genes. However, the link between genetic mutations and autism is complex:

- Most people with autism have different mutations and combinations of mutations. Not everyone with autism has changes in every gene that scientists have linked to ASD.

- Many people without autism or autism symptoms also have some of these genetic mutations that scientists have linked to autism.

This evidence means that different genetic mutations probably play different roles in ASD. For example, certain mutations or combinations of mutations might:

- Cause-specific symptoms of ASD

- Control how mild or severe those symptoms are

- Increase susceptibility to autism. This means someone with one of these gene mutations is at greater risk for autism than someone without the mutation.

Interactions between Genes and the Environment

If someone is susceptible to ASD because of genetic mutations, then certain situations might cause autism in that person.

For instance, an infection or contact with chemicals in the environment could cause autism in someone who is susceptible because of genetic mutations. However, someone who is genetically susceptible might not get an ASD even if she or he has the same experiences.

Other Biological Causes

Researchers are also looking into biological factors other than genes that might be involved in ASD. Some of these include:

- Problems with brain connections
- Problems with growth or overgrowth in certain areas of the brain
- Problems with metabolism (the body's energy production system)
- Problems in the body's immune system, which protects against infections

What Are the Risk Factors for Autism?

Autism spectrum disorders (ASDs) are a group of developmental disabilities defined by significant social, communication, and behavioral impairments. The term "spectrum disorders" refers to the fact that although people with ASDs share some common symptoms, ASDs affect different people in different ways, with some experiencing very mild symptoms and others experiencing severe symptoms. ASDs encompass autistic disorder and the generally less severe forms, Asperger syndrome (AS) and pervasive developmental disorder-not otherwise specified (PDD-NOS). Children with ASDs may lack interest in other people, have trouble showing or talking about feelings, and avoid or resist physical contact.

A range of communication problems is seen in children with ASDs: some speak very well, while many children with an ASD do not speak at all. Another hallmark characteristic of ASDs is the demonstration of restrictive or repetitive interests or behaviors, such as lining up toys, flapping hands, rocking his or her body, or spinning in circles.

To date, no single risk factor sufficient to cause ASD has been identified; rather each case is likely to be caused by the combination of multiple genetic and environmental risk factors. Several ASD research findings and hypotheses may imply an important role for environmental contaminants. First, there has been a sharp upward trend in reported prevalence that cannot be fully explained by factors such as younger ages at diagnosis, migration patterns, changes in diagnostic criteria, inclusion of milder cases, or increased parental age.

Also, the neurological signaling systems that are impaired in children with ASDs can be affected by certain environmental chemicals. For example, several pesticides are known to interfere with acetylcholine (ACh) and γ-aminobutyric acid (GABA) neurotransmission, chemical messenger systems that have been altered in certain subsets of autistic individuals. Some studies have reported associations between certain pharmaceuticals taken by pregnant women and increased incidence of autism, which may suggest that there are biological pathways by which other chemical exposures during pregnancy could increase the risk of autism.

Furthermore, some of the identified genetic risk factors for autism are *de novo* mutations, meaning that the genetic defect is not present in either of the parents' genes, yet can be found in the genes of the child when a new genetic mutation forms in a parent's germ cells (egg or sperm), potentially from exposure to contaminants. Many environmental contaminants have been identified as agents capable of causing mutations in deoxyribonucleic acid, by leading to oxidative deoxyribonucleic acid (DNA) damage and by inhibiting the body's normal ability to repair DNA damage. Some children with autism have been shown to display markers of increased oxidative stress, which may strengthen this line of reasoning. Many studies have linked increasing paternal and maternal age with increased risk of ASDs. The role of parental age in increased autism risk might be explained by evidence that shows advanced parental age can contribute significantly to the frequency of *de novo* mutations in a parent's germ cells. Advanced parental age signifies a longer period of time when environmental exposures may act on germ cells and cause DNA damage and *de novo* mutations. Finally, a study concluded that the role of genetic factors in ASDs has been overestimated, and that environmental factors play a greater role than genetic factors in contributing to autism. This study did not evaluate the role of any particular environmental factors, and in this context "environmental factors" are defined broadly to include any influence that is not genetic.

Studies, limited in number and often limited in research design, have examined the possible role that certain environmental contaminants may play in the development of ASDs. A number of these studies have focused on mercury exposures. Earlier studies reported higher levels of mercury in the blood, baby teeth, and urine of children with ASDs compared with control children; however, another study reported no difference in the blood mercury levels of children with autism and typically developing children. Proximity to industrial and power plant sources of environmental mercury was reported to be associated with increased autism prevalence in a study conducted in Texas.

Thimerosal is a mercury-containing preservative that is used in some vaccines to prevent contamination and growth of harmful bacteria in vaccine vials. Since 2001, thimerosal has not been used in routinely administered childhood vaccines, with the exception of some influenza vaccines. The Institute of Medicine (IOM) has rejected the hypothesis of a causal relationship between thimerosal-containing vaccines and autism.

Some studies have also considered air pollutants as possible contributors to autism. A study conducted in the San Francisco Bay Area reported an association between the amount of certain airborne pollutants at a child's place of birth (mercury, cadmium, nickel, trichloroethylene (TCE), and vinyl chloride) and the risk for autism, but a similar study in North Carolina and West Virginia did not find such a relationship. Another study in California reported that mothers who lived near a freeway at the time of delivery were more likely to have children diagnosed with autism, suggesting that exposure to traffic-related air pollutants may play a role in contributing to ASDs.

Finally, a study in Sweden reported an increased risk of ASDs in children born to families living in homes with polyvinyl chloride (PVC) flooring, which is a source of certain phthalates in indoor environments.

Chapter 7

Early Brain Development and ASD

The early years of a child's life are very important for later health and development. One of the main reasons is how fast the brain grows starting before birth and continuing into early childhood. Although the brain continues to develop and change into adulthood, the first eight years can build a foundation for future learning, health and life success.

How well a brain develops depends on many factors in addition to genes, such as:

- Proper nutrition starting in pregnancy

- Exposure to toxins or infections

- The child's experiences with other people and the world

Nurturing and responsive care for the child's body and mind is the key to supporting healthy brain development. Positive or negative experiences can add up to shape a child's development and can have lifelong effects. To nurture their child's body and mind, parents and caregivers need support and the right resources. The right care

---

This chapter contains text excerpted from the following sources: Text in this chapter begins with excerpts from "Early Brain Development and Health," Centers for Disease Control and Prevention (CDC), May 23, 2018; Text under the heading "Brain Scans Show Early Signs of Autism Spectrum Disorder" is excerpted from "Brain Scans Show Early Signs of Autism Spectrum Disorder," National Institutes of Health (NIH), February 21, 2017.

33

for children, starting before birth and continuing through childhood, ensures that the child's brain grows well and reaches its full potential. Centers for Disease Control and Prevention (CDC) is working to protect children so that their brains have a healthy start.

The Importance of Early Childhood Experiences for Brain Development

Children are born ready to learn, and have many skills to learn over many years. They depend on parents, family members, and other caregivers as their first teachers to develop the right skills to become independent and lead healthy and successful lives. How the brain grows is strongly affected by the child's experiences with other people and the world. Nurturing care for the mind is critical for brain growth. Children grow and learn best in a safe environment where they are protected from neglect and from extreme or chronic stress with plenty of opportunities to play and explore.

Parents and other caregivers can support healthy brain growth by speaking to, playing with, and caring for their child. Children learn best when parents take turns when talking and playing, and build on their child's skills and interests. Nurturing a child by understanding their needs and responding sensitively helps to protect children's brains from stress. Speaking with children and exposing them to books, stories, and songs helps strengthen children's language and communication, which puts them on a path towards learning and succeeding in school.

Exposure to stress and trauma can have long-term negative consequences for the child's brain, whereas talking, reading, and playing can stimulate brain growth. Ensuring that parents, caregivers, and early childhood care providers have the resources and skills to provide safe, stable, nurturing, and stimulating care is an important public health goal.

When children are at risk, tracking children's development and making sure they reach developmental milestones can help ensure that any problems are detected early and children can receive the intervention they may need.

Brain Scans Show Early Signs of Autism Spectrum Disorder

For children with autism spectrum disorder (ASD), early diagnosis is critical to allow for possible interventions at a time when the brain is most amenable to change. But that's been tough to implement for

a simple reason: the symptoms of ASD, such as communication difficulties, social deficits, and repetitive behaviors, often do not show up
until a child turns two or even three years old.

Now, a National Institutes of Health (NIH)-funded research team
has news that may pave the way for earlier detection of ASD. The
key is to shift the diagnostic focus from how kids act to how their
brains grow. In their brain imaging study, the researchers found that,
compared to other children, youngsters with ASD showed unusually
rapid brain growth from infancy to age two. In fact, the growth differences were already evident by their first birthdays, well before autistic
behaviors typically emerge.

Autism spectrum disorder includes a range of developmental conditions, such as autism and Asperger syndrome (AS), that are characterized by challenges in social skills and communication. Scientists
have long known that teens and adults with ASD have unusually large
brain volumes. Researchers, including Heather Hazlett and Joseph
Piven of the University of North Carolina (UNC), Chapel Hill, found
more than a decade ago that those differences in brain size emerge
by about age two. However, no one had ever visually tracked those
developmental differences.

In the study reported in *Nature*, Hazlett, Piven, and their colleagues
set out to collect that visual evidence. They examined 106 infants at
high risk of ASD, based on an older sibling with that diagnosis. Fifteen
of the study's high-risk infants went on to be diagnosed with ASD at
age 2. The study also included another 42 infants with no family history of ASD and a low risk for the disorder. In all groups, the infants
were mostly white, had similar birth weights, and comparable family
backgrounds.

Each infant underwent detailed behavioral assessments for early
signs of ASD, such as trouble babbling or making eye contact, at 6,
12, and 24 months of age. At each visit, the researchers also used a
magnetic resonance imaging (MRI) scanner to capture detailed images
of each child's brain while napping.

Between the first and second scans, or just 6 to 12 months into
the study, the MRIs showed something remarkable. There was a significant increase in the surface area of the brains of kids who would
later develop ASD compared to other children. By age 2, the brains
of these kids were obviously larger. The researchers found that kids
whose brains grew the fastest also had the most severe social deficits.

But could these observations be translated into early diagnosis? To
begin looking for an answer, the researchers turned to machine learning. They wanted to find out whether a computer could use features

captured in those MRI scans, including the surface area and volume of the brain, to predict accurately which kids would develop ASD and which ones wouldn't. They found that 8 times out of 10, the computer got it right. Importantly, the computer-derived algorithm relied primarily on the changes in brain surface area between the ages of 6 months and 1 year to make those calls.

If the findings can be confirmed in more children, it may lead to a much-needed new approach to early diagnosis for kids at high risk of ASD. Piven says the findings also highlight that ASD doesn't occur suddenly and spontaneously, as sometimes incorrectly thought. Rather, the disorder develops over time—beginning in the first year of life or likely earlier—from genetic and environmental influences that the North Carolina team and others are working hard to understand.

Why should the development of a larger brain lead to ASD? The answer is not known yet. Perhaps in the process of molding the brain for optimum function, it's not just the expansion of neurons and synaptic junctions that matter, but also the "pruning" that allows this complex network—the most complicated structure in the known universe—to achieve maximum efficacy for human abilities and social interactions. The findings also add to evidence from studies in mice that ASD may be related to abnormalities in the progenitor cells that allow the brain to grow. The hope is that, as more is learned about ASD's underlying biology, researchers will make even greater strides toward improving its diagnosis and discovering entirely new kinds of treatments to help these kids and their parents.

Chapter 8

Genetics Impact Autism Spectrum Disorder

Chapter Contents

Section 8.1

Is Autism Inherited?

This section contains text excerpted from the following sources: Text under the heading "Autism and Genes" is excerpted from "Autism Awareness Month: Genes and Development in Autism Spectrum Disorder," National Institute of Mental Health (NIMH), April 4, 2017; Text under the heading "Causes of Autism" is excerpted from "Learning about Autism," National Human Genome Research Institute (NHGRI), January 18, 2017.

Autism and Genes

For some time, we have known that autism spectrum disorder (ASD) is a heritable condition—that is, it runs in families. We know this from a variety of studies—including twin studies, which demonstrate that if one identical twin has ASD, the other twin almost always does also. Indeed, studies suggest that up to 90 percent of the variation in developing ASD is due to genetic factors. Nonetheless, as with all complex genetic conditions, environment also plays a role.

Early efforts to identify genetic factors associated with ASD were largely unsuccessful. As little as five years ago, only a handful of genes had been identified, all of which caused complex genetic syndromes, like fragile X, Rett, and Down syndromes, of which ASD is one of several possible comorbid features. At present, however, the situation has changed dramatically. We now know dozens of genes that contribute to ASD, with more being discovered seemingly every day. How many of these genes are there? The estimates suggest that hundreds of genes contribute to the likelihood of developing ASD.

Causes of Autism

Scientists are not certain what causes autism, but it's likely that both genetics and environment play a role.

The causes of autism may be divided into 'idiopathic,' (of unknown cause) which is the majority of cases, and 'secondary,' in which a chromosome abnormality, single-gene disorder or environmental agent can be identified. Approximately 15 percent of individuals with autism can be diagnosed with secondary autism; the remaining 85 percent have idiopathic autism.

Exposure during pregnancy to rubella (German measles), valproic acid, and thalidomide, are recognized causes of secondary autism;

however, it remains unclear whether those who develop autism after such an exposure are also genetically predisposed.

The search for new environmental causes of secondary autism has centered primarily on childhood immunizations given around the time that regressive-onset autism is recognized. Both childhood immunizations and mercury in thimerosal, which was used as a preservative in some routine immunizations until 2001, have both been under scrutiny; however, no scientific evidence for a relationship between vaccines and autism has been identified.

Researchers have identified a number of genes associated with autism. Studies of people with autism have found irregularities in several regions of the brain. Other studies suggest that people with autism have abnormal levels of serotonin or other neurotransmitters in the brain. These abnormalities indicate that autism usually results from the disruption of normal brain development early in fetal development caused by defects in genes that control brain growth and that regulate how neurons communicate with each other. These are preliminary findings and require further study.

The risk that a brother or sister of an individual who has idiopathic autism will also develop autism is around four percent, plus an additional four to six percent risk for a milder condition that includes language, social or behavioral symptoms. Brothers have a higher risk (about 7%) of developing autism, plus the additional seven percent risk of milder autism spectrum symptoms, over sisters whose risk is only about one to two percent.

When the cause of autism is a chromosome abnormality or a single-gene alteration, the risk that other brothers and sisters will also have autism depends on the specific genetic cause.

Section 8.2

Genes Involved with Autism

This section includes text excerpted from "Autism Awareness Month: Genes and Development in Autism Spectrum Disorder," National Institute of Mental Health (NIMH), April 4, 2017.

Gene mutations that raise the risk for ASD come in two basic types—common variants with small effects, and rare variants with large effects. Common variants are, well, common. Many people in the population carry these and most of them do not have ASD. However, each of these genetic variants raises the risk for developing ASD very slightly—often by as little as 5 percent, meaning that if you have any one of these variants, your risk of ASD is 1.05 times that of someone who doesn't carry it. We know from family and population studies that common variation explains a large portion of risk for ASD. Identifying the genes in which common variants play a role in ASD is difficult, however, and we have very few as yet. Ultimately, common variants can give clues about the biology underlying ASD. Even then, however, any single common variant can't really predict with any great certainty whether an individual will develop ASD. Rare variants are bigger deals—they can confer significant risk on their own for ASD. For some of these variants, carriers are 30–50 times more likely to develop ASD than noncarriers.

Understanding how these genetic variants lead to ASD may help us understand particular features of risk. For example, we've known for a while that a child of older parents (mothers older than 35 or fathers older than 40) seem to be at higher risk for developing ASD. At least part of this increased risk appears to be due to the fact that new mutations—especially mutations that disrupt the function of genes—are found more often in the sperm of older men. Scientists have also found that girls with ASD have more frequent and more damaging mutations than boys, suggesting that girls are more resilient and boys more susceptible to ASD-related genetic variation, an insight that may help clarify why ASD is diagnosed much more often in boys. Finally, genetic factors that increase the risk for ASD also influence normal differences in cognitive, social, and communication abilities in individuals in the general population, suggesting that these factors are important for normal development as well as for explaining ASD.

ASD Begins in Early Neural Development

Another way in which understanding the genetic basis of ASD helps us clarify its origins is by helping to specify when during development ASD first arises. National Institute of Mental Health (NIMH)-funded research has revealed that ASD risk genes are most likely to be activated in specific brain cells—pyramidal neurons in the cortex—during mid-fetal development. A prenatal timeframe for the neurodevelopmental origins of ASD is also consistent with evidence from epidemiological studies suggesting links between prenatal infections and the later development of the disorder.

If the developmental process that leads to ASD starts in the womb, one might expect that signs of the disorder would be discoverable even in early infancy. In fact, considerable evidence has emerged that subtle signs and symptoms of ASD are present as early as the first few months of life, long before the diagnosis is typically made. Subtle differences in behavior and motor skills can distinguish between children who will develop ASD and typically developing children. These include delays in motor development that can be found as early as six months of age. Early social behavior can also be affected; researchers have reported a decline in attention to others' eyes within the first two to six months of life in infants who go on to be diagnosed with ASD. In a separate study, ASD experts identified combinations of vocal communication behaviors at 18 months that could predict a later diagnosis of ASD.

A National Institutes of Health (NIH)-funded brain imaging study supports and extends these behavioral findings. Using magnetic resonance imaging (MRI) scans to image brain growth over time in a high-risk group of siblings of children with ASD, researchers showed an increase in the growth of the cerebral cortex area between 6 and 12 months of age in infants who were diagnosed with ASD at 24 months. Researchers in the study were able to predict 88 percent of those infants who would later meet criteria for ASD at age two.

Collectively, the genetic, behavioral and neuroimaging findings clarify that the period of risk for ASD is earlier than the age when symptoms may first be noticed by families and caregivers. Attempts to understand how ASD arises—and particularly any environmental exposures that may moderate genetic risk—should be directed at the prenatal and very early postnatal period. The findings also suggest that early detection of ASD might be feasible, in order to link affected children with appropriate interventions as soon as possible. Indeed, straightforward screening of children in primary care settings can identify individuals who are at high risk for developing ASD, enabling early intervention, which we know from numerous studies improves long-term outcomes.

Section 8.3

Common Gene Variants Account for Most Genetic Risk for Autism

This section includes text excerpted from "Common Gene Variants Account for Most Genetic Risk for Autism," National Institutes of Health (NIH), July 20, 2014. Reviewed October 2018.

Most of the genetic risk for autism comes from versions of genes that are common in the population rather than from rare variants or spontaneous glitches, researchers funded by the National Institutes of Health (NIH) have found. Heritability also outweighed other risk factors in this largest study of its kind to date.

About 52 percent of the risk for autism was traced to common and rare inherited variation, with spontaneous mutations contributing a modest 2.6 percent of the total risk.

"Genetic variation likely accounts for roughly 60 percent of the liability for autism, with common variants comprising the bulk of its genetic architecture," explained Joseph Buxbaum, Ph.D., of the Icahn School of Medicine at Mount Sinai (ISMMS), New York City. "Although each exerts just a tiny effect individually, these common variations in the genetic code add up to substantial impact, taken together."

Buxbaum, and colleagues of the Population-Based Autism Genetics and Environment Study (PAGES) Consortium, report on their findings in a unique Swedish sample in the journal *Nature Genetics*.

"Thanks to the boost in statistical power that comes with ample sample size, autism geneticists can now detect common as well as rare genetic variation associated with risk," said Thomas R. Insel, M.D., director of the NIH's National Institute of Mental Health (NIMH). "Knowing the nature of the genetic risk will reveal clues to the molecular roots of the disorder. Common variation may be more important than we thought."

Although autism is thought to be caused by an interplay of genetic and other factors, including environmental, consensus on their relative contributions and the outlines of its genetic architecture has remained elusive. Evidence has been mounting that genomes of people with autism are prone to harboring rare mutations, often spontaneous, that exert strong effects and can largely account for particular cases of the disease.

More challenging is to gauge the collective impact on autism risk of numerous variations in the genetic code shared by most people, which are individually much subtler in effect. Limitations of sample size and composition made it difficult to detect these effects and to estimate the relative influence of such common, rare inherited, and rare spontaneous variation.

Differences in methods and statistical models also resulted in sometimes wildly discrepant estimates of autism's heritability—ranging from 17–50 percent.

Meanwhile, genome-wide studies of schizophrenia have achieved large enough sample sizes to reveal the involvement of well over 100 common gene variants in that disorder. These promise improved understanding of the underlying biology—and even development of risk-scores, which could help predict who might benefit from early interventions to nip psychotic episodes in the bud.

With their new study, autism genetics is beginning to catch up, say the researchers. It was made possible by Sweden's universal health registry, which allowed investigators to compare a very large sample of about 3,000 people with autism with matched controls. Researchers also brought to bear statistical methods that allowed them to more reliably sort out the heritability of the disorder. In addition, they were able to compare their results with a parallel study in 1.6 million Swedish families, which took into account data from twins and cousins, and factors like age of the father at birth and parents' psychiatric history. A best-fit statistical model took form, based mostly on combined effects of multiple genes and nonshared environmental factors.

"This is a different kind of analysis than employed in previous studies," explained Thomas Lehner, Ph.D., chief of NIMH's Genomics Research Branch. "Data from genome-wide association studies was used to identify a genetic model instead of focusing just on pinpointing genetic risk factors. The researchers were able to pick from all of the cases of illness within a population-based registry."

Now that the genetic architecture is better understood, the researchers are identifying specific genetic risk factors detected in the sample, such as deletions and duplications of genetic material and spontaneous mutations. Even though such rare spontaneous mutations accounted for only a small fraction of autism risk, the potentially large effects of these glitches makes them important clues to understanding the molecular underpinnings of the disorder, say the researchers.

"Within a given family, the mutations could be a critical determinant that leads to the manifestation of autism spectrum disorder (ASD) in a particular family member," said Buxbaum. "The family may have a common variation that puts it at risk, but if there is also a *de novo* (spontaneous) mutation on top of that, it could push an individual over the edge. So for many families, the interplay between common and spontaneous genetic factors could be the underlying genetic architecture of the disorder."

Section 8.4

Oxytocin Affects Facial Recognition

This section includes text excerpted from "Oxytocin Affects Facial Recognition," National Institutes of Health (NIH), January 13, 2014. Reviewed October 2018.

A genetic variation in the receptor for oxytocin, a hormone involved in social bonding, affects the ability to remember faces in families with a child who has autism. The finding points the way to a better understanding of oxytocin's role in social behavior.

Animals that live in social groups need to be able to recognize individuals from their own species. Rodents and many others rely on smells or pheromones to identify each other. Humans and other primates rely more on sights and sounds. Evidence has been building that the hormones oxytocin and vasopressin are involved in social recognition. Studies in mice, for example, show that oxytocin receptors are essential for recognizing individuals.

The ability to remember faces varies among people, and these differences are partly heritable. Researchers from Emory University, University College London, and the University of Tampere (UTA) in Finland explored whether variations in the genes for oxytocin and vasopressin receptors play a role. Their study was supported primarily by the National Institutes of Health's (NIH) National Institute of Mental Health (NIMH). The findings appeared online in *Proceedings of the National Academy of Sciences (NAS)*.

The scientists analyzed 198 families from the United Kingdom and Finland in which a single child had been diagnosed with autism spectrum disorder (ASD). Included in the study were 153 nonautistic siblings and 311 parents (178 mothers and 133 fathers), none of whom had significant autistic traits. The scientists chose such families because of their wide variation in face recognition memory and other social skills.

The researchers first created unique standardized "growth charts" from general population data for three social characteristics that are often impaired in people with ASD: face recognition memory, gaze fixation, and facial emotion recognition. These charts allowed the team to derive and assign standardized scores for these skills to all the participants, regardless of age or gender.

The children with ASD scored lower on each skill than did either of their parents or siblings. The scientists next searched for associations between test performance and variations in the vasopressin receptor (*AVPR1a*) and oxytocin receptor (*OXTR*) genes. The analysis revealed a single genetic variation in the oxytocin receptor that was strongly associated with facial recognition memory. The researchers estimate that this variation accounted for 2 to 10 percent of the test performance variance in both groups studied.

"It's definitely not fully predictive of face recognition memory," says study coauthor Dr. Larry Young of Emory. "But the important thing is that it suggests that the oxytocin receptor and oxytocin itself plays some role in face recognition memory."

Although rodents and primates rely on different sensory cues to recognize each other, the same gene appears to be involved in processing that social information. The researchers are now working to manipulate the oxytocin system to further explore how it affects social cue processing. This information may be useful for developing approaches to improve social cognition in people with autism.

Section 8.5

Gene Disruptions Associated with Autism Risk

This section includes text excerpted from "Gene Disruptions Associated with Autism Risk," National Institutes of Health (NIH), November 24, 2014. Reviewed October 2018.

Autism is a complex brain disorder characterized by difficulties with social interactions and communication. The symptoms and levels of disability can range from mild to severe. The wide range of disorders is collectively referred to as autism spectrum disorder (ASD). ASD affects about 1 in 68 American children.

Researchers previously linked less than a dozen genes to ASD. To further uncover genes that might be associated with the disorder, a large international team led by Dr. Joseph D. Buxbaum at the Icahn School of Medicine at Mount Sinai (ISMMS), Dr. Mark J. Daly at Broad Institute of Harvard and Massachusetts Institute of Technology (MIT), and the Autism Sequencing Consortium (ASC) analyzed more than 14,000 deoxyribonucleic acid (DNA) samples. More than 3,800 were from children with autism. The others were from parents and control samples of unrelated people. The study was funded in part by the National Institutes of Health's (NIH) National Human Genome Research Institute (NHGRI) and the National Institute of Mental Health (NIMH). Results were published in *Nature*.

The scientists looked for genetic lesions that were either inherited or *de novo*—spontaneous variations found in a child's DNA but not in either parent's. The team sequenced the exome regions of DNA, which comprise one percent of the human genome that codes for proteins. This is in contrast to whole-genome sequencing, which analyzes the entire three billion DNA base pairs of the human genome.

The researchers identified changes in 107 genes that are likely to contribute to the risk for ASD. More than five percent of the people with ASD had *de novo* loss-of-function mutations, which prevent the production of a normal protein. The researchers predicted that more than 1,000 genes may be involved in the risk for ASD, many of which will only have a modest impact on risk.

Among the genes found to be associated with a risk for ASD, many coded for proteins involved in three pathways important for normal development. One involves the structure of synapses, the connections between nerve cells across which brain signals travel. A second involves the remodeling of chromatin—the way DNA is packaged in cells, which can affect whether genes are turned on or off. A third pathway involves transcription, the process by which instructions in genes are read to build proteins.

Together, the findings provide a better understanding of some of the genetic and cellular changes in the pathways and processes thought to be involved in ASD. Eventually, this knowledge may help lead to potential therapies.

"The steps we added to our analysis over past studies provide the most complete theoretical picture to date of how many genetic changes pile up to affect the brains of children with autism," Buxbaum says. "While we have very strong findings in these genetic analyses, new-found genetic discoveries must next be moved into molecular, cell, and animal studies to realize future benefits for families."

Section 8.6

Autism Shares Genetic Roots with Other Mental Disorders

This section includes text excerpted from "Five Major Mental Disorders Share Genetic Roots," National Institute of Mental Health (NIMH), March 1, 2013. Reviewed October 2018.

Five major mental disorders share some of the same genetic risk factors, the largest genome-wide study of its kind has found. Evidence for such genetic overlap had previously been limited to pairs of disorders.

National Institutes of Health (NIH)-funded researchers discovered that people with disorders traditionally thought to be distinct—autism, attention deficit hyperactivity disorder (ADHD), bipolar disorder, major depression, and schizophrenia—were more likely to have suspect genetic variation at the same four chromosomal sites. These included risk versions of two genes that regulate the flow of calcium into cells.

"These results will help us move toward diagnostic classification informed by disease cause," said Jordan Smoller, M.D., of Massachusetts General Hospital (MGH), Boston, a coordinator of the study, which was supported by NIH's National Institute of Mental Health (NIMH). "Although statistically significant, each of these genetic associations individually can account for only a small amount of risk for mental illness, making them insufficient for predictive or diagnostic usefulness by themselves."

Smoller, Kenneth Kendler, M.D., Virginia Commonwealth University, Richmond; Nicholas Craddock, PhD., Cardiff University, England; Stephan Ripke, M.D., Massachusetts General, Patrick Sullivan, M.D., University of North Carolina at Chapel Hill, and colleagues in the Cross-Disorder Group of the Psychiatric Genomics Consortium (PGC), report on their findings February 28, 2013 in *The Lancet.*

Prior to the study, researchers had turned up evidence of shared genetic risk factors for pairs of disorders, such as schizophrenia and bipolar disorder, autism and schizophrenia, and depression and bipolar disorder. Such evidence of overlap at the genetic level has blurred the boundaries of traditional diagnostic categories and given rise to research domain criteria, or RDoC, an NIMH initiative to develop new ways of classifying psychopathology for research based on neuroscience and genetics as well as observed behavior.

To learn more, the consortium researchers analyzed the five key disorders as if they were the same illness. They screened for evidence of illness-associated genetic variation across the genomes of 33,332 patients with all five disorders and 27,888 controls, drawing on samples from previous consortium mega-analyses.

For the first time, specific variations significantly associated with all five disorders were among several suspect genomic sites that turned up. These included variation in two genes that code for the cellular machinery for regulating the flow of calcium into neurons. Variation in one of these, called *CACNA1C*, which had previously been implicated in susceptibility to bipolar disorder, schizophrenia, and major depression, is known to impact brain circuitry involved in emotion, thinking, attention and memory—functions disrupted in mental illnesses. Variation in another calcium channel gene, called *CACNB2*, was also linked to the disorders.

Alterations in calcium-channel signaling could represent a fundamental mechanism contributing to a broad vulnerability to psychopathology, suggest the researchers.

They also discovered illness-linked variation for all five disorders in certain regions of chromosomes 3 and 10. Each of these sites spans several genes, and the specific causal factors within them remain elusive. However, one region, called 3p21, which produced the strongest signal of illness association, harbors suspect variations identified in previous genome-wide studies of bipolar disorder and schizophrenia.

Section 8.7

Where Toddlers Look Is Affected by Genes and Altered in Autism

This section includes text excerpted from "Where Toddlers Look Is Affected by Genes and Altered in Autism," National Institutes of Health (NIH), July 25, 2017.

Where babies look helps them learn about and engage with the world. They give particular attention to social stimuli like people's faces. Reduced attention to people's eyes and faces is a behavior associated with autism spectrum disorder (ASD), and is often used to screen for and help diagnose the disorder. Reduced eye contact often appears by the first six months of age and persists as children grow older. ASD affects how a person acts, communicates, and learns.

Researchers have identified a number of genes associated with autism spectrum disorder. To explore whether there is a genetic foundation for a child's gaze, a team of scientists conducted eye-tracking experiments in nearly 340 toddlers, ages 18–24 months. The group was led by Drs. John N. Constantino at Washington University and Ami Klin and Warren Jones at Marcus Autism Center and Emory University School of Medicine. Their work was funded in part by the National Institutes of Health's (NIH) *Eunice Kennedy Shriver* National Institute of Child Health and Human Development (NICHD) and the National Institute of Mental Health (NIMH). Results appeared online on July 12, 2017, in *Nature*.

The researchers examined 250 typically developing children: 82 identical twins (41 pairs), 84 nonidentical twins (42 pairs), and 84 non-siblings (42 randomized pairs). They also evaluated 88 nontwin children diagnosed with autism. Each child watched videos that showed either an actress speaking directly to the viewer or scenes of children interacting in daycare. Special software captured the timing and direction of the children's eye movements, including how often they looked at the onscreen characters' eyes, mouth, body, or surrounding objects.

The team found that identical twins had much more similar visual patterns than those of nonidentical twins and nonsibling pairs. Identical twins tended to shift their eyes at the same times and in the same direction. They were also more likely to look at the subject's eyes or mouth at the same moments. Nonidentical twins matched when they looked at a person's eyes and mouth far less. Nonsibling pairs had very little similarity. The scientists also found that children with autism looked at people's eye and mouth areas much less than the other children.

When the children were tested again 15 months later, these effects persisted. Identical twins continued to look in nearly the same places. The gazes of nonidentical twins diverged slightly more than the previous year.

With these findings, researchers can now explore which genes are involved in social visual engagement and how these genetic pathways are disrupted in neurodevelopmental disorders such as autism.

"This is a mechanism by which genes actually modify a child's life experience," Constantino says. "And, because of that, this creates a new opportunity to design interventions to ensure that children at risk for autism acquire the kind of social environmental inputs that they need."

Chapter 9

Diseases, Vaccines, and Autism Spectrum Disorder

Chapter Contents

Section 9.1

Can Diseases and Vaccines Cause ASD?

This section contains text excerpted from the following sources:
Text beginning with the heading "Do Vaccines Cause Autism
Spectrum Disorder (ASD)" is excerpted from "Autism Spectrum
Disorder (ASD)—Related Topics," Centers for Disease Control and
Prevention (CDC), April 26, 2018; Text beginning with the heading
"Vaccines and Autism" is excerpted from "Vaccines Do Not Cause
Autism," Centers for Disease Control and Prevention (CDC),
October 27, 2015. Reviewed October 2018.

Do Vaccines Cause Autism Spectrum Disorder?

Many studies that have looked at whether there is a relationship
between vaccines and autism spectrum disorder (ASD). To date,
the studies continue to show that vaccines are not associated with
ASD.

However, the Centers for Disease Control and Prevention (CDC)
knows that some parents and others still have concerns. To address
these concerns, the CDC is part of the Interagency Autism Coordinating Committee (IACC) (www.iacc.hhs.gov), which is working with the
National Vaccine Advisory Committee (NVAC) (www.hhs.gov/nvpo/
nvac/index.html) on this issue. The job of the NVAC is to advise and
make recommendations regarding the National Vaccine Program.
Communication between the IACC and NVAC will allow each group to
share skills and knowledge, improve coordination, and promote better
use of research resources on vaccine topics.

Is There an Autism Spectrum Disorder Epidemic?

More people than ever before are being diagnosed with an ASD. It is
unclear exactly how much of this increase is due to a broader definition
of ASD and better efforts in diagnosis. However, a true increase in the
number of people with an ASD cannot be ruled out. The CDC believes
the increase in the diagnosis of ASD is likely due to a combination of
these factors.

The CDC is working with partners to study the prevalence of ASD
over time, so that we can find out if the number of children with these
disorders is rising, dropping, or staying the same.

We do know that ASD are more common than we thought before
and should be considered an important public health concern.

There is still a lot to learn about ASD. In addition, increased concern in the communities, continued demand for services, and reports estimating a prevalence of about 1.7 percent show the need for a coordinated and serious national response to improve the lives of people with ASD.

Can Adults Be Diagnosed with an ASD?

Yes, adults can be diagnosed with an ASD. Diagnosis includes looking at the person's medical history, watching the person's behavior, and giving the person some psychological tests. But, it can be more challenging to diagnose an adult because it is not always possible to know about the person's development during the first few years of life, and a long history of other diagnoses may complicate an ASD diagnosis. Because the focus of ASD has been on children, we still have much to learn about the prevalence and causes of ASD across the lifespan. Behavioral interventions can be effective for adults coping with a new diagnosis of autism.

What Are Mitochondrial Diseases?

Mitochondria are tiny parts of almost every cell in your body. Mitochondria are like the powerhouse of the cells. They turn sugar and oxygen into energy that the cells need to work. In mitochondrial diseases, the mitochondria cannot efficiently turn sugar and oxygen into energy, so the cells do not work the way they should.

There are many types of mitochondrial disease, and they can affect different parts of the body: the brain, kidneys, muscles, heart, eyes, ears, and others. Mitochondrial diseases can affect one part of the body or many parts. The effects can be mild or very serious.

Not everyone with a mitochondrial disease will show symptoms. However, among the mitochondrial diseases that tend to affect children, symptoms usually appear in the toddler and preschool years.

Is There a Link between Mitochondrial Diseases and Autism Spectrum Disorder?

A child with an ASD may or may not have a mitochondrial disease. When children have both an ASD and a mitochondrial disease, they sometimes have other problems too, including epilepsy, problems with muscle tone, or movement disorders.

More research is needed to find out how common it is for people to have an ASD and a mitochondrial disease. Right now, it seems rare. In general, more research on mitochondrial disease and ASDs is needed.

Vaccines and Autism

There is no link between vaccines and autism. Some people have had concerns that ASD might be linked to the vaccines children receive, but studies have shown that there is no link between receiving vaccines and developing ASD. In 2011, an Institute of Medicine (IOM) report on eight vaccines given to children and adults found that with rare exceptions, these vaccines are very safe.

A 2013 CDC study added to the research showing that vaccines do not cause ASD. The study looked at the number of antigens (substances in vaccines that cause the body's immune system to produce disease-fighting antibodies) from vaccines during the first two years of life. The results showed that the total amount of antigen from vaccines received was the same between children with ASD and those that did not have ASD.

Vaccine Ingredients and Autism

Vaccine ingredients do not cause autism. One vaccine ingredient that has been studied specifically is thimerosal, a mercury-based preservative used to prevent contamination of multidose vials of vaccines. Research shows that thimerosal does not cause ASD. In fact, a 2004 scientific review by the IOM concluded that "the evidence favors rejection of a causal relationship between thimerosal-containing vaccines and autism." Since 2003, there have been nine CDC-funded or conducted studies that have found no link between thimerosal-containing vaccines and ASD, as well as no link between the measles, mumps, and rubella (MMR) vaccine and ASD in children.

Between 1999 and 2001, thimerosal was removed or reduced to trace amounts in all childhood vaccines except for some flu vaccines. This was done as part of a broader national effort to reduce all types of mercury exposure in children before studies were conducted that determined that thimerosal was not harmful. It was done as a precaution. Currently, the only childhood vaccines that contain thimerosal are flu vaccines packaged in multidose vials. Thimerosal-free alternatives are also available for flu vaccine.

Besides thimerosal, some people have had concerns about other vaccine ingredients in relation to ASD as well. However, no links have been found between any vaccine ingredients and ASD.

Section 9.2

The Facts on Thimerosal, Mercury, and Vaccine Safety

This section includes text excerpted from "Understanding Thimerosal, Mercury, and Vaccine Safety," Centers for Disease Control and Prevention (CDC), February 2013. Reviewed October 2018.

What Is Thimerosal? Is It the Same as Mercury?

Thimerosal is a compound that contains mercury. Mercury is a metal found naturally in the environment.

Why Is Thimerosal Used in Some Vaccines?

Because it prevents the growth of dangerous microbes, thimerosal is used as a preservative in multidose vials of flu vaccines, and in two other childhood vaccines, it is used in the manufacturing process. When each new needle is inserted into the multidose vial, it is possible for microbes to get into the vial. The preservative, thimerosal, prevents contamination in the multidose vial when individual doses are drawn from it. Receiving a vaccine contaminated with bacteria can be deadly. For two childhood vaccines, thimerosal is used to prevent the growth of microbes during the manufacturing process. When thimerosal is used this way, it is removed later in the process. Only trace (very tiny) amounts remain. The only childhood vaccines that have trace amounts of thimerosal are one Diphtheria, Pertussis, and Tetanus (DTaP) and one DTaP-Hib (Diphtheria, Pertussis, and Tetanus-Haemophilus B) combination vaccine.

Why Was Thimerosal Removed from Vaccines Given to Children?

In 1999, the U.S. Food and Drug Administration (FDA) was required by law to assess the amount of mercury in all the products the agency oversees, not just vaccines. The U.S. Public Health Service (USPHS) decided that as much mercury as possible should be removed from vaccines, and thimerosal was the only source of mercury in vaccines. Even though there was no evidence that thimerosal in vaccines was dangerous, the decision to remove it was a made as a precautionary measure to decrease overall exposure to mercury among young infants.

55

This decision was possible because childhood vaccines could be reformulated to leave out thimerosal without threatening their safety, effectiveness, and purity. At present, no childhood vaccine used in the United States—except some formulations of flu vaccine in multidose vials—use thimerosal as a preservative.

Why Is Thimerosal Still in Some Flu Vaccines That Children May Receive?

To produce enough flu vaccine for the entire country, some of it must be put into multidose vials. When each individual vaccine dose is drawn from the vial with a fresh needle, it is possible for microbes to get into the vial. So, this preservative is needed to prevent contamination of the vial when individual doses are drawn from it. Children can safely receive flu vaccine that contains thimerosal. Flu vaccine in single-dose vials that does not contain thimerosal also is available.

Was Thimerosal in Vaccines a Cause of Autism?

Reputable scientific studies have shown that mercury in vaccines given to young children is not a cause of autism. The studies used different methods. Some examined rates of autism in a state or a country, comparing autism rates before and after thimerosal was removed as a preservative from vaccines. In the United States and other countries, the number of children diagnosed with autism has not gone down since thimerosal was removed from vaccines.

What Keeps Childhood Vaccines from Becoming Contaminated If They Do Not Contain Thimerosal as a Preservative?

The childhood vaccines that used to contain thimerosal as a preservative are now put into single-dose vials, so no preservative is needed. In the past, the vaccines were put into multidose vials, which could become contaminated when new needles were used to get the vaccine out of the vial for each dose.

Was Thimerosal Used in All Childhood Vaccines?

No. A few vaccines contained other preservatives, and they still do. Some other vaccines, including the measles, mumps, and rubella vaccine (MMR) never contained any preservative or any mercury.

56

Section 9.3

No Link between MMR Vaccine and Autism

This section includes text excerpted from "No Link between MMR Vaccine and Autism, Even in High-Risk Kids," National Institutes of Health (NIH), April 28, 2015. Reviewed October 2018.

Study after study has found no link between autism spectrum disorders (ASD) and the measles-mumps-rubella (MMR) vaccine—or any vaccine for that matter. Yet many parents still refuse or delay vaccinations for their young children based on misplaced fear of ASD, which can be traced back to a small 1998 study that's since been debunked and retracted. Such decisions can have a major negative impact on public health. With vaccination rates in decline, there is a resurgence of measles and other potentially fatal childhood infectious diseases.

Among the parents most likely to avoid getting their kids vaccinated are those who already have a child with ASD. So, it's especially important and timely news that researchers have once again found no link between MMR vaccines and ASD—even among children known to be at greater risk for autism because an older sibling has the developmental brain disorder (DBD).

In the new study published in *The Journal of the American Medical Association* (*JAMA*), an NIH-funded team, led by Anjali Jain of The Lewin Group, Falls Church, U.S. Department of Veterans Affairs, and Craig Newschaffer of Drexel University, Philadelphia, analyzed 2001–2012 health insurance claims for more than 95,000 children, ages birth to 5, plus their older siblings. More than 1,900 of the children studied had an older sibling with ASD, which is known to place them at greater risk of being diagnosed with ASD themselves.

Overall, about one percent of the children were diagnosed with ASD during the time period studied. The rate was significantly higher—nearly seven percent—among the children with an older sibling with ASD, but the risk did not increase if they had received the MMR vaccine. In fact, in families that had an older child with ASD, a vaccinated younger sibling was actually somewhat less likely to receive an autism diagnosis.

U.S. recommendations call for two doses of MMR vaccine in children at ages 12 to 15 months and then again at ages 4 to 6. Given the distressing resurgence of measles in California and elsewhere, and this study showing once again the lack of any connection of MMR vaccine and ASD, it's more critical than ever that parents protect their children against measles and other infectious diseases by staying current with vaccinations.

The consequences of not vaccinating children are serious: last year, in the United States, 668 people contracted measles in 27 states. That's no small matter because measles can lead to ear infections, pneumonia, seizures, brain damage, and even death. Furthermore, parents have a responsibility not only to their own children, but to the community— it's only by achieving a very high level of population immunity that outbreaks can be prevented. That's particularly crucial for those children with cancer and other diseases that cause immunosuppression. They cannot be vaccinated and depend on the so-called herd immunity of the community for protection against a potentially fatal infection.

As for ASD, the condition remains a major challenge for scientists and families alike. The research is just one part of a much larger effort by the National Institutes of Health (NIH) and its partners to understand the genetic and environmental risk factors for ASD, as well as to develop more effective pharmacological and behavioral interventions for affected children.

Chapter 10

Autism and the Environment

Research has shown that environmental factors likely play a role in autism. Studies also indicate that genetics contribute to the disorder. The National Institute of Environmental Health Sciences (NIEHS) supports research to discover how the environment may influence autism. This important environmental research offers real promise for prevention—because you can't change your genes, but you can change your environment.

What Is Autism?

Autism is a group of developmental brain disorders, known as autism spectrum disorders (ASDs), that begin early in life and affect how a person acts and interacts with others, communicates, and learns.

What Are the Symptoms?

Although people with autism have a variety of symptoms that vary in severity, they all have difficulties communicating and interacting with others, and show restricted and repetitive patterns of behavior and interests. Most symptoms are noticeable by the time a child is two to three years old, but many children are not diagnosed until later.

This chapter contains text excerpted from the following sources: Text in this chapter begins with excerpts from "Autism and the Environment," National Institute of Environmental Health Sciences (NIEHS), July 2014. Reviewed October 2018; Text under the heading "Prenatal Inflammation Linked to Autism Risk" is excerpted from "Prenatal Inflammation Linked to Autism Risk," National Institutes of Health (NIH), January 24, 2013. Reviewed October 2018.

59

Early intensive behavioral intervention can improve communication, learning, and social skills in children with autism.

Autism affects people for their entire lives, and often comes with other conditions, such as epilepsy, sleep disturbances, and gastrointestinal (GI) problems. At present, no drugs have proven effective for treating core autism symptoms.

The Impact of Autism

- Autism affects about one in 68 children.

- The number of children with autism more than doubled from 2000–2010.

- Autism is nearly five times more common in boys, one in 42, than girls, one in 189.

- People with autism had average medical expenses of $4,110 to $6,200 more per year than people without autism.

- Nearly half of children with autism, 46 percent, have average or above average intellectual ability.

Environmental Factors Play a Role in Autism

Air Pollution

Work supported by NIEHS indicates that early-life exposure to air pollution is a risk factor for autism.

- A 2011 study reported that children living within 1,014 feet, or a little less than 3.5 football fields, of a freeway, at birth, were twice as likely to develop autism.

- Building on those findings, in 2013, researchers reported an association between exposure to traffic-related air pollution, as well as components of regional air pollution, and an increased risk of autism.

- A 2014 study pointed to a likely gene-environment interaction. Children whose genetic makeup causes them to be more susceptible to the health effects of high levels of air pollution showed the highest risk for autism.

Nutrition

According to NIEHS-funded research, prenatal vitamins may help lower autism risk.

- Women who took a daily prenatal vitamin during the three months before and during the first month of pregnancy, were less likely to have a child with autism than women not taking the supplements. This was more evident in genetically susceptible women or children, suggesting that a gene-environment interaction could be responsible.

- A later study identified folic acid as the source of the protective effects of prenatal vitamins. Women who consumed the daily recommended dosage during the first month of pregnancy had a reduced risk of having a child with autism.

Mercury and Other Contaminants

There continues to be concern about autism and mercury exposure. NIEHS funds research examining this and exposures to other contaminants.

- Eating fish is the primary way that we are exposed to organic mercury. A study examined people in the Republic of Seychelles, where fish consumption is high. The study found no association between prenatal organic mercury exposure and autism behaviors.

- Scientists can test for recent exposure to organic mercury with blood tests. Researchers found that after adjusting for dietary and other mercury sources, children with autism had blood mercury levels that were similar to those found in children without autism.

- Researchers are also studying other contaminants, such as bisphenol A (BPA), phthalates, heavy metals, flame retardants, polychlorinated biphenyls (PCBs), and pesticides, to see if they affect early brain development and play a role in autism.

Prenatal Inflammation Linked to Autism Risk

Maternal inflammation during early pregnancy may be related to an increased risk of autism in children, according to the findings supported by the National Institute of Environmental Health Sciences (NIEHS), part of the National Institutes of Health (NIH). Researchers found this in children of mothers with elevated C-reactive protein (CRP), a well-established marker of systemic inflammation.

The risk of autism among children in the study was increased by 43 percent among mothers with CRP levels in the top twentieth

61

percentile, and by 80 percent for maternal CRP in the top tenth percentile. The findings appear in the journal *Molecular Psychiatry* and add to mounting evidence that an overactive immune response can alter the development of the central nervous system in the fetus.

"Elevated CRP is a signal that the body is undergoing a response to inflammation from, for example, a viral or bacterial infection," said lead scientist on the study, Alan Brown, M.D., professor of clinical psychiatry and epidemiology at Columbia University College of Physicians and Surgeons (P&S), New York State Psychiatric Institute (NYSPI), and Mailman School of Public Health. "The higher the level of CRP in the mother, the greater the risk of autism in the child."

Brown cautioned that the results should be viewed in perspective since the prevalence of inflammation during pregnancy is substantially higher than the prevalence of autism.

"The vast majority of mothers with increased CRP levels will not give birth to children with autism," Brown said. "We don't know enough yet to suggest routine testing of pregnant mothers for CRP for this reason alone; however, exercising precautionary measures to prevent infections during pregnancy may be of considerable value."

"The brain develops rapidly throughout pregnancy," said Linda Birnbaum, Ph.D., director of NIEHS, which funds a broad portfolio of autism and neurodevelopmental-related research. "This has important implications for understanding how the environment and our genes interact to cause autism and other neurodevelopmental disorders."

The study capitalized on a unique national birth cohort known as the Finnish Maternity Cohort (FMC), which contains an archive of samples collected from pregnant women in Finland, where a component of whole blood, referred to as serum, is systematically collected during the early part of pregnancy. The FMC consists of 1.6 million specimens from about 810,000 women, archived in a single, centralized biorepository. Finland also maintains diagnoses of virtually all childhood autism cases from national registries of both hospital admissions and outpatient treatment.

From this large national sample, the researchers analyzed CRP in archived maternal serum corresponding to 677 childhood autism cases and an equal number of matched controls. The findings were not explained by maternal age, paternal age, gender, previous births, socioeconomic status, preterm birth, or birth weight. The work was conducted in collaboration with investigators in Finland, including the University of Turku and the National Institute for Health and Welfare (THL) in Oulu and Helsinki.

"Studying autism can be challenging, because symptoms may not be apparent in children until certain brain functions, such as language, come on line," said Cindy Lawler, Ph.D., head of the NIEHS Cellular, Organ, and Systems Pathobiology Branch (COSPB) and program lead for the Institute's extramural portfolio of autism research. "This study is remarkable, because it uses biomarker data to give us a glimpse back to a critical time in early pregnancy."

This work is expected to stimulate further research on autism, which is complex and challenging to identify causes. Future studies may help define how infections, other inflammatory insults, and the body's immune response interact with genes to elevate the risk for autism and other neurodevelopmental disorders. Preventative approaches addressing environmental causes of autism may also benefit from additional research.

Chapter 11

Premature Birth and Autism

Preterm Birth (PB)—A Growing Global Healthcare Crisis

Preterm birth (PB) is the leading cause of death in the first month of life and a contributing factor in more than a third of all infant deaths. Moreover, infants who survive an early birth face the risk of serious lifelong health problems. Even late preterm infants have a greater risk of respiratory problems, feeding difficulties, temperature instability, delayed brain development and an increased risk of autism, cerebral palsy (CP), and mental retardation. In fact, according to an analysis of nearly 7 million U.S. live births, preterm infants are more than twice as likely to have major birth defects as full-term infants.

In a report on the topic of child health, from the Institute of Medicine (IOM) of the National Academies, it is stated that in 2005, 12.5 percent of births in the United States were preterm (less than 37 weeks gestation). The high rate of premature births in the United States alone constitutes a public health concern that costs society at least $26 billion a year. The heartbreaking toll in terms of human and family suffering cannot be calculated. For the underprivileged and those in underdeveloped and developing countries, additional tens of millions are even more devastated—as the families and children

---

This chapter includes text excerpted from "Preterm Birth: A Growing Human Healthcare Crisis," National Institute of Standards and Technology (NIST), November 13, 2009. Reviewed October 2018.

struggling with this condition and suffering these outcomes are unable to obtain medical assistance and are also often outcast by their societies.

The report, "Preterm Birth: Causes, Consequences, and Prevention," notes that despite great strides in improving the survival of infants born preterm, little is known about how preterm births can be prevented (a primary focus to the research and development underway at TechDyne/ViaTechMD). Nevertheless, survival very often comes at the great cost of serious lifelong health problems. The report goes on to recommend a multidisciplinary research agenda aimed at improving the prediction and prevention of preterm labor and better understanding the health and developmental problems to which preterm infants are more vulnerable. With layer upon layer of bureaucracy complicating matters, little is being accomplished.

The increasing prevalence of PB, related mortality, and lifelong disability is a complex public health issue that requires multifaceted solutions. The subject of PB is described by a confused cluster of datum, with a complex set of overlapping factors of influence. Its causes may include individual-level behavioral and psychosocial factors, sociodemographic and neighborhood characteristics, environmental exposure, medical conditions, infertility treatments, and biological factors. Many of these factors co-occur, particularly in those who are socioeconomically disadvantaged or who are members of racial and ethnic minority groups, further complicating the equation.

While advances in perinatal and neonatal care have improved survival for preterm infants, those infants who do survive have a greater risk than infants born at full term for developmental disabilities, health problems, and poor growth. The birth of a preterm two infant can also bring considerable emotional and economic costs to families and have implications for public sector services, such as health insurance, educational, and other social support systems.

Autism—Directly Related to Preterm Birth

Autism is a brain development disorder characterized by impaired social interaction and communication, and by restricted and repetitive behavior. According to the fact-findings, compiled from sources including the National Institutes of Health (NIH), the Centers for Disease Control and Prevention (CDC), the U.S. Department of Education (ED), and the Autism Society of America (ASA), autism is the fastest growing developmental disease (which correlates with the growing incidence of PB birth due specifically to insufficient cervix (IC)).

While research in this critical area is limited, a U.S. study (released by *The Journal of Pediatrics*) focused on children born more than three months prematurely provided fresh evidence supporting the thesis of this paper—including the link between PB birth and autism. Those children were found to be two to three times more likely to show signs of autism at age two (as measured in a standard screening tool compared to other children).

Autism refers to a group of developmental problems known as autism spectrum disorders that appear in early childhood and impair the ability to communicate and interact with others. Early research suggesting a link between PB and autism followed 988 U.S. children born very prematurely, at least three months before their due date. At age two, the children were evaluated using a screening method in which they are rated on a checklist of 23 behaviors for signs of autism. This tool flags children who may have autism but is not considered a definitive diagnosis. While more typically, a formal diagnosis of autism does not occur until around age 3, in this study, less than 6 percent of infants born full-term screened positive for possible autism, while 21 percent of infants born preterm scored positive.

Even with this dramatic evidence, researchers remain confused, partially because preterm infants may also demonstrate certain developmental problems unrelated to autism that could trigger a positive score. For example, researchers typically excluded children with motor, vision and hearing impairments. Even after doing that, 16 percent of the preterm infants scored positive for possible autism. Moreover, after also excluding infants with cognitive impairment on the premise that it may not be full-term, about 10 percent of the preterm children still had a positive screening score. What researchers are likely missing is the fact that multiple disorders are possible as a result of PB (just as multiple injuries to an individual are possible as a result of a single automobile accident). Confused research or not, it is very clear that PB is associated with a long list of health risks for infants.

About 1 in 150 U.S. children has an autism spectrum disorder, according to U.S. government figures. The socioeconomic consequences of autism, all told exceed $90 billion annually (U.S. only).

Chapter 12

Early Development Risk Factors for ASD

Study to Explore Early Development (SEED)

The Study to Explore Early Development (SEED) is a multiyear study funded by the Centers for Disease Control and Prevention (CDC). It is one of the largest studies of its kind that will help identify factors that might put children at risk for autism spectrum disorder (ASD).

- SEED continues to invite children, ages two through five years, and their parents into the study. Thousands of families have participated. It is one of the largest studies of ASD in the United States.

- There are three study groups in SEED:

  - Children with ASD

  - Children with their developmental disabilities

  - Children without developmental disabilities

This chapter contains text excerpted from the following sources: Text beginning with the heading "Study to Explore Early Development (SEED)" is excerpted from "CDC's Study to Explore Early Development," Centers for Disease Control and Prevention (CDC), March 27, 2014. Reviewed October 2018; Text beginning with the heading "Understanding Autism Spectrum Disorders and Other Developmental Disabilities" is excerpted from "Study to Explore Early Development," Centers for Disease Control and Prevention (CDC), March 30, 2012. Reviewed October 2018.

- It collects in-depth information from participants to answer questions about many factors that might put children at risk for ASD, including genetic, environmental, pregnancy, and behavioral factors.

Building the Public Health Infrastructure for Autism Spectrum Disorder

To better characterize factors that put children at risk for ASD, the Children's Health Act of 2000 authorized the CDC to create regional centers of excellence for autism and other developmental disabilities. These centers make up the Centers for Autism and Developmental Disabilities Research and Epidemiology (CADDRE) Network. At present, the CADDRE Network is working on the Study to Explore Early Development (SEED). The SEED research study sites are located in Colorado, Georgia, Maryland, Missouri, North Carolina, and Wisconsin. The Data Coordinating Center (DCC) is in Michigan and it is responsible for data information systems and technology. CADDRE also supports a laboratory at the Maryland SEED site where SEED biological samples are processed and stored.

Research Goals for SEED

- Physical and behavioral characteristics of children with ASD, children with other developmental disabilities, and children without a developmental delay or disability.

  ASD is complex. The CDC wants to learn more about children with ASD—how they behave, grow, think, and interact with the world around them. It also wants to know the same things about children with other developmental disabilities and those with typical development.

- Health conditions among children with ASD, children with other developmental disabilities, and children with typical development.

  SEED provides an opportunity to compare health conditions and health-related issues (such as sleeping and eating patterns) among children with ASD, among children with other developmental disabilities, and among children without a developmental delay or disability.

- Factors that might affect a child's risk for ASD.

  It is expected that SEED will give a better idea which of the many possible factors that will be evaluated seem to be associated with or related to ASD. The factors might be related, for example, to genes, health conditions, experiences of the mother during pregnancy, or the health and development of the child during infancy and the first few years of life.

Understanding Autism Spectrum Disorders and Other Developmental Disabilities

- The CDC estimates that 1 in 88 children has been identified with an ASD.
- ASDs occur among all racial, ethnic, and socioeconomic groups.
- ASDs are almost five times more common among boys than among girls.
- Medical costs for children with ASDs are estimated to be six times higher than for children without ASDs.
- In addition to medical costs, intensive behavioral interventions for children with ASDs can cost $40,000 to $60,000 per child per year.

Identifying Risk Factors for Autism Spectrum Disorders and Other Developmental Disabilities

There is still a lot to learn about ASDs. Research on ASDs has increased and the CDC is part of the larger group of public and private organizations working to better understand ASDs through research. The CDC is undertaking efforts to find out how many children have ASDs, discover the risk factors for and causes of ASDs, and raise awareness of the signs and symptoms of ASDs.

- The Study to Explore Early Development (SEED) is a multiyear, multisite study in six diverse areas that looks at possible causes of and risks for ASDs and other developmental delays.
- SEED is the largest multisite study in the United States to help identify factors that might put children at risk for ASDs and other developmental disabilities.
- SEED is looking at many possible risk factors for ASDs, including genetic, environmental, pregnancy, and behavioral factors.

Chapter 13

Assisted Reproductive Technology and Risk for Autism Spectrum Disorder

What Is Assisted Reproductive Technology?

Although various definitions have been used for assisted reproductive technology (ART), the definition used by the Centers for Disease Control and Prevention (CDC) is based on the 1992 Fertility Clinic Success Rate and Certification Act (FCSRCA) that requires the CDC to publish the annual ART Success Rates Report. According to this definition, ART includes all fertility treatments in which both eggs and embryos are handled. In general, ART procedures involve surgically removing eggs from a woman's ovaries, combining them with sperm in the laboratory, and returning them to the woman's body or donating them to another woman. They do NOT include treatments in which only sperm are handled (i.e., intrauterine—or artificial—insemination)

This chapter contains text excerpted from the following sources: Text beginning with the heading "What Is Assisted Reproductive Technology (ART)?" is excerpted from "What Is Assisted Reproductive Technology?" Centers for Disease Control and Prevention (CDC), February 7, 2017; Text beginning with the heading "The Association between Assisted Reproductive Technology and Autism Spectrum Disorder" is excerpted from "Key Findings: The Association between Assisted Reproductive Technology and Autism Spectrum Disorder," Centers for Disease Control and Prevention (CDC), April 28, 2017.

or procedures in which a woman takes medicine only to stimulate egg production without the intention of having eggs retrieved.

More than 20 Years of ART Surveillance

ART can alleviate the burden of infertility on individuals and families, but it can also present challenges to public health as evidenced by the high rates of multiple delivery, preterm delivery, and low birth-weight delivery experienced with ART. Monitoring the outcomes of technologies that affect reproduction, such as contraception and ART, has become an important public health activity.

The CDC's Division of Reproductive Health (DRH) has a long history of surveillance and research in women's health and fertility, adolescent reproductive health, and safe motherhood. In response to congressional mandate, the CDC began work to strengthen existing data collection efforts initiated by the American Society for Reproductive Medicine (ASRM) and the Society for Assisted Reproductive Technology (SART) and to develop a national system for monitoring ART use and outcomes.

In 1997, the CDC submitted to Congress the first annual report, titled *Assisted Reproductive Technology Success Rates: National Summary and Fertility Clinic Reports*. This report gained a wide audience, including potential ART patients and their families, policymakers, researchers, and healthcare providers. Maternal and child health professionals, as well as state and local public health departments, also began requesting data on birth outcomes among infants born using ART technologies in their localities. In 2002, the CDC prepared the first ART surveillance report on ART use and outcomes by state. The ART Surveillance Summary is published as a supplement to the CDC's Morbidity and Mortality Weekly Report (MMWR).

Expanding the Scope of ART Outcomes Research

The National ART Surveillance System (NASS) does not contain information on long-term outcomes of ART. This information can be obtained by linking ART surveillance data with other surveillance systems and registries, while paying close attention to confidentiality protection. Since 2001, the CDC has collaborated with health departments of three states (Massachusetts, and later Michigan and Florida), to link NASS with vital records, hospital discharge data, birth defects registries, cancer registries, and other surveillance systems of these states. This project, called States Monitoring ART (SMART)

Collaborative, provides a unique opportunity for federal and state public health agencies to work together on establishing state-based public health surveillance of ART, infertility, and related issues.

The Association between Assisted Reproductive Technology and Autism Spectrum Disorder

Researchers have published new studies looking at the relationship between assisted reproductive technology (ART) and autism spectrum disorder (ASD) among a group of children born in California between 1997 and 2007. The key findings from each study are highlighted below.

Does Assisted Reproductive Technology Increase the Risk for Autism Spectrum Disorder?

- Overall, children conceived using ART were about two times more likely to be diagnosed with ASD compared to children conceived without using ART.

- Evidence suggests that for pregnancies conceived with ART, the increased risk for ASD is, in large part, due to the higher likelihood of adverse pregnancy and delivery outcomes. In other words, using ART may lead to factors that are known to put children at risk for ASD, such as being born a twin or multiple (triplets, quadruplets, etc.), being born too early, or being born too small.

- More research is needed to explore what exactly underlies the observed relationship between ART and ASD.

- However, these findings suggest that single embryo transfer, where appropriate, may reduce the risk of ASD among children conceived using ART.

Does Type of ART Procedure Impact the Relationship between Assisted Reproductive Technology and Autism Spectrum Disorder?

- Among children conceived using ART, about 0.8 percent of those born as singletons (only one baby carried during the pregnancy) and about 1.2 percent of those born as a twin or multiple were diagnosed with ASD.

- Children conceived using ART were more likely to be diagnosed with ASD if intracytoplasmic sperm injection (ICSI) was used compared to conventional in vitro fertilization. ICSI and in vitro fertilization are procedures in which fertilization (a sperm entering an egg) occurs outside of the body; ICSI occurs by injecting a sperm directly into an egg while in vitro fertilization involves mixing sperm with eggs in a laboratory dish and allowing fertilization to occur.

- More research is needed to explore what exactly underlies the observed relationship between ICSI and ASD.

Part Three

Identifying and Diagnosing Autism Spectrum Disorders

Chapter 14

Symptoms of Autism Spectrum Disorder

Chapter Contents

Section 14.1

Range of Symptoms

This section includes text excerpted from "Autism
Spectrum Disorder (ASD)—Signs and Symptoms," Centers for
Disease Control and Prevention (CDC), April 26, 2018.

Autism spectrum disorder (ASD) is a developmental disability caused by differences in the brain. Scientists do not know yet exactly what causes these differences for most people with ASD. However, some people with ASD have a known difference, such as a genetic condition. There are multiple causes of ASD, although most are not yet known.

There is often nothing about how people with ASD look that sets them apart from other people, but they may communicate, interact, behave, and learn in ways that are different from most other people. The learning, thinking, and problem-solving abilities of people with ASD can range from gifted to severely challenged. Some people with ASD need a lot of help in their daily lives; others need less.

A diagnosis of ASD now includes several conditions that used to be diagnosed separately: autistic disorder, pervasive developmental disorder not otherwise specified (PDD-NOS), and Asperger syndrome. These conditions are now all called autism spectrum disorder.

ASD begins before the age of 3 and lasts throughout a person's life, although symptoms may improve over time. Some children with ASD show hints of future problems within the first few months of life. In others, symptoms may not show up until 24 months or later. Some children with an ASD seem to develop normally until around 18–24 months of age and then they stop gaining new skills, or they lose the skills they once had. Studies have shown that one third to half of the parents of children with an ASD noticed a problem before their child's first birthday, and nearly 80–90 percent saw problems by 24 months of age.

It is important to note that some people without ASD might also have some of these symptoms. But for people with ASD, the impairments make life very challenging.

Possible "Red Flags"

A person with ASD might:

- Not respond to their name by 12 months of age

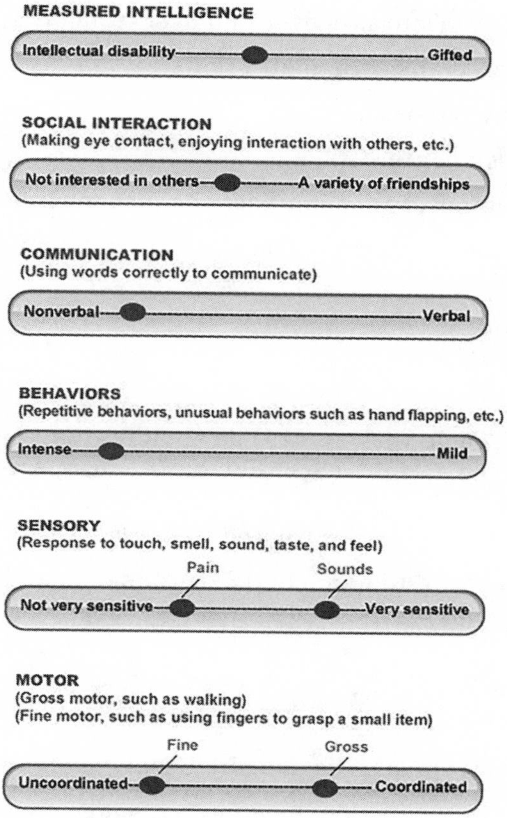

MEASURED INTELLIGENCE

Intellectual disability————●————————Gifted

SOCIAL INTERACTION
(Making eye contact, enjoying interaction with others, etc.)

Not interested in others—●————A variety of friendships

COMMUNICATION
(Using words correctly to communicate)

Nonverbal—●————————————Verbal

BEHAVIORS
(Repetitive behaviors, unusual behaviors such as hand flapping, etc.)

Intense—●————————————Mild

SENSORY
(Response to touch, smell, sound, taste, and feel)

Pain   Sounds

Not very sensitive—●————————●—Very sensitive

MOTOR
(Gross motor, such as walking)
(Fine motor, such as using fingers to grasp a small item)

Fine   Gross

Uncoordinated—●————————●—Coordinated

Figure 14.1. *Example of Range of Symptoms*

The above chart—a person might have average intelligence, have little interest in other people, use limited verbal language, experience intense self-stimulatory behaviors such as hand-flapping, under-react to pain and over-react to sounds, have very good gross motor skills, and have weaknesses in fine motor skills. These symptoms may vary widely from person to person.

- Not point at objects to show interest (point at an airplane flying over) by 14 months
- Not play "pretend" games (pretend to "feed" a doll) by 18 months
- Avoid eye contact and want to be alone
- Have trouble understanding other people's feelings or talking about their own feelings
- Have delayed speech and language skills

81

- Repeat words or phrases over and over (echolalia)
- Give unrelated answers to questions
- Get upset by minor changes
- Have obsessive interests
- Flap their hands, rock their body, or spin in circles
- Have unusual reactions to the way things sound, smell, taste, look, or feel

Social Skills

Social issues are one of the most common symptoms in all of the types of ASD. People with an ASD do not have just social "difficulties" like shyness. The social issues they have cause serious problems in everyday life.

Examples of social issues related to ASD:

- Does not respond to name by 12 months of age
- Avoids eye contact
- Prefers to play alone
- Does not share interests with others
- Only interacts to achieve a desired goal
- Has flat or inappropriate facial expressions
- Does not understand personal space boundaries
- Avoids or resists physical contact
- Is not comforted by others during distress
- Has trouble understanding other people's feelings or talking about own feelings

Typical infants are very interested in the world and people around them. By the first birthday, a typical toddler interacts with others by looking people in the eye, copying words and actions, and using simple gestures such as clapping and waving "bye bye." Typical toddlers also show interests in social games like peek-a-boo and pat-a-cake. But a young child with an ASD might have a very hard time learning to interact with other people.

Some people with an ASD might not be interested in other people at all. Others might want friends, but not understand how to develop friendships. Many children with an ASD have a very hard time learning to take turns and share—much more so than other children. This can make other children not want to play with them.

People with an ASD might have problems with showing or talking about their feelings. They might also have trouble understanding other people's feelings. Many people with an ASD are very sensitive to being touched and might not want to be held or cuddled. Self-stimulatory behaviors (e.g., flapping arms over and over) are common among people with an ASD. Anxiety and depression also affect some people with an ASD. All of these symptoms can make other social problems even harder to manage.

Communication

Each person with ASD has different communication skills. Some people can speak well. Others can't speak at all or only very little. About 40 percent of children with an ASD do not talk at all. About 25–30 percent of children with ASD have some words at 12–18 months of age and then lose them. Others might speak, but not until later in childhood.

Examples of communication issues related to ASD:

- Delayed speech and language skills

- Repeats words or phrases over and over (echolalia)

- Reverses pronouns (e.g., says "you" instead of "I")

- Gives unrelated answers to questions

- Does not point or respond to pointing

- Uses few or no gestures (e.g., does not wave goodbye)

- Talks in a flat, robot-like, or singsong voice

- Does not pretend in play (e.g., does not pretend to "feed" a doll)

- Does not understand jokes, sarcasm, or teasing

People with ASD who do speak might use language in unusual ways. They might not be able to put words into real sentences. Some people with ASD say only one word at a time. Others repeat the same words or phrases over and over. Some children repeat what others say, a condition called echolalia. The repeated words might be said right away or at a later time. For example, if you ask someone with ASD, "Do you want some juice?" she or he might repeat "Do you want some juice?" instead of answering your question. Although many children without an ASD go through a stage where they repeat what they hear, it normally passes by three years of age. Some people with an ASD can speak well but might have a hard time listening to what other people say.

People with ASD might have a hard time using and understanding gestures, body language, or tone of voice. For example, people with ASD might not understand what it means to wave goodbye. Facial expressions, movements, and gestures may not match what they are saying. For instance, people with an ASD might smile while saying something sad.

People with ASD might say "I" when they mean "you," or vice versa. Their voices might sound flat, robot-like, or high-pitched. People with an ASD might stand too close to the person they are talking to, or might stick with one topic of conversation for too long. They might talk a lot about something they really like, rather than have a back-and-forth conversation with someone. Some children with fairly good language skills speak like little adults, failing to pick up on the "kid-speak" that is common with other children.

Unusual Interests and Behaviors

Many people with ASD have unusual interest or behaviors. Examples of unusual interests and behaviors related to ASD:

- Lines up toys or other objects
- Plays with toys the same way every time
- Likes parts of objects (e.g., wheels)
- Is very organized
- Gets upset by minor changes
- Has obsessive interests
- Has to follow certain routines
- Flaps hands, rocks body, or spins self in circles

Repetitive motions are actions repeated over and over again. They can involve one part of the body or the entire body or even an object or toy. For instance, people with an ASD might spend a lot of time repeatedly flapping their arms or rocking from side to side. They might repeatedly turn a light on and off or spin the wheels of a toy car. These types of activities are known as self-stimulation or "stimming."

People with ASD often thrive on routine. A change in the normal pattern of the day—like a stop on the way home from school—can be very upsetting to people with ASD. They might "lose control" and have a "meltdown" or tantrum, especially if in a strange place.

Some people with ASD also may develop routines that might seem unusual or unnecessary. For example, a person might try to look in every window she or he walks by a building or might always want to watch a video from beginning to end, including the previews and the credits. Not being allowed to do these types of routines might cause severe frustration and tantrums.

Other Symptoms

Some people with ASD have other symptoms. These might include:

- Hyperactivity (very active)

- Impulsivity (acting without thinking)

- Short attention span

- Aggression

- Causing self-injury

- Temper tantrums

- Unusual eating and sleeping habits

- Unusual mood or emotional reactions

- Lack of fear or more fear than expected

- Unusual reactions to the way things sound, smell, taste, look, or feel

People with ASD might have unusual responses to touch, smell, sounds, sights, and taste, and feel. For example, they might over- or under-react to pain or to a loud noise. They might have abnormal eating habits. For instance, some people with an ASD limit their diet to only a few foods. Others might eat nonfood items like dirt or rocks (this is called pica). They might also have issues like chronic constipation or diarrhea.

People with ASD might have odd sleeping habits. They also might have abnormal moods or emotional reactions. For instance, they might laugh or cry at unusual times or show no emotional response at times you would expect one. In addition, they might not be afraid of dangerous things, and they could be fearful of harmless objects or events.

85

Development

Children with ASD develop at different rates in different areas. They may have delays in language, social, and learning skills, while their ability to walk and move around are about the same as other children their age. They might be very good at putting puzzles together or solving computer problems, but they might have trouble with social activities like talking or making friends. Children with an ASD might also learn a hard skill before they learn an easy one. For example, a child might be able to read long words but not be able to tell you what sound a "b" makes.

Children develop at their own pace, so it can be difficult to tell exactly when a child will learn a particular skill. But, there are age-specific developmental milestones used to measure a child's social and emotional progress in the first few years of life.

Section 14.2

Autism Symptoms Emerge in Infancy

This section includes text excerpted from "When Do Children Usually Show Symptoms of Autism?" *Eunice Kennedy Shriver* National Institute of Child Health and Human Development (NICHD), January 31, 2017.

The behavioral symptoms of autism spectrum disorder (ASD) often appear early in development. Many children show symptoms of autism by 12 months to 18 months of age or earlier. Some early signs of autism include:

- Problems with eye contact

- No response to his or her name

- Problems following another person's gaze or pointed finger to an object (or "joint attention")

- Poor skills in pretend play and imitation

- Problems with nonverbal communication

Many parents are not aware of these "early" signs of autism and don't start thinking about autism until their children do not start talking at a typical age.

Most children with autism are not diagnosed until after age three, even though healthcare providers can often see developmental problems before that age.

Research shows that early detection and early intervention greatly improve outcomes, so it's important to look for these symptoms when a child is as young as possible.

Regression

Some children with autism regress, meaning they stop using language, play, or social skills that they've already learned. This regression may happen between ages one year and two years. It might happen earlier for some social behaviors, such as looking at faces and sharing a smile. Researchers don't know why some children regress into autism or which children are likely to regress.

Other Early Signs

There also may be early biological signs of ASD. Some studies have shown that:

- People with autism have unique brain activity, structures, and connections even at very young ages.

- There are differences in brain growth in ASD as early as six months of age.

Section 14.3

Eye Response during Infancy for Autism

This section includes text excerpted from "Earliest
Marker for Autism Found in Young Infants," National
Institutes of Health (NIH), November 6, 2013.
Reviewed October 2018.

Eye contact during early infancy may be a key to early identification of autism, according to a study funded by the National Institute of Mental Health (NIMH), part of the National Institutes of Health (NIH). Published in the journal *Nature*, the study reveals the earliest sign of developing autism ever observed—a steady decline in attention to others' eyes within the first two to six months of life.

"Autism isn't usually diagnosed until after age 2, when delays in a child's social behavior and language skills become apparent. This study shows that children exhibit clear signs of autism at a much younger age," said Thomas R. Insel, M.D., director of NIMH. "The sooner we are able to identify early markers for autism, the more effective our treatment interventions can be."

Typically developing children begin to focus on human faces within the first few hours of life, and they learn to pick up social cues by paying special attention to other people's eyes. Children with autism, however, do not exhibit this sort of interest in eye-looking. In fact, a lack of eye contact is one of the diagnostic features of the disorder.

To find out how this deficit in eye-looking emerges in children with autism, Warren Jones, Ph.D., and Ami Klin, Ph.D., of the Marcus Autism Center (MAC), Children's Healthcare of Atlanta, and Emory University School of Medicine followed infants from birth to age three. The infants were divided into two groups, based on their risk for developing an autism spectrum disorder (ASD). Those in the high-risk group had an older sibling already diagnosed with autism; those in the low-risk group did not.

Jones and Klin used eye-tracking equipment to measure each child's eye movements as they watched video scenes of a caregiver. The researchers calculated the percentage of time each child fixated on the caregiver's eyes, mouth, and body, as well as the nonhuman spaces in the images. Children were tested at 10 different times between 2 and 24 months of age.

By age 3, some of the children—nearly all from the high-risk group—had received a clinical diagnosis of an autism spectrum disorder. The researchers then reviewed the eye-tracking data to determine what factors differed between those children who received an autism diagnosis and those who did not.

"In infants later diagnosed with autism, we see a steady decline in how much they look at mom's eyes," said Jones. This drop in eye-looking began between two and six months and continued throughout the course of the study. By 24 months, the children later diagnosed with autism focused on the caregiver's eyes only about half as long as did their typically developing counterparts.

This decline in attention to others' eyes was somewhat surprising to the researchers. In opposition to a long-standing theory in the field— that social behaviors are entirely absent in children with autism— these results suggest that social engagement skills are intact shortly after birth in children with autism. If clinicians can identify this sort of marker for autism in a young infant, interventions may be better able to keep the child's social development on track.

"This insight, the preservation of some early eye-looking, is important," explained Jones. "In the future, if we were able to use similar technologies to identify early signs of social disability, we could then consider interventions to build on that early eye-looking and help reduce some of the associated disabilities that often accompany autism."

The next step for Jones and Klin is to translate this finding into a viable tool for use in the clinic. With support from the NIH Autism Centers of Excellence (ACE) program, the research team has already started to extend this research by enrolling many more babies and their families into related long-term studies. They also plan to examine additional markers for autism in infancy in order to give clinicians more tools for the early identification and treatment of autism.

Chapter 15

Developmental Screening

Chapter Contents

Section 15.1

Developmental Milestones

This section contains text excerpted from the following
sources: Text in this section begins with excerpts from "Autism
Spectrum Disorder (ASD)—Screening and Diagnosis," Centers
for Disease Control and Prevention (CDC), April 26, 2018; Text
beginning with the heading "Your Child by One Year" is excerpted
from "Important Milestones: Your Child by One Year," Centers for
Disease Control and Prevention (CDC), June 19, 2018.

Diagnosing autism spectrum disorder (ASD) can be difficult, since there is no medical test, like a blood test, to diagnose the disorders. Doctors look at the child's behavior and development to make a diagnosis.

ASD can sometimes be detected at 18 months or younger. By age two, a diagnosis by an experienced professional can be considered very reliable. However, many children do not receive a final diagnosis until much older. This delay means that children with an ASD might not get the help they need.

Diagnosing an ASD takes two steps:

1. Developmental screening

2. Comprehensive diagnostic evaluation

Developmental Screening

Developmental screening is a short test to tell if children are learning basic skills when they should, or if they might have delays. During developmental screening, the doctor might ask the parent some questions or talk and play with the child during an exam to see how she learns, speaks, behaves, and moves. A delay in any of these areas could be a sign of a problem.

All children should be screened for developmental delays and disabilities during regular well-child doctor visits at:

- 9 months

- 18 months

- 24 or 30 months

- Additional screening might be needed if a child is at high risk for developmental problems due to preterm birth, low birth weight or other reasons

In addition, all children should be screened specifically for ASD during regular well-child doctor visits at:

- 18 months

- 24 months

- Additional screening might be needed if a child is at high risk for ASD (e.g., having a sister, brother, or other family member with an ASD) or if behaviors sometimes associated with ASD are present

It is important for doctors to screen all children for developmental delays, but especially to monitor those who are at a higher risk for developmental problems due to preterm birth, low birth weight, or having a brother or sister with an ASD.

If your child's doctor does not routinely check your child with this type of developmental screening test, ask that it be done.

If the doctor sees any signs of a problem, a comprehensive diagnostic evaluation is needed.

Comprehensive Diagnostic Evaluation

The second step of diagnosis is a comprehensive evaluation. This thorough review may include looking at the child's behavior and development and interviewing the parents. It may also include a hearing and vision screening, genetic testing, neurological testing, and other medical testing.

In some cases, the primary care doctor might choose to refer the child and family to a specialist for further assessment and diagnosis. Specialists who can do this type of evaluation include:

- Developmental Pediatricians (doctors who have special training in child development and children with special needs)

- Child Neurologists (doctors who work on the brain, spine, and nerves)

- Child Psychologists or Psychiatrists (doctors who know about the human mind)

Your Child by One Year

How your child plays, learns, speaks, acts, and moves offer important clues about your child's development. Developmental milestones are things most children can do by a certain age.

Check the milestones your child has reached by his or her 1st birthday. Take this with you and talk with your child's doctor at every visit about the milestones your child has reached and what to expect next.

What Most Children Do by This Age
Social and Emotional

- Is shy or nervous with strangers
- Cries when mom or dad leaves
- Has favorite things and people
- Shows fear in some situations
- Hands you a book when he wants to hear a story
- Repeats sounds or actions to get attention
- Puts out arm or leg to help with dressing
- Plays games such as "peek-a-boo" and "pat-a-cake"

Language/Communication

- Responds to simple spoken requests
- Uses simple gestures, like shaking head "no" or waving "bye-bye"
- Makes sounds with changes in tone (sounds more like speech)
- Says "mama" and "dada" and exclamations like "uh-oh!"
- Tries to say words you say

Cognitive (Learning, Thinking, Problem-Solving)

- Explores things in different ways, like shaking, banging, throwing
- Finds hidden things easily
- Looks at the right picture or thing when it's named
- Copies gestures
- Starts to use things correctly; for example, drinks from a cup, brushes hair
- Bangs two things together
- Puts things in a container, takes things out of a container

- Lets things go without help
- Pokes with index (pointer) finger
- Follows simple directions like "pick up the toy"

Movement / Physical Development

- Gets to a sitting position without help
- Pulls up to stand, walks holding on to furniture ("cruising")
- May take a few steps without holding on
- May stand alone

When to Contact Doctor

Act early by talking to your child's doctor if your child:

- Doesn't crawl
- Can't stand when supported
- Doesn't search for things that she sees you hide
- Doesn't say single words like "mama" or "dada"
- Doesn't learn gestures like waving or shaking head
- Doesn't point to things
- Loses skills he once had

Section 15.2

Recommendations for Routine Healthcare Developmental Screening

This section includes text excerpted from "Autism Spectrum Disorder (ASD)—Recommendations and Guidelines," Centers for Disease Control and Prevention (CDC), April 26, 2018.

Autism A.L.A.R.M. Guidelines

The Autism is prevalent, Listen to parents, Act early, Refer, and Monitor (A.L.A.R.M.) guidelines, adapted from key policy statements of the American Academy of Pediatrics (AAP) and American Academy of Neurology (AAN), were developed to establish standard practices among physicians, simplify the screening process, and ensure that all children receive routine and appropriate screenings and timely interventions.

Developmental Surveillance and Screening

Early identification of developmental disorders is critical to the well-being of children and their families. It is an integral function of medical primary care and an appropriate responsibility of all pediatric healthcare professionals.

The American Academy of Pediatrics (AAP) recommends that developmental surveillance be incorporated at every well-child preventive care visit. Any concerns raised during surveillance should be addressed promptly with standardized developmental screening tests. In addition, screening tests should be administered regularly at the 9-, 18-, and 24- or 30-month visits.

The early identification of developmental problems should lead to further developmental and medical evaluation, diagnosis, and treatment, including early developmental intervention. Children diagnosed with developmental disorders should be identified as children with special healthcare needs, and chronic-condition management should be initiated. Identification of a developmental disorder and its underlying etiology may also drive a range of treatment planning, from medical treatment of the child to genetic counseling for the parents.

Developmental Surveillance and Screening for Autism Spectrum Disorder

1. Developmental surveillance should be performed at all well-child visits from infancy through school age, and at any age thereafter if concerns are raised about social acceptance, learning, or behavior.

2. Recommended developmental screening tools include the Ages and Stages Questionnaire, the BRIGANCE® Screens, the Child Development Inventories, and the Parents' Evaluations of Developmental Status.

3. Because of the lack of sensitivity and specificity, the Denver-II (DDST-II) and the Revised Denver Pre-Screening Developmental Questionnaire (R-DPDQ) are not recommended for appropriate primary-care developmental surveillance.

4. Further developmental evaluation is required whenever a child fails to meet any of the following milestones: babbling by 12 months; gesturing (e.g., pointing, waving bye-bye) by 12 months; single words by 16 months; two-word spontaneous (not just echolalic) phrases by 24 months; loss of any language or social skills at any age.

5. Siblings of children with autism should be monitored carefully for acquisition of social, communication, and play skills, and the occurrence of maladaptive behaviors. Screening should be performed not only for autism-related symptoms but also for language delays, learning difficulties, social problems, and anxiety or depressive symptoms.

6. For all children failing routine developmental surveillance procedures, screening specifically for autism should be performed using one of the validated instruments.

7. Laboratory investigations, including audiologic assessment and lead screening, are recommended for any child with developmental delay and/or autism. Early referral for a formal audiologic assessment should include behavioral audiometric measures, assessment of middle ear function, and electrophysiologic procedures using experienced pediatric audiologists with current audiologic testing methods and technologies. Lead screening should be performed in any

child with developmental delay and pica. Additional periodic screening should be considered if the pica persists.

Diagnosis and Evaluation for Autism Spectrum Disorder

1. Genetic testing in children with autism, specifically high-resolution chromosome studies (karyotype) and deoxyribonucleic acid (DNA) analysis for fragile X, should be performed in the presence of intellectual disability (or if intellectual disability cannot be excluded), if there is a family history of fragile X or undiagnosed intellectual disability, or if dysmorphic features are present. However, there is little likelihood of positive karyotype or fragile X testing in the presence of high-functioning autism.

2. Selective metabolic testing should be initiated by the presence of suggestive clinical and physical findings such as the following: evidence of lethargy, cyclic vomiting, or early seizures; presence of dysmorphic or coarse features; evidence of intellectual disability cannot be ruled out; or if occurrence or adequacy of newborn screening is questionable.

3. There is inadequate evidence to recommend an electroencephalogram study in all individuals with autism. Indications for an adequate sleep-deprived electroencephalogram (EEG) with appropriate sampling of slow wave sleep include clinical seizures or suspicion of subclinical seizures and a history of regression (clinically significant loss of social and communicative function) at any age, but especially in toddlers and preschoolers.

4. Recording of event-related potentials and magnetoencephalography are research tools at the present time, without evidence of routine clinical utility.

5. There is no clinical evidence to support the role of routine clinical neuroimaging in the diagnostic evaluation of autism, even in the presence of megalencephaly.

6. There is inadequate supporting evidence for hair analysis, celiac antibodies, allergy testing (particularly food allergies for gluten, casein, Candida, and other molds), immunologic or neurochemical abnormalities, micronutrients such as

vitamin levels, intestinal permeability studies, stool analysis, urinary peptides, mitochondrial disorders (including lactate and pyruvate), thyroid function tests (TFTs), or erythrocyte glutathione peroxidase (GPx) studies.

Section 15.3

Screening Tools for Early Identification of Children with ASD

This section includes text excerpted from "Autism Spectrum Disorder (ASD)—Screening and Diagnosis for Healthcare Providers," Centers for Disease Control and Prevention (CDC), April 26, 2018.

Developmental Screening Tools

Screening tools are designed to help identify children who might have developmental delays. Screening tools can be specific to a disorder (for example, autism) or an area (for example, cognitive development, language, or gross motor skills), or they may be general, encompassing multiple areas of concern. Some screening tools are used primarily in pediatric practices, while others are used by school systems or in other community settings.

Screening tools do not provide conclusive evidence of developmental delays and do not result in diagnoses. A positive screening result should be followed by a thorough assessment. Screening tools do not provide in-depth information about an area of development.

Selecting a Screening Tool

When selecting a developmental screening tool, take the following into consideration:

- Domain(s) the Screening Tool Covers
  - What are the questions that need to be answered?
  - What types of delays or conditions do you want to detect?
- Psychometric Properties

These affect the overall ability of the test to do what it is meant to do.

- The sensitivity of a screening tool is the probability that it will correctly identify children who exhibit developmental delays or disorders.

- The specificity of a screening tool is the probability that it will correctly identify children who are developing normally.

- Characteristics of the Child

For example, age and presence of risk factors.

- Setting in which the Screening Tool will be Administered

Will the tool be used in a physician's office, daycare setting, or community setting? Screening can be performed by professionals, such as nurses or teachers, or by trained paraprofessionals.

Types of Screening Tools

There are many different developmental screening tools. The CDC does not approve or endorse any specific tools for screening purposes. This list is not exhaustive, and other tests may be available.

Selected examples of screening tools for general development and ASD:

- Ages and Stages Questionnaires (ASQ) (agesandstages.com)

- This is a general developmental screening tool. Parent-completed questionnaire; series of 19 age-specific questionnaires screening communication, gross motor, fine motor, problem-solving, and personal adaptive skills; results in a pass/fail score for domains.

- Communication and Symbolic Behavior Scales (CSBS) (words. fsu.edu/pdf/checklist.pdf)

- Standardized tool for screening of communication and symbolic abilities up to the 24-month level; the Infant-Toddler Checklist (ITC) is a one-page, parent-completed screening tool.

- Parents' Evaluation of Developmental Status (PEDS) (www. pedstest.com/default.aspx)

- This is a general developmental screening tool. Parent-interview form; screens for developmental and behavioral problems needing further evaluation; single response form used for all ages; may be useful as a surveillance tool.

- Modified Checklist for Autism in Toddlers (MCHAT) (mchatscreen.com)

- Parent-completed questionnaire designed to identify children at risk for autism in the general population.

- Screening Tool for Autism in Toddlers and Young Children (STAT) (vkc.mc.vanderbilt.edu/vkc/triad/stat)

- This is an interactive screening tool designed for children when developmental concerns are suspected. It consists of 12 activities assessing play, communication, and imitation skills and takes 20 minutes to administer.

Diagnostic Tools

There are many tools to assess ASD in young children, but no single tool should be used as the basis for diagnosis. Diagnostic tools usually rely on two main sources of information—parents' or caregivers' descriptions of their child's development and a professional's observation of the child's behavior.

In some cases, the primary care provider might choose to refer the child and family to a specialist for further assessment and diagnosis. Such specialists include neurodevelopmental pediatricians, developmental-behavioral pediatricians, child neurologists, geneticists, and early intervention programs that provide assessment services.

Selected examples of diagnostic tools:

- Autism Diagnosis Interview—Revised (ADI-R) (www.ncbi.nlm.nih.gov/pubmed/7814313)

  A clinical diagnostic instrument for assessing autism in children and adults. The instrument focuses on behavior in three main areas: reciprocal social interaction; communication and language; and restricted and repetitive, stereotyped interests and behaviors. The ADI-R is appropriate for children and adults with mental ages about 18 months and above.

- Autism Diagnostic Observation Schedule—Generic (ADOS-G) (www.ncbi.nlm.nih.gov/pubmed/11055457)

  A semi-structured, standardized assessment of social interaction, communication, play, and imaginative use of materials for individuals suspected of having ASD. The observational schedule consists of four 30-minute modules, each designed to be administered to different individuals according to their level of expressive language.

- Childhood Autism Rating Scale (CARS)

  Brief assessment suitable for use with any child over two years of age. CARS includes items drawn from five prominent systems for diagnosing autism; each item covers a particular characteristic, ability, or behavior.

- Gilliam Autism Rating Scale—Second Edition (GARS-2) (www.pearsonclinical.co.uk/Psychology/ChildMentalHealth/ ChildAutisticSpectrumDisorders/GilliamAutismRatingScale-SecondEdition(GARS-2)/GilliamAutismRatingScale-SecondEdition(GARS-2).aspx)

  Assists teachers, parents, and clinicians in identifying and diagnosing autism in individuals ages 3 through 22. It also helps estimate the severity of the child's disorder.

In addition to the tools above, the American Psychiatric Association's (APA) *Diagnostic and Statistical Manual, Fifth Edition (DSM-5)* provides standardized criteria to help diagnose ASD.

Myths about Developmental Screening

Myth #1

There are no adequate screening tools for preschoolers.

Fact

Although this may have been true decades ago, today sound screening measures exist. Many screening measures have sensitivities and specificities greater than 70 percent.

Myth #2

A great deal of training is needed to administer screening correctly.

Fact

Training requirements are not extensive for most screening tools. Many can be administered by paraprofessionals.

Myth #3

Screening takes a lot of time.

Fact

Many screening instruments take less than 15 minutes to administer, and some require only about 2 minutes of professional time.

Myth #4

Tools that incorporate information from the parents are not valid.

Fact

Parents' concerns are generally valid and are predictive of developmental delays. Research has shown that parental concerns detect 70–80 percent of children with disabilities.

Section 15.4

Audiological Screening

This section includes text excerpted from "Your Baby's
Hearing Screening," National Institute on Deafness and Other
Communication Disorders (NIDCD), June 19, 2017.

Most children hear and listen to sounds at birth. They learn to talk by imitating the sounds they hear around them and the voices of their parents and caregivers. But that's not true for all children. In fact, about two or three out of every 1,000 children in the United States are born with detectable hearing loss in one or both ears. More lose hearing later during childhood. Children who have hearing loss may not learn speech and language as well as children who can hear. For this reason, it's important to detect deafness or hearing loss as early as possible.

Because of the need for prompt identification of and intervention for childhood hearing loss, universal newborn hearing screening programs operate in all U.S. states and most U.S. territories. With help from the federal government, every state has established an Early Hearing Detection and Intervention program. As a result, more than 96 percent of babies have their hearing screened within one month of birth.

Why Is It Important to Have My Baby's Hearing Screened Early?

The most important time for a child to learn language is in the first three years of life, when the brain is developing and maturing. In fact, children begin learning speech and language in the first six months of life. Research suggests that children with hearing loss who get help early develop better language skills than those who don't.

When Will My Baby's Hearing Be Screened?

Your baby's hearing should be screened before she or he leaves the hospital or birthing center. If your baby's hearing was not tested within the first month of life, or if you haven't been told the results of the hearing screening, ask your child's doctor today. Quick action will be important if the screening shows a possible problem.

How Will My Baby's Hearing Be Screened?

Two different tests are used to screen for hearing loss in babies. Your baby can rest or sleep during both tests.

- **Otoacoustic emissions (OAE)** test whether some parts of the ear respond to sound. During this test, a soft earphone is inserted into your baby's ear canal. It plays sounds and measures an "echo" response that occurs in ears with normal hearing. If there is no echo, your baby might have hearing loss.

- **The auditory brainstem response (ABR)** tests how the auditory nerve and brain stem (which carry sound from the ear to the brain) respond to sound. During this test, your baby wears small earphones and has electrodes painlessly placed on his or her head. The electrodes adhere and come off like stickers, and should not cause discomfort.

Section 15.5

Observing Child's Development through Play

This section includes text excerpted from "Go Out and Play! Kit," Centers for Disease Control and Prevention (CDC), June 22, 2009. Reviewed October 2018.

Play isn't just healthy and fun. It's also how your child learns! Time spent playing can be a chance to observe your child's development—how she or he plays, learns, speaks, and acts. You can even look for milestones during playtime. Milestones are the things your child should be doing at different ages. Keeping track of milestones is really important. It helps you to see if your child is developing typically for his or her age or if your child could be at risk for a developmental delay. Noticing a delay and getting help for your child as early as possible can help ensure that your child reaches his or her full potential. If you are concerned about your child's development, don't wait. Talk with your child's doctor about your concerns.

Children often will adapt the game themselves; following their lead can be an easy way to make sure they like what they are doing and get the most from the activity.

1. **Scavenger Hunt**—A traditional scavenger hunt easily can be adapted according to the age of the children. It also can be adapted so you can track milestones you normally might not be able to track during a traditional hunt.

   • Sorts objects by shape and color: Tell the children to collect something green, something blue, and something red. When they bring the objects to you, have them make piles of the items according to color. You also can substitute shapes for colors.

   • Understands concept of "2": Instruct half the class to find two of one thing and half to find two of another. While they are looking, start a pile for each object. When students return, have them place their objects in the correct pile.

   • Recognizes common objects or pictures: Show children pictures of items to collect, but do not tell them what the item is. For example, hold up a picture of a flower and say, "Find one of these" instead of saying, "Find a flower."

- Follows two- to three-step command: Before the children begin their search, tell them what items to find and where to put the items once they've been found. When the children begin to return, do not repeat where they are supposed to place their items.

- Cooperates with other children: Pair the children or place them in small groups before sending them on their search. If you have pictures of the items they are looking for, give all the pictures to one child in each group and tell these children to give pictures to their team members.

2. **People to People**—This is a game for kids who are learning their body parts.

   - Divide the children into pairs. Call out, or have a child call out, a body part in the following manner: "toes to toes," "arm to arm," "knee to knee," etc. Children then stand with their partner with these body parts touching. At any time, the caller can call out "people to people," when that happens, the children should all run together into a group. Divide the children into new teams, and start over.

3. **Three Little Pigs**—You can engage children's skills in imitation, pretend play, and storytelling with this role-playing game.

   - Divide the class into roles from the story "The Three Little Pigs." Several children might need to perform the same role. While the teacher or another student tells the story, the children act it out, using areas designated by the teacher as the three houses (e.g., an area behind a bench could be the house of straw, behind a tree could be the house of sticks, and so on). Each time the wolf "blows down" the "house," all the little pigs run to the next house with the wolf chasing them. Each child caught by the wolf becomes another wolf. At the end of the story, the pigs can chase the wolves away.

4. **Follow the Leader**—This classic game builds on a child's ability to imitate the development of the concepts of "same" and "different."

   - Put a new spin on this familiar game by instructing the children to do something different than the child in front of them.

106

5. **Crazy Ball**—This game helps children demonstrate and develop skills such as direction following, imitating, turn-taking, and being able to differentiate between concepts.

   - Have the children form a line, leaving a few feet between each child. Using one playground-sized ball, have each child do something silly with the ball while passing it down the line. You can change the direction to alter whether the child with the ball does the same thing or something different than the child before him or her.

6. **Playground Equipment**—The playground provides many opportunities to see children engaging in imitating, taking turns, engaging in fantasy play, wanting to please and be like friends, and cooperating with friends.

   - A great time to encourage children to use their imagination is when they are playing on playground equipment. Children on swings can fly to the moon; children on slides can sled down a hill; and children on a jungle gym can be monkeys in trees. Pull out your milestones lists, put on your thinking cap, and give children some hints that will start games that allow you to see if they are meeting their milestones.

7. **Hide and Seek**—This is a favorite game of many children. It is a great game that demonstrates a child's ability to understand placement in space, follow directions, and cooperate with others.

   - Hide and Seek is a wonderful way to observe how children change their manner of play over time. Younger children often hide in obvious places—sometimes in plain view—and often hide in the same place a friend was just hiding. They also tend to give away their hiding place by saying things like, "You can't find me" or giggling while they are being looked for. As children get older, their hiding skills become more advanced, and they begin to develop strategies to reach home base without being caught.

   - You can track milestones by adding a little more structure to the game. For example, tell children to hide under or behind something, or have the seeker call out where they see their friends (e.g., "Joe is behind the tree."). Place children in pairs or small groups and have them decide where the group will hide before the counting begins. Have the children

107

choose and pretend to be characters who might look for each other (e.g., a knight searching for dragons or a mother duck looking for her ducklings).

8. **Animal Tag**—A few changes can turn this traditional game of tag into an easy way to monitor milestones. During this game, children will show their ability to follow directions and recognize common objects or pictures, and their awareness of which sex they are.

    *   Separate the children into small teams. Assign a different animal to each small team and instruct the children to act and make sounds like the animal throughout the game. When a child is tagged, they are "frozen" (must stand completely still). Only another child of the same "species" can unfreeze a frozen child. Children can identify their teammates by the noises they are making.

    *   Check on object or picture recognition by giving each child a picture of an animal instead of telling the child what animal to be.

    *   Tag also can be altered to include identifying which sex a child is by allowing only a child of the same (or opposite) sex to be the "unfreezer" (e.g., only boys can unfreeze girls, or only boys can unfreeze other boys, depending on how you establish the rules).

9. **Dance Party**—Grab a CD player and head outside for a dance party! Dance Party will showcase children's ability to imitate and cooperate with others and dress themselves.

Section 15.6

Early Brain Changes May Help Predict Autism among High-Risk Infants

This section includes text excerpted from "Early Brain Changes May Help Predict Autism among High-Risk Infants," *Eunice Kennedy Shriver* National Institute of Child Health and Human Development (NICHD), February 15, 2017.

Brain changes at age 6 or 12 months may help predict the development of autism spectrum disorder by age 2 years among infants with a high family risk, according to a study funded by the National Institutes of Health (NIH). At present, autism can be diagnosed as early as age 2 years, based on certain behaviors and communication difficulties. The study, funded by the NIH Autism Centers of Excellence (ACE) Program, is published in the February 16, 2017, issue of *Nature*.

Approximately 1 out of every 68 children in the United States has autism, according to the Centers for Disease Control and Prevention (CDC). Siblings of children diagnosed with autism have a higher risk of developing the disorder, compared to those in the general population. While there is no cure for autism, early diagnosis and intervention can ease symptoms and improve social, emotional and cognitive skills.

Previous studies have shown that people with autism have larger brains, which can be detected during early childhood. In the new study, a team led by researchers from the University of North Carolina, Chapel Hill, used magnetic resonance imaging (MRI) to look for differences in brain development among three groups: infants with a high family risk (i.e., older sibling with autism) who were later diagnosed with autism at age 2 years (15), infants with a high family risk who did not have autism at age 2 years (91), and infants with a low family risk who did not have autism at age 2 years (42).

The researchers evaluated the infants at 6, 12 and 24 months. Children with autism had a faster brain surface growth rate between 6 and 12 months, as well as a faster growth rate of overall brain size between 12 and 24 months, compared to children without autism. Next, the team analyzed the MRI data using a computer-based technology called machine learning to see if early brain differences at 6 and 12 months can predict autism at age 2 years. Among children with a high family risk, the computer program identified approximately 8 out of 10 infants who later developed autism. While the findings are

109

promising, the researchers caution that more studies are needed before this tool can be used for predicting autism development.

Section 15.7

Neuroimaging Technique May Help Predict Autism among High-Risk Infants

This section includes text excerpted from "Neuroimaging Technique May Help Predict Autism among High-Risk Infants," National Institutes of Health (NIH), June 7, 2017.

Functional connectivity magnetic resonance imaging (fcMRI) may predict which high-risk, six-month-old infants will develop autism spectrum disorder (ASD) by age two years, according to a study funded by the *Eunice Kennedy Shriver* National Institute of Child Health and Human Development (NICHD) and the National Institute of Mental Health (NIMH), two components of the National Institutes of Health (NIH). The study is published in the June 7, 2017, issue of *Science Translational Medicine.*

Autism affects roughly 1 out of every 68 children in the United States. Siblings of children diagnosed with autism are at higher risk of developing the disorder. Although early diagnosis and intervention can help improve outcomes for children with autism, there currently is no method to diagnose the disease before children show symptoms.

"Previous findings suggest that brain-related changes occur in autism before behavioral symptoms emerge," said Diana Bianchi, M.D., NICHD Director. "If future studies confirm these results, detecting brain differences may enable physicians to diagnose and treat autism earlier than they do today."

In the study, a research team led by NIH-funded investigators at the University of North Carolina (UNC) at Chapel Hill and Washington University School of Medicine (WUSM) in St. Louis focused on the brain's functional connectivity—how regions of the brain work together during different tasks and during rest. Using fcMRI, the researchers scanned 59 high-risk, 6-month-old infants while they slept naturally. The children were deemed high-risk because they have older siblings with autism. At age 2 years, 11 of the 59 infants in this group were diagnosed with autism.

The researchers used a computer-based technology called machine learning, which trains itself to look for differences that can separate the neuroimaging results into two groups—autism or nonautism—and predict future diagnoses. One analysis predicted each infant's future diagnosis by using the other 58 infants' data to train the computer program. This method identified 82 percent of the infants who would go on to have autism (9 out of 11), and it correctly identified all of the infants who did not develop autism. In another analysis that tested how well the results could apply to other cases, the computer program predicted diagnoses for groups of 10 infants, at an accuracy rate of 93 percent.

"Although the findings are early-stage, the study suggests that in the future, neuroimaging may be a useful tool to diagnose autism or help healthcare providers evaluate a child's risk of developing the disorder," said Joshua Gordon, M.D., Ph.D., NIMH Director.

Overall, the team found 974 functional connections in the brains of six-month-olds that were associated with autism-related behaviors. The authors propose that a single neuroimaging scan may accurately predict autism among high-risk infants, but caution that the findings need to be replicated in a larger group.

Section 15.8

Progress toward Earlier Diagnosis

This section includes text excerpted from "Autism Spectrum Disorder: Progress toward Earlier Diagnosis," National Institutes of Health (NIH), June 13, 2017.

Research shows that the roots of autism spectrum disorder (ASD) generally start early—most likely in the womb. That's one more reason, on top of a large number of epidemiological studies, why current claims about the role of vaccines in causing autism can't be right. But how early is ASD detectable? It's a critical question, since early intervention has been shown to help limit the effects of autism. The problem is there's currently no reliable way to detect ASD until around 18–24 months, when the social deficits and repetitive behaviors associated with the condition begin to appear.

Several months ago, a National Institutes of Health (NIH)-funded team offered promising evidence that it may be possible to detect ASD in high-risk one-year-olds by shifting attention from how kids act to how their brains have grown. Now, new evidence from that same team suggests that neurological signs of ASD might be detectable even earlier.

That evidence comes from a study of children at high risk of ASD, who as babies underwent specialized brain scans while asleep to measure connectivity between different regions of the brain. Using a sophisticated computer algorithm to analyze the scans, researchers could predict accurately which infants would receive a diagnosis of ASD 18 months later—and which would not. While the results need to be confirmed in larger groups of babies, these findings suggest that neuroimaging may be a valuable tool for early detection of ASD.

In the new study, researchers enrolled 59 babies who were 6 months old and had an older sibling diagnosed with ASD. That gave each a 20 percent chance of also developing the condition. The team, including Robert Emerson and Joseph Piven at the University of North Carolina (UNC) at Chapel Hill and John Pruett at Washington University School of Medicine (WUSM), St. Louis, then performed brain scans of each infant while napping, using functional magnetic resonance imaging (fMRI). That's an imaging technique specially designed to measure neural activity.

With the scans in hand, the team created maps that, like a wiring diagram, showed the interconnections between 230 defined brain regions. All told, the researchers mapped out 26,335 brain connections spanning the entire brain.

Eighteen months later, the now-2 year-olds returned for a follow-up visit, where they underwent a series of cognitive, behavioral, and diagnostic assessments. Eleven of the 59 toddlers were determined to have ASD, or just over the predicted 20 percent.

The researchers wondered whether they could find clues as to those outcomes in the children's brain connectivity maps. In an exciting sign of research progress, they could. Of the 26,335 functional brain connections measured at age 6 months, the researchers identified 974 that were related to the later development of ASD.

But were those differences enough to accurately predict which kids would develop ASD? To get the answer, the researchers used a special algorithm to allow a standard computer to process the original brain scans and "train" itself to distinguish between kids with ASD and those without. As part of this machine-learning process, the computer held out one baby's scan at a time and then attempted to predict, based on the connectivity data for the other 58 children, whether or not that infant had ASD.

For 9 of the 11 babies who developed ASD, the computer predicted correctly. Based on data from just one brain scan at 6 months of age, that's pretty extraordinary. Better yet, the computer never mistook a normally developing infant for one who developed ASD.

The researchers will now try to confirm their findings in larger groups of children. But they already have provided proof of principle that it's possible to detect ASD long before children show the first visible signs of the condition. The findings could pave the way for developing more cost-effective mobile neuroimaging tools, which might be used in early ASD screening.

For those parents who still find themselves worrying about a possible connection between ASD and vaccines, despite study after study showing there's no link, these new findings come as further reassurance. The biological foundations for ASD are present in the brains of children who will develop ASD-related behaviors from very early in life. The best way to keep all kids healthy and protected is to have them vaccinated on schedule.

Chapter 16

Getting Help for Developmental Delay

Chapter Contents

Section 16.1

If You Are Concerned, Act Early

This section includes text excerpted from "If You're
Concerned," Centers for Disease Control and
Prevention (CDC), July 6, 2018.

Talk to Your Child's Doctor

As a parent, you know your child best. If your child is not meeting
the milestones for his or her age, or if you think there could be a problem with the way your child plays, learns, speaks, acts, and moves,
talk to your child's doctor and share your concerns. Don't wait. Acting
early can make a real difference!

Complete a Milestone Checklist for Your Child's Age

Use the Milestone Tracker app (www.cdc.gov/ncbddd/actearly/
milestones-app.html) or fill out a milestone checklist (www.cdc.gov/
ncbddd/actearly/pdf/checklists/all_checklists.pdf) to track your child's
development. Share the completed checklist or milestone summary
with your child's healthcare provider.

Note: These checklists are not a substitute for standardized, validated, developmental screening tools.

Ask about Developmental Screening

The American Academy of Pediatrics (AAP) recommends that children be screened for general development using standardized, validated tools at 9, 18, and 24 or 30 months and for autism at 18 and 24
months or whenever a parent or provider has a concern. Ask the doctor
about your child's developmental screening.

Easterseals provides parents with FREE access to the Ages &
Stages Questionnaires®, Third Edition, one of many general developmental screening tools.

Ask for a Referral

If you or the doctor thinks there might be a delay, ask the doctor
for a referral to a specialist who can do a more in-depth evaluation of
your child.

Doctors your child might be referred to include:

- **Developmental pediatricians.** These doctors have special training in child development and children with special needs.

- **Child neurologists.** These doctors work on the brain, spine, and nerves.

- **Child psychologists or psychiatrists.** These doctors know about the human mind.

Get an Evaluation

At the same time as you ask the doctor for a referral to a specialist, call your state's public early childhood system to request a free evaluation to find out if your child qualifies for intervention services. This is sometimes called a Child Find evaluation. You do not need to wait for a doctor's referral or a medical diagnosis to make this call. Where to call for a free evaluation from the state depends on your child's age:

Children 0–3 Years Old

If your child is younger than three years old, contact your local early intervention system.

Children 3 Years Old or Older

If your child is age three or older, call any local public elementary school (even if your child does not go to school there) and say: "I have concerns about my child's development and I would like to have my child evaluated through the school system for preschool special education services."

- If the person who answers is unfamiliar with preschool special education, ask to speak with the school or district's special education director.

Section 16.2

Sharing Concerns with Your Child's Physician

This section includes text excerpted from "Concerned about Development? How to Help Your Child," Centers for Disease Control and Prevention (CDC), October 5, 2014. Reviewed October 2018.

How to Talk with the Doctor

A first step toward getting help for your child when you are concerned about his or her development (how your child plays, learns, speaks, acts and moves) is to talk with your child's doctor.

Here are some tips for talking with your child's doctor:

1. Prepare for your visit.

   - When you make the appointment, tell the doctor's staff you have concerns about your child's development that you want to discuss.

   - Write down your questions, concerns, and some examples; take these to the appointment.

   - Fill out a milestones checklist for your child's age from www.cdc.gov/milestones and take it with you to share with the doctor.

   - Have other adults who know your child well fill out a milestone checklist, too.

   - If you can, take another adult with you to play with your child so you can better focus on what the doctor says.

2. Ask all of your questions during the visit; you know your child best and your concerns are important!

   - Tell the doctor you have concerns at the start of the visit and share the milestones checklist and any questions you might have written down. If the doctor seems to be in a hurry, ask if you should schedule another visit.

   - Ask about your child's most recent developmental screening results. If a screening has not been done, ask for one. For information about developmental screening, go to www.cdc.gov/devscreening.

- Take notes to help you remember what the doctor says and what to do next.

3. Make sure you understand what the doctor says and what to do next.

   - Before you leave, make sure all of your questions have been answered.

   - If you do not understand something, ask the doctor to explain it again or in a different way.

   - Review your notes and ask the doctor, nurse, or office staff for any information you will need to do what the doctor has told you. For example, "What is the phone number for my local early intervention program?"

   - When you get home, review your notes and call the doctor's office if you have any questions.

   - Take the steps the doctor has told you and remember to follow up with the doctor about how it went.

Chapter 17

ASD Assessment

Children who have been diagnosed with an autism spectrum disorder (ASD) typically undergo a series of assessments to help parents and educators gain a better understanding of the children's abilities and deficits. Autism specialists analyze the results of various assessments and use the information to organize interventions, services, and resources to maximize the children's growth and development. The assessment process can be complicated, time-consuming, stressful, and often disheartening for parents, since the results tend to focus on the children's disabilities. Yet such evaluations are critical to understanding the social and communication challenges children with ASDs must overcome in order to reach their potential.

It is important to keep in mind that each type of assessment has different strengths and weaknesses, which has implications for accurately interpreting and applying the results. Parents should make an effort to understand the purpose and goals of the various types of ASD assessments so that they can use the results proactively to benefit their children. A thorough knowledge of the assessment process enables parents to glean relevant and useful information to help them serve as effective advocates for their children.

What Is Assessment?

Assessment is a comprehensive process that involves various methods of gathering information about a child's skills, abilities, challenges,

"ASD Assessment," © 2016 Omnigraphics. Reviewed October 2018.

and deficits across multiple functional areas. This information is typically used by autism specialists to determine the type of treatment and services that would most benefit the child. There are many different types of assessment tools, instruments, and methods available to measure different aspects of a child's level of functioning, performance, and progress toward meeting developmental goals. The results of the various assessments can help parents, teachers, and medical professionals determine the following in relation to a child with an ASD:

- The accuracy of an initial diagnosis;
- Strengths, deficits, and levels of functioning across skill areas;
- Performance as compared to other children of a similar age;
- Performance in relation to goals, standards, or desired outcomes;
- Needs or problem areas in terms of development;
- Measures of progress at home or at school;
- Effectiveness of intervention, instruction, or behavior support strategies;
- Objectives to include in the Individualized Education Program (IEP), a written document that outlines the special education services provided by a school district under the Individuals with Disabilities Education Act of 2004 (IDEA);
- Eligibility for other services.

Ideally, the assessments should be conducted by a team of professionals from various disciplines working in collaboration in order to provide a full evaluation of the child. This team may include psychologists, neurologists, speech-language pathologists, occupational and physical therapists, and behavior analysts. To ensure accurate results, the individuals performing the assessments should have expertise and experience evaluating children with ASDs. Parents can locate qualified professionals through searchable databases on autism-related websites or through recommendations from parents of children with ASDs.

Purpose of Assessment

The main purpose of ASD assessment is gathering detailed information about a child's abilities and deficits in order to tailor goals and interventions to his or her individual needs. The initial diagnostic assessment is the most comprehensive, and it is used to diagnose an ASD and provide a baseline that can be refined through further testing. In order to receive a diagnosis of ASD, the child must meet the criteria established by the American Psychiatric Association (APA) in its *Diagnostic and Statistical Manual of Mental Disorders* (DSM).

Following the formal diagnosis, different types of assessments are used to evaluate a child's level of functioning in specific areas, such as speech and language abilities, social skills, independent living skills, and emotional well-being. It is important to note that any assessment provides a snapshot of a child's strengths and challenges at a specific point in time. As the child develops, additional assessments should be used to reevaluate skills and abilities and track progress toward meeting objectives. The results of these assessments can then be used to review and revise goals and design new treatments and interventions.

Reevaluation assessments are typically conducted every three years under the IEP review process to enable school districts to target special education programming to a child's needs. Such assessments can occur more frequently, however, at the request of parents or on the recommendation of medical professionals, teachers, or the IEP team. Reevaluation assessments are often conducted to answer emerging questions about a child's skills in a specific area of functioning, such as reading comprehension or ability to ride a bus independently.

Types of Assessment
Initial Diagnostic Assessment

When a child shows signs of having an ASD, the first step in the assessment process is getting a referral for a formal diagnostic assessment. The diagnostic assessment involves a variety of methods of gathering information and measuring abilities, and it can be a long and complex process for families. Parents may be asked to provide a complete developmental history of their child, including social skills, communication skills, and behavioral development. They may also be asked to bring medical records and questionnaires completed by the child's pediatrician, teachers, and caregivers.

The next part of the diagnostic assessment is likely to involve extensive interviews with a psychologist for both the parents and the child. The psychologist may also observe the child as she or he performs everyday tasks in several settings, such as the home, the classroom, or the playground. The diagnostic assessment may also include a standardized test, such as the Autism Diagnostic Observation Schedule (ADOS) or the Autism Diagnostic Interview-Revised (ADI-R).

The following additional assessments may be conducted as part of the initial diagnostic assessment or later as part of an effort to evaluate a specific skill set:

Cognitive

A cognitive assessment evaluates the child's strengths and difficulties in such areas as problem solving, memory, attention, and concentration. Many children with ASDs have deficits in these areas, which are important to identify and address in educational planning.

Speech and Language

Deficits in verbal and nonverbal communication are central to the diagnosis of ASD. A speech and language assessment evaluates the child's communication skills, including his or her abilities to use and understand language as well as communicate with gestures and symbols. The results of the speech and language assessment are used to develop interventions to increase the child's ability to communicate.

Adaptive Behavior

An adaptive behavior assessment examines skills related to daily living and independent functioning, such as eating, dressing, using the toilet, and riding a bus. Although the skills will vary depending on the age of the child, the assessment provides information about the level of supervision the child requires at home and at school, as well as areas of deficit that should be targeted for improvement.

Functional Behavior

This type of assessment attempts to determine the purpose of challenging or unwanted behavior in order to develop interventions to decrease its occurrence and replace it with appropriate behavior. A trained behavior specialist conducts the assessment by observing the child in various settings over time and recording information about the circumstances that lead to unwanted behavior and the results the child gets from the behavior.

Occupational or Physical Therapy

This type of assessment is designed to identify deficits in motor skills, visual perception, and sensory modulation that may limit the child's ability to function independently. The results are used to design interventions to improve physical strength, hand-eye coordination, and other skills needed in daily life.

Social–Emotional

Since children with ASDs may experience depression, bipolar disorder, or anxiety disorder, social–emotional assessments look for symptoms of mood disorders and measure emotional well-being. The results of these assessments are useful in developing behavior support plans.

The Assessment Process

Sometimes parents seek ASD assessments due to concerns about their child not reaching age-appropriate social or developmental milestones. In other cases, the process begins after a pediatrician raises questions about a child's development and provides a referral for an ASD assessment. Teachers or schools may also suggest that a child be evaluated for an ASD based on his or her behavior or educational progress. Whatever the source of the referral, parents should make sure they understand why the assessment is being recommended and what information it is intended to provide.

Although the process varies depending on the type of assessment being conducted, most assessments include interviews, a review of school and medical records, a developmental history, the completion of behavior checklists, and standardized measures of adaptive behavior, social functioning, or emotional status. Many assessments also involve a period of observation by the professional as the child completes tasks. Some assessments may take a few hours, while others may last several days.

At the end of the assessment, the professional will interpret the results of the testing and offer a diagnosis. Parents are encouraged to ask questions if there is anything they do not understand. Finally, the professional will provide a written report of the results and observations, along with treatment recommendations. After receiving the written report, parents should schedule a meeting with the evaluation team to discuss the recommendations and clarify the next steps in the process. Parental input is important in establishing behavioral and educational goals for the child and determining what interventions and support services are needed to reach them.

References

1. "Life Journey through Autism: A Parent's Guide to Assessment," Organization for Autism Research (OAR), 2008.

2. "A Parent's Guide to Psychological Assessments for ASD," Vanderbilt Kennedy Center (VKC), 2013.

Chapter 18

Diagnostic Criteria for ASD

The American Psychiatric Association's (APA) *Diagnostic and Statistical Manual, Fifth Edition (DSM-5)* provides standardized criteria to help diagnose autism spectrum disorder (ASD).

1. Persistent deficits in social communication and social interaction across multiple contexts, as manifested by the following, currently or by history:

    i. Deficits in social-emotional reciprocity, ranging, for example, from abnormal social approach and failure of normal back-and-forth conversation; to reduced sharing of interests, emotions, or affect; to failure to initiate or respond to social interactions.

    ii. Deficits in nonverbal communicative behaviors used for social interaction, ranging, for example, from poorly integrated verbal and nonverbal communication; to abnormalities in eye contact and body language or deficits in understanding and use of gestures; to a total lack of facial expressions and nonverbal communication.

    iii. Deficits in developing, maintaining, and understand relationships, ranging, for example, from difficulties adjusting behavior to suit various social contexts; to

---

This chapter includes text excerpted from "Autism Spectrum Disorder (ASD)—Diagnostic Criteria," Centers for Disease Control and Prevention (CDC), April 26, 2018.

difficulties in sharing imaginative play or in making friends; to absence of interest in peers.

Specify current severity:

Severity is based on social communication impairments and restricted, repetitive patterns of behavior.

2. Restricted, repetitive patterns of behavior, interests, or activities, as manifested by at least two of the following, currently or by history:

    i.   Stereotyped or repetitive motor movements, use of objects, or speech (e.g., simple motor stereotypes, lining up toys or flipping objects, echolalia, idiosyncratic phrases).

    ii. Insistence on sameness, inflexible adherence to routines, or ritualized patterns of verbal or nonverbal behavior (e.g., extreme distress at small changes, difficulties with transitions, rigid thinking patterns, greeting rituals, need to take the same route or eat the same food every day).

    iii. Highly restricted, fixated interests that are abnormal in intensity or focus (e.g., strong attachment to or preoccupation with unusual objects, excessively circumscribed or perseverative interests).

    iv. Hyper- or hyporeactivity to sensory input or unusual interest in sensory aspects of the environment (e.g., apparent indifference to pain/temperature, adverse response to specific sounds or textures, excessive smelling or touching of objects, visual fascination with lights or movement).

    Specify current severity:

    Severity is based on social communication impairments and restricted, repetitive patterns of behavior.

3. Symptoms must be present in the early developmental period (but may not become fully manifest until social demands exceed limited capacities, or may be masked by learned strategies in later life).

4. Symptoms cause clinically significant impairment in social, occupational, or other important areas of current functioning.

5. These disturbances are not better explained by intellectual disability (ID) (intellectual developmental disorder) or global

developmental delay. Intellectual disability and autism spectrum disorder frequently co-occur; to make comorbid diagnoses of autism spectrum disorder and intellectual disability, social communication should be below that expected for general developmental level.

Note: Individuals with a well-established *Diagnostic and Statistical Manual of Mental Disorders 4th Edition (DSM-IV)* diagnosis of autistic disorder, Asperger disorder, or pervasive developmental disorder not otherwise specified (PDD-NOS) should be given the diagnosis of autism spectrum disorder. Individuals who have marked deficits in social communication, but whose symptoms do not otherwise meet criteria for autism spectrum disorder, should be evaluated for social (pragmatic) communication disorder.

Specify if:

- With or without accompanying intellectual impairment
- With or without accompanying language impairment
- Associated with a known medical or genetic condition or environmental factor
- Associated with another neurodevelopmental, mental, or behavioral disorder
- With catatonia

Chapter 19

Medical Tests and Evaluations Used to Diagnose ASD

The first signs of an autism spectrum disorder (ASD) often appear before a child reaches the age of two. These signs usually take the form of developmental delays in early-language skills and social interactions. If a baby does not point or use other intentional gestures by 12 months, for instance, or use two-word spontaneous phrases by 24 months, she or he should be evaluated for an ASD. Identifying these signs as soon as possible is key to early diagnosis and treatment, which can improve skill and language development and help the child reach her or his full potential.

Under recommendations issued by the American Academy of Pediatrics (AAP), pediatricians and other healthcare providers are trained to screen children for ASDs during regular well-child visits. If they notice signs of developmental delays or symptoms of an ASD, they will usually refer the child to a specialist—such as a developmental pediatrician, child psychologist, pediatric neurologist, psychiatrist, or speech pathologist—for a complete evaluation.

Since autism is a spectrum disorder with varying degrees of severity, it can be difficult to diagnose. No single medical test can

"Medical Tests and Evaluations Used to Diagnose ASD," © 2016 Omnigraphics. Reviewed October 2018.

determine whether a child has an ASD. Instead, specialists typically conduct a series of assessments to figure out whether the developmental delays they have identified in a child are caused by an ASD or another condition that may present similar symptoms, such as a personality disorder, hearing problems, lead poisoning, or fragile X syndrome (FXS).

Medical Tests to Diagnose Autism Spectrum Disorders

Specialists use various types of behavioral evaluations and physical assessments to gather the information needed to make a diagnosis of ASD. Some of the common types of behavioral evaluations include:

- Application of the American Association of Childhood and Adolescent Psychiatry (AACAP) guidelines for assessing whether a child's behavior indicates an ASD

- Compilation of a complete medical and developmental history through interviews or questionnaires with parents or other caregivers

- Observations of the child's behavior, social interactions, and communication skills in different situations over time

- Administration of structured tests covering developmental-level intelligence, communication, behavior, and social interaction to determine whether the child's developmental delays affect his or her thinking, problem-solving, and decision-making abilities

Specialists may also perform physical examinations and laboratory tests to help determine whether a child's symptoms indicate ASD or may be related to a physical problem. Some of these assessments include:

- A complete physical examination—including height, weight, and head measurements—to see whether the child's growth is following a normal pattern

- An ear examination and hearing tests to see whether speech and language delays or issues with social skills and behavior may be caused by a hearing problem

- Blood tests for lead poisoning, which can cause developmental delays

- Chromosomal analysis to determine whether signs of intellectual disability may be related to a genetic disorder, such as fragile X syndrome (FXS)

- Brain scans, such as an electroencephalograph (EEG) or magnetic resonance imaging (MRI), to see whether differences in brain structure may be causing regression in the child's development or behavior

All of these medical tests and evaluations are intended to rule out other conditions and pinpoint ASD as the cause of the child's developmental delays. Once the diagnosis has been made, ASD specialists can design a program of treatments and interventions to help address any deficits and enable the child to reach his or her full potential.

Reference

"Autism: Exams and Tests," WebMD, November 14, 2014.

Chapter 20

Genetic Test for Autism

Genetic abnormalities have been linked to many developmental disabilities (DDs). Studies suggest that up to 40 percent of DDs may be caused by some genetic aberration. Conventional G-banded karyotyping has been used for decades to confirm the diagnosis of DDs (e.g., aneuploidies) that have a well-defined genetic etiology. At present, new genetic methods (e.g., microarray-based comparative genomic hybridization (aCGH), whole genome or exome sequencing) have been developed and used to detect genetic abnormalities associated with DDs. These newer tests support the examination of genetic information at a higher resolution and may show genetic abnormalities not seen on G-band karyotyping (GBK).

As previously discussed, clinical diagnosis of intellectual disability (ID), autism spectrum disorder (ASD), or global developmental delay (GDD) is typically based on clinical manifestations and cognitive and developmental assessment using standardized measures. ID, ASD, and GDD are "functional diagnoses," which are phenotype-oriented descriptions of DDs. Each of these functional diagnoses includes multiple disorders of different etiologies (e.g., Angelman syndrome (AS), fragile X syndrome (FXS), Prader-Willi syndrome (PWS), Rett syndrome (RTT), Rubinstein Taybi syndrome (RTS), Smith-Magenis syndrome (SMS), velocardiofacial syndrome (VCFS), and Williams syndrome (WS)).

This chapter includes text excerpted from "Genetic Testing for Developmental Disabilities, Intellectual Disability, and Autism Spectrum Disorder," Effective Health Care Program, Agency for Healthcare Research and Quality (AHRQ), June 2015. Reviewed October 2018.

When genetic tests are used to assess patients diagnosed with ID, ASD, or GDD, they are not used to confirm these functional diagnoses. Instead, these tests are used to establish an "etiologic diagnosis," that is, whether a patient who has an apparent functional diagnosis carries a specific genetic variant.

Etiologic diagnosis is a genotype-oriented description of genetic disorders and may be viewed as an early stage of defining a clinical disorder that has not yet been well understood or defined. A new etiologic diagnosis (i.e., the new genetic variant identified) can be further evaluated among individuals with the genotype in common to determine whether or not they share a common phenotype. If they share a common phenotype, a new genetic disorder may be defined and the genotype becomes part of the clinical definition of the disorder (e.g., fragile X syndrome).

Proposed benefits of establishing an etiologic diagnosis in patients with ID, ASD, or GDD include the following:

- Clarifying a genetic cause and improving the psychosocial outcomes (e.g., improved knowledge and sense of empowerment) for patients and their families

- Providing prognosis or expected clinical course

- Evaluating recurrence risks and helping families in reproductive decision-making

- Refining treatment options

- Avoiding unnecessary and redundant diagnostic tests

- Identifying associated medical risks to prevent morbidity

- Providing condition-specific family support

- Facilitating acquisition of needed services and improving access to research treatment protocols

Because of these potential benefits, genetic tests are being used at an increasingly rapid rate. Medical genetics groups now recommend chromosomal microarray analysis (CMA) as a first-line genetic test to identify genetic mutations in children with multiple anomalies not specific to well-delineated syndromes, nonsyndromic DD/ID, and ASD. Payers have seen a significant number of claims for genetic testing in children with suspected or proven DDs.

However, little evidence from controlled studies exists to directly link genetic testing to health outcomes. Published studies have reported superior diagnostic yields of newer genetic tests (e.g., aCGH) in identifying DD-related genetic abnormalities, and some have identified the impact of the tests on medical management (e.g., medical referrals, diagnostic imaging, further laboratory testing). However, these findings are not sufficient for drawing a conclusion that use of the tests will lead to improved health outcomes.

The impact of increased use of genetic tests, such as CMA, on healthcare costs is unclear. Advanced genetic tests are generally more expensive to perform than conventional G-banded karyotyping or other clinical tests. Identification of genetic abnormalities on germline cells may also lead to genetic testing in patients' relatives, which further expands the pool of children for testing and magnifies the potential cost impact. Conversely, the potential increased diagnostic yield of advanced genetic tests may reduce the number of other clinical tests or services used to identify genetic causes of DDs. Besides the uncertain clinical utility and concerns about economic impact, ethical issues— such as how to deal with genetic abnormalities unrelated to DD that are detected in genome-wide CMA—also remain controversial.

Availability of Genetic Tests for Developmental Disabilities in the United States

Genetic tests become clinically available in the United States via one of two pathways. A genetic test may reach the market as a commercially distributed test kit approved or cleared by the U.S. Food and Drug Administration (FDA) or as a laboratory-developed test (LDT). Test kits cleared or approved by FDA include all reagents and instructions needed to complete the test procedure and interpret the results. These test kits can be used in multiple laboratories. LDTs are developed in laboratories using either FDA-regulated or self-developed analyte-specific reagents and are intended for performance solely in the test developer's laboratory.

The U.S. Centers for Medicare and Medicaid Services (CMS) regulates laboratories that perform LDTs under the Clinical Laboratory Improvement Amendments of 1988 (CLIA). Under CLIA regulations, facilities that perform tests on "materials derived from the human body for the purpose of providing information for the diagnosis, prevention, or treatment of any disease or impairment of, or the assessment of the health of, human beings" must obtain a certificate from the CLIA program. The requirements for CLIA certification are based on the complexity of the tests. LDTs compose the majority of the genetic tests that have become available to clinical practice. Laboratories offering

LDTs must be licensed as high-complexity clinical laboratories under CLIA regulations. A technology-assessment report suggested that genetic tests for diagnosing DDs are primarily available as LDTs.

Historically, the FDA has exercised regulatory enforcement discretion over LDTs because they were relatively simple lab tests. As LDTs become more complex and proliferate in clinical use, the agency is taking steps to actively regulate LDTs. On October 3, 2014, the FDA published two draft guidance documents regarding oversight of LDTs, titled "Framework for Regulatory Oversight of Laboratory Developed Tests (LDTs)" and "FDA Notification and Medical Device Reporting for Laboratory Developed Tests (LDTs)." Under the proposed regulatory framework, LDTs will fall into one of the three categories: LDTs subject to full enforcement discretion; LDTs subject to partial enforcement discretion; and LDTs subject to full FDA regulation. Once the proposed FDA guidance documents are finalized, it will become clearer how genetic tests for DDs will be regulated.

Chapter 21

Speech and Language Developmental Milestones

How Do Speech and Language Develop?

The first three years of life, when the brain is developing and maturing, is the most intensive period for acquiring speech and language skills. These skills develop best in a world that is rich with sounds, sights, and consistent exposure to the speech and language of others.

There appear to be critical periods for speech and language development in infants and young children when the brain is best able to absorb language. If these critical periods are allowed to pass without exposure to language, it will be more difficult to learn.

What Are the Milestones for Speech and Language Development?

The first signs of communication occur when an infant learns that a cry will bring food, comfort, and companionship. Newborns also begin to recognize important sounds in their environment, such as the voice of their mother or primary caretaker. As they grow, babies begin to sort out the speech sounds that compose the words of their language.

This chapter includes text excerpted from "Speech and Language Developmental Milestones," National Institute on Deafness and Other Communication Disorders (NIDCD), March 6, 2017.

By six months of age, most babies recognize the basic sounds of their native language.

Children vary in their development of speech and language skills. However, they follow a natural progression or timetable for mastering the skills of language. A checklist of milestones for the normal development of speech and language skills in children from birth to five years of age is included below. These milestones help doctors and other health professionals determine if a child is on track or if she or he may need extra help. Sometimes a delay may be caused by hearing loss, while other times it may be due to a speech or language disorder.

What Is the Difference between Speech and Language Disorders?

Children who have trouble understanding what others say (receptive language) or difficulty sharing their thoughts (expressive language) may have a language disorder. Specific language impairment (SLI) is a language disorder that delays the mastery of language skills. Some children with SLI may not begin to talk until their third or fourth year.

Children who have trouble producing speech sounds correctly or who hesitate or stutter when talking may have a speech disorder. Apraxia of speech (AOS) is a speech disorder that makes it difficult to put sounds and syllables together in the correct order to form words.

What Should I Do If My Child's Speech or Language Appears to Be Delayed?

Talk to your child's doctor if you have any concerns. Your doctor may refer you to a speech-language pathologist, who is a health professional trained to evaluate and treat people with speech or language disorders. The speech-language pathologist will talk to you about your child's communication and general development. She or he will also use special spoken tests to evaluate your child. A hearing test is often included in the evaluation because a hearing problem can affect speech and language development. Depending on the result of the evaluation, the speech-language pathologist may suggest activities you can do at home to stimulate your child's development. They might also recommend group or individual therapy or suggest further evaluation by an audiologist (a healthcare professional trained to identify and measure hearing loss), or a developmental psychologist (a healthcare professional with special expertise in the psychological development of infants and children).

What Research Is Being Conducted on Developmental Speech and Language Problems?

The National Institute on Deafness and Other Communication Disorders (NIDCD) sponsors a broad range of research to better understand the development of speech and language disorders, improve diagnostic capabilities, and fine-tune more effective treatments. An ongoing area of study is the search for better ways to diagnose and differentiate among the various types of speech delay. A large study following approximately 4,000 children is gathering data as the children grow to establish reliable signs and symptoms for specific speech disorders, which can then be used to develop accurate diagnostic tests. Additional genetic studies are looking for matches between different genetic variations and specific speech deficits.

Researchers sponsored by the NIDCD have discovered one genetic variant, in particular, that is linked to specific language impairment (SLI), a disorder that delays children's use of words and slows their mastery of language skills throughout their school years. The finding is the first to tie the presence of a distinct genetic mutation to any kind of inherited language impairment. Further research is exploring the role this genetic variant may also play in dyslexia, autism, and speech-sound disorders.

A long-term study looking at how deafness impacts the brain is exploring how the brain "rewires" itself to accommodate deafness. So far, the research has shown that adults who are deaf react faster and more accurately than hearing adults when they observe objects in motion. This ongoing research continues to explore the concept of "brain plasticity"—the ways in which the brain is influenced by health conditions or life experiences—and how it can be used to develop learning strategies that encourage healthy language and speech development in early childhood.

A workshop convened by the NIDCD drew together a group of experts to explore issues related to a subgroup of children with autism spectrum disorders who do not have functional verbal language by the age of five. Because these children are so different from one another, with no set of defining characteristics or patterns of cognitive strengths or weaknesses, development of standard assessment tests or effective treatments has been difficult. The workshop featured a series of presentations to familiarize participants with the challenges facing these

141

children and helped them to identify a number of research gaps and opportunities that could be addressed in future research studies.

Your Baby's Hearing and Communicative Development Checklist

Birth to 3 Months

- Reacts to loud sounds
- Calms down or smiles when spoken to
- Recognizes your voice and calms down if crying
- When feeding, starts or stops sucking in response to sound
- Coos and makes pleasure sounds
- Has a special way of crying for different needs
- Smiles when she or he sees you

4 to 6 Months

- Follows sounds with her or his eyes
- Responds to changes in the tone of your voice
- Notices toys that make sounds
- Pays attention to music
- Babbles in a speech-like way and uses many different sounds, including sounds that begin with p, b, and m
- Laughs
- Babbles when excited or unhappy
- Makes gurgling sounds when alone or playing with you

7 Months to 1 Year

- Enjoys playing peek-a-boo and pat-a-cake
- Turns and looks in the direction of sounds
- Listens when spoken to
- Understands words for common items such as "cup," "shoe," or "juice"
- Responds to requests ("Come here")

- Babbles using long and short groups of sounds ("tata, upup, bibibi")

- Babbles to get and keep attention

- Communicates using gestures such as waving or holding up arms

- Imitates different speech sounds

- Has one or two words ("Hi," "dog," "Dada," or "Mama") by first birthday

1 to 2 Years

- Knows a few parts of the body and can point to them when asked

- Follows simple commands ("Roll the ball") and understands simple questions ("Where's your shoe?")

- Enjoys simple stories, songs, and rhymes

- Points to pictures, when named, in books

- Acquires new words on a regular basis

- Uses some one- or two-word questions ("Where kitty?" or "Go bye-bye?")

- Puts two words together ("More cookie")

- Uses many different consonant sounds at the beginning of words

2 to 3 Years

- Has a word for almost everything

- Uses two- or three-word phrases to talk about and ask for things

- Uses k, g, f, t, d, and n sounds

- Speaks in a way that is understood by family members and friends

- Names objects to ask for them or to direct attention to them

3 to 4 Years

- Hears you when you call from another room

- Hears the television or radio at the same sound level as other family members

- Answers simple "Who?" "What?" "Where?" and "Why?" questions
- Talks about activities at daycare, preschool, or friends' homes
- Uses sentences with four or more words
- Speaks easily without having to repeat syllables or words

4 to 5 Years

- Pays attention to a short story and answers simple questions about it
- Hears and understands most of what is said at home and in school
- Uses sentences that give many details
- Tells stories that stay on topic
- Communicates easily with other children and adults
- Says most sounds correctly except for a few (l, s, r, v, z, ch, sh, and th)
- Uses rhyming words
- Names some letters and numbers
- Uses adult grammar

Chapter 22

Measuring Autistic Intelligence

People with autism spectrum disorders (ASDs) were once widely thought to have below-average intellectual abilities. Doctors came to this conclusion based on their generally poor performance on the standard intelligence quotient (IQ) tests used to measure intelligence. However, research has shown that the common symptoms of ASD—including difficulties with social interaction, verbal and nonverbal communication, sensory processing, and motor skills—complicate the process of measuring the intelligence of people on the autism spectrum. As a result, their IQ scores do not necessarily reflect their true intellectual potential.

IQ tests such as the Stanford-Binet and the Wechsler Scales are often used in psychological assessments to determine whether a person has a developmental disorder or learning disability. The administration of these tests can be problematic for people with ASD, however, because they might have trouble understanding and responding quickly to verbal questions asked by a stranger. They also might have sensory-processing challenges that make it hard for them to tolerate a testing room with bright fluorescent lights, or behavioral issues that make it tough for them to sit still long enough to complete the test. IQ test results thus may not provide an accurate measure of their cognitive abilities.

"Measuring Autistic Intelligence," © 2016 Omnigraphics. Reviewed October 2018.

Adaptive Functioning

Given the difficulties of measuring autistic intelligence using standard IQ tests, the American Psychiatric Association's (APA) *Diagnostic and Statistical Manual of Mental Disorders* (DSM) recommends that assessments of intellectual ability also consider adaptive functioning. Adaptive functioning refers to the practical skills needed for daily living and personal independence, such as the ability to bathe, dress, take medicine, prepare food, cross the street safely, or ride a bus. IQ tests, on the other hand, focus on the sort of intelligence required in an academic setting, such as problem-solving and abstract reasoning.

Although adaptive skills vary depending on a person's age and culture, they usually correspond with IQ scores, so that people with high IQ scores would also be expected to score highly in adaptive skills. In people with ASD, however, the opposite may be true. Research suggests that people with higher cognitive abilities and autism tend to have more problems with daily living tasks than expected for their age and IQ. In fact, their adaptive skills are more similar to those of people with mild to moderate intellectual disability.

Researchers are not sure why there appears to be a disconnect between IQ and adaptive skills in people with ASD. This situation can clearly be frustrating, however, for people with autism who have higher cognitive abilities yet struggle with seemingly easier adaptive skills. In fact, they may not function as well in school or work settings as people with intellectual disability but good adaptive skills. Assessing adaptive skills in addition to IQ can lead to interventions that improve functioning in these areas.

Increasing Intelligence Quotient Scores with Autism Spectrum Disorders

Despite the difficulties in measuring autistic intelligence, studies have shown that the average IQ scores of people with ASD have increased dramatically over time. A 1999 study found that only 20 percent of people with ASD had scored in the normal range of intelligence during the previous three decades. In 2014, however, a study found that nearly 50 percent of children with ASD had average or above-average intelligence, and only about 30 percent had intellectual disability.

Researchers have put forth several possible explanations for the increase in IQ scores among people with ASD. Some believe the change reflects an expansion of ASD diagnosis to include people with milder forms of autism, such as Asperger Syndrome. Others credit earlier diagnosis and treatment, along with the development of more effective interventions, with reducing developmental delays and improving cognitive and communication skills among children with ASD.

As researchers increase their understanding of ASD, they may develop new, more accurate methods of measuring intellectual ability. In the meantime, experts recommend using comprehensive assessments that measure adaptive skills, behavior, attention, and social-emotional functioning in addition to IQ in order to compile a complete picture of the abilities and challenges of people with ASD.

References

1. Sarris, Marina. "Measuring Intelligence in Autism," Interactive Autism Network (IAN), October 20, 2015.

2. Sicile-Kira, Chantal. "What IQ Tests Really Tell Us about Children with Autism," *Psychology Today*, March 2011.

Part Four

Conditions That May Accompany Autism Spectrum Disorders

Chapter 23

Autism Spectrum Disorder and Communication Difficulties

Chapter Contents

Section 23.1

Communication Problems Associated with Autism

This section contains text excerpted from the following sources: Text beginning with the heading "What Is Autism Spectrum Disorder (ASD)?" is excerpted from "Autism Spectrum Disorder: Communication Problems in Children," National Institute on Deafness and Other Communication Disorders (NIDCD), March 23, 2018; Text beginning with the heading "Statistics on Voice, Speech, and Language" is excerpted from "Statistics on Voice, Speech, and Language," National Institute on Deafness and Other Communication Disorders (NIDCD), July 11, 2016.

What Is Autism Spectrum Disorder and Who Gets Affected?

Autism spectrum disorder (ASD) is a developmental disability that can cause significant social, communication, and behavioral challenges. The term "spectrum" refers to the wide range of symptoms, skills, and levels of impairment that people with ASD can have.

ASD affects people of every race, ethnic group, and socioeconomic background. It is five times more common among boys than among girls. The Centers for Disease Control and Prevention (CDC) estimates that about 1 in every 68 children in the United States has been identified as having ASD.

ASD affects people in different ways and can range from mild to severe. People with ASD share some symptoms, such as difficulties with social interaction, but there are differences in when the symptoms start, how severe they are, the number of symptoms, and whether other problems are present. The symptoms and their severity can change over time.

How Does Autism Spectrum Disorder Affect Communication?

The word "autism" has its origin in the Greek word "autos," which means "self." Children with ASD are often self-absorbed and seem to exist in a private world in which they have limited ability to successfully communicate and interact with others. Children with ASD may have difficulty developing language skills and understanding what others say to them. They also often have difficulty communicating nonverbally, such as through hand gestures, eye contact, and facial expressions.

The ability of children with ASD to communicate and use language depends on their intellectual and social development. Some children with ASD may not be able to communicate using speech or language, and some may have very limited speaking skills. Others may have rich vocabularies and be able to talk about specific subjects in great detail. Many have problems with the meaning and rhythm of words and sentences. They also may be unable to understand body language and the meanings of different vocal tones. Taken together, these difficulties affect the ability of children with ASD to interact with others, especially people their own age.

Below are some patterns of language use and behaviors that are often found in children with ASD.

- **Repetitive or rigid language.** Often, children with ASD who can speak will say things that have no meaning or that do not relate to the conversations they are having with others. For example, a child may count from one to five repeatedly amid a conversation that is not related to numbers. Or a child may continuously repeat words she or he has heard—a condition called echolalia. Immediate echolalia occurs when the child repeats words someone has just said. For example, the child may respond to a question by asking the same question. In delayed echolalia, the child repeats words heard at an earlier time. The child may say "Do you want something to drink?" whenever she or he asks for a drink. Some children with ASD speak in a high-pitched or sing-song voice or use robot-like speech. Other children may use stock phrases to start a conversation. For example, a child may say, "My name is Tom," even when he talks with friends or family. Still, others may repeat what they hear on television programs or commercials.

- **Narrow interests and exceptional abilities.** Some children may be able to deliver an in-depth monologue about a topic that holds their interest, even though they may not be able to carry on a two-way conversation about the same topic. Others may have musical talents or an advanced ability to count and do math calculations. Approximately 10 percent of children with ASD show "savant" skills, or extremely high abilities in specific areas, such as memorization, calendar calculation, music, or math.

- **Uneven language development.** Many children with ASD develop some speech and language skills, but not to a normal

153

level of ability, and their progress is usually uneven. For example, they may develop a strong vocabulary in a particular area of interest very quickly. Many children have good memories for information just heard or seen. Some may be able to read words before age five, but may not comprehend what they have read. They often do not respond to the speech of others and may not respond to their own names. As a result, these children are sometimes mistakenly thought to have a hearing problem.

- **Poor nonverbal conversation skills.** Children with ASD are often unable to use gestures—such as pointing to an object—to give meaning to their speech. They often avoid eye contact, which can make them seem rude, uninterested, or inattentive. Without meaningful gestures or other nonverbal skills to enhance their oral language skills, many children with ASD become frustrated in their attempts to make their feelings, thoughts, and needs known. They may act out their frustrations through vocal outbursts or other inappropriate behaviors.

How Are the Speech and Language Problems of Autism Spectrum Disorder Treated?

If a doctor suspects a child has ASD or another developmental disability, she or he usually will refer the child to a variety of specialists, including a speech-language pathologist (SLP). This is a health professional trained to treat individuals with voice, speech, and language disorders. The speech-language pathologist will perform a comprehensive evaluation of the child's ability to communicate, and will design an appropriate treatment program. In addition, the speech-language pathologist might make a referral for a hearing test to make sure the child's hearing is normal.

Teaching children with ASD to improve their communication skills is essential for helping them reach their full potential. There are many different approaches, but the best treatment program begins early, during the preschool years, and is tailored to the child's age and interests. It should address both the child's behavior and communication skills and offer regular reinforcement of positive actions. Most children with ASD respond well to highly structured, specialized programs. Parents or primary caregivers, as well as other family members, should be involved in the treatment program so that it becomes part of the child's daily life.

For some younger children with ASD, improving speech and language skills is a realistic goal of treatment. Parents and caregivers can increase a child's chance of reaching this goal by paying attention to his or her language development early on. Just as toddlers learn to crawl before they walk, children first develop prelanguage skills before they begin to use words. These skills include using eye contact, gestures, body movements, imitation, and babbling and other vocalizations to help them communicate. Children who lack these skills may be evaluated and treated by a speech-language pathologist to prevent further developmental delays.

For slightly older children with ASD, communication training teaches basic speech and language skills, such as single words and phrases. Advanced training emphasizes the way language can serve a purpose, such as learning to hold a conversation with another person, which includes staying on topic and taking turns speaking.

Some children with ASD may never develop oral speech and language skills. For these children, the goal may be learning to communicate using gestures, such as sign language. For others, the goal may be to communicate by means of a symbol system in which pictures are used to convey thoughts. Symbol systems can range from picture boards or cards to sophisticated electronic devices that generate speech through the use of buttons to represent common items or actions.

Statistics on Voice, Speech, and Language

The functions, skills and abilities of voice, speech, and language are related. Some dictionaries and textbooks use the terms almost interchangeably. But, for scientists and medical professionals, it is important to distinguish among them.

Head trauma can have an adverse effect on all three. Males who are between 15 and 24 years of age tend to be more vulnerable because of their high-risk lifestyles. Young children and individuals over 75 years of age are also more susceptible to head injury. Falls around the home are the leading cause of injury for infants, toddlers, and elderly people. Violent shaking of an infant or toddler is another significant cause. The leading causes for adolescents and adults are automobile and motorcycle accidents, but injuries that occur during violent crimes are also a major source. Approximately 200,000 Americans die each year from their injuries. An additional half million or more are hospitalized. About 10 percent of the surviving individuals have mild to moderate problems that threaten their ability to live independently. Another

200,000 have serious problems that may require institutionalization or some other form of close supervision.

Speech Statistics

- The prevalence of speech sound disorder in young children is eight to nine percent. By the first grade, roughly five percent of children have noticeable speech disorders; the majority of these speech disorders have no known cause.

- Usually, by 6 months of age an infant babbles or produces repetitive syllables such as "ba, ba, ba" or "da, da, da." Babbling soon turns into a type of nonsense speech called jargon that often has the tone and cadence of human speech but does not contain real words. By the end of their first year, most children have mastered the ability to say a few simple words. By 18 months of age most children can say 8–10 words and, by age 2, are putting words together in crude sentences such as "more milk." At ages 3, 4, and 5 a child's vocabulary rapidly increases, and she or he begins to master the rules of language.

- It is estimated that more than three million Americans stutter. Stuttering affects individuals of all ages but occurs most frequently in young children between the ages of two and six who are developing language. Boys are three times more likely to stutter than girls. Most children, however, outgrow their stuttering, and it is estimated that fewer than one percent of adults stutter.

- Autism is one of the most common developmental disabilities, affecting individuals of all races and ethnic and socioeconomic backgrounds. Current estimates suggest that approximately 400,000 individuals in the United States have autism. Autism is 3–4 times more likely to affect boys than girls and occurs in individuals of all levels of intelligence. Approximately 75 percent are of low intelligence while 10 percent may demonstrate high intelligence in specific areas such as math.

Language Statistics

- Between six and eight million people in the United States have some form of language impairment.

- Research suggests that the first six months are the most crucial to a child's development of language skills. For a person to become fully competent in any language, exposure must begin as early as possible, preferably before school age.

- Anyone can acquire aphasia (a loss of the ability to use or understand language), but most people who have aphasia are in their middle to late years. Men and women are equally affected. It is estimated that approximately 80,000 individuals acquire aphasia each year. About 1 million persons in the United States currently have aphasia.

- More than 160 cases of Landau-Kleffner syndrome (LKS)—a childhood disorder involving loss of the ability to understand and use spoken language—have been reported from 1957 through 1990. Approximately 80 percent of children with LKS have one or more epileptic seizures that usually occur at night. Most children outgrow the seizures, and electrical brain activity on the electroencephalogram (EEG) usually returns to normal by age 15.

Section 23.2

Auditory Processing Disorder in Children

This section contains text excerpted from the following sources: Text in this section begins with excerpts from "Auditory Processing Disorder," National Institute on Deafness and Other Communication Disorders (NIDCD), June 7, 2010. Reviewed October 2018; Text under the heading "Variety of Approaches Help Children Overcome Auditory Processing and Language Problems" is excerpted from "Study Shows Variety of Approaches Help Children Overcome Auditory Processing and Language Problems," National Institute on Deafness and Other Communication Disorders (NIDCD), January 30, 2008. Reviewed October 2018.

Auditory processing disorder (APD) is a condition in which people have trouble making sense of the sounds around them.

Variety of Approaches Help Children Overcome Auditory Processing and Language Problems

For children who struggle to learn a language, the choice between various interventions may matter less than the intensity and format of the intervention, a new study sponsored by the National Institute on Deafness and Other Communication Disorders (NIDCD) suggests. The study, led by Ronald B. Gillam, Ph.D., of Utah State University is online in the February 2008 *Journal of Speech, Language, and Hearing Research*. NIDCD is one of the National Institutes of Health (NIH).

The study compared four intervention strategies in children who have unusual difficulty understanding and using language, and found that all four methods resulted in significant, long-term improvements in the children's language abilities. The aim of the study was to assess whether children who used commercially available language software program Fast ForWord-Language had greater improvement in language skills than children using other methods. This program was specifically designed to improve auditory processing deficits which may underlie some language impairments. Children who have auditory processing deficits can jumble the order of sounds that are heard in close sequence. Researchers believe that this deficit can interfere with vocabulary and grammar development.

"These results show that any of a number of intensive educational approaches can make a tremendous difference for children whose language and auditory processing skills are lagging," says NIDCD director James F. Battey, Jr., M.D., Ph.D. "Even play with peers seemed to support the improvements the children in this study made."

"We had a very positive outcome," says Dr. Gillam. "Our results tell us that a variety of intensive interventions that we can provide kids will improve auditory processing and language learning."

While most children are chattering easily by the time they are toddlers, about seven percent struggle to speak, read and understand language despite having adequate hearing, intelligence, and motor skills. Children with language impairment have trouble learning language or expressing their thoughts through language. They often have difficulty learning new vocabulary words or sentence structures, comprehending what's said to them, holding conversations, or telling stories. These children tend to perform poorly on measures of auditory processing and standardized tests of language development. Many of these children are hindered academically throughout their formal education, explains Dr. Gillam.

To address auditory processing problems, a different group of language researchers developed the computer software package called Fast ForWord-Language several years ago. The program uses slow and exaggerated speech to improve a child's ability to process spoken language. As children advance through the program, subsequent language exercises use gradually faster and less exaggerated speech.

Dr. Gillam's team designed a study that would compare Fast ForWord-Language to three other interventions. He and colleagues at the University of Kansas, the University of Texas at Austin and the University of Texas at Dallas enrolled 216 children in the trial. All were between ages 6 and 9 and had been diagnosed with language impairment.

The children, from Northeast Kansas, Central Texas or North Texas, were randomly assigned to receive one of four possible interventions. In addition to Fast ForWord-Language, the trial included another computer-assisted language intervention, an individual language intervention with a speech-language pathologist (SLP), and a nonlanguage academic enrichment intervention that focused only on math, science, and geography.

The other computer-assisted language intervention, which used Earobics and Laureate Learning Systems software, differed from Fast ForWord-Language in not using slow or exaggerated speech. Groups of children worked on the computer intervention exercises at their own pace wearing headphones and supervised by a speech-language pathologist.

Children assigned to the individual language intervention worked one-on-one with a speech-language pathologist for the duration of the trial. In their sessions, the children read picture books that contained a variety of age-appropriate vocabulary words.

In the academic enrichment intervention, children worked on educational computer games designed to teach math, science, and geography. This intervention was delivered in the same way as the language-focused computer interventions. It served as a comparison group against which the researchers could measure the results of the language interventions.

All of the interventions were delivered in an intensive, six-week, summer program that also included day camp activities such as arts and crafts, outdoor games, board games and snack time. The children attended the program five days per week for three and a half hours per day. They practiced their assigned interventions for an hour and forty minutes each day. The children took a standard language test—the Comprehensive Test of Spoken Language—and completed a variety of auditory processing measures at the beginning and end of the program as well as three and six months afterward. The children in all four groups demonstrated statistically significant improvement on the auditory processing measures and the language measures immediately after their six-week program.

The children showed even greater improvement when their language skills were tested again six months later. Even a subgroup of children with very poor auditory processing skills made improvements on the auditory processing tasks and the language measures. About 74 percent of children in the Fast ForWord-Language group made large improvements on the language measures. Sixty-three percent of children in the computer-assisted language intervention group made large improvements. Of those who worked with a speech-language pathologist, 80 percent made large gains, and in the general academic enrichment group, almost 69 percent made large gains. These gains are much larger than the improvements that have been reported in long-term studies of children who have received language therapy in public school settings.

The researchers were surprised that such a large percentage of the children who worked on the math, science, and geography computer games improved their auditory processing and language skills. They speculate that all the children may have benefited from the opportunities to listen carefully, to decide on an appropriate response based on what they heard, and to practice language skills with each other. The recreation and play time built into each day of the six-week program gave the children the chance to form friendships with peers who were functioning at similar language levels.

The intensive delivery of the interventions—500 minutes per week—may also have benefited kids in every intervention group. In comparison, school systems typically offer speech-language pathology services to students with language impairment for 30 minutes twice per week.

"I urge speech-language pathologists to engage children with auditory processing problems and language impairments in activities in which they have to listen carefully, attend closely and respond quickly, and to do it in an intense manner," says Dr. Gillam. "And clinicians should provide children with ample opportunity to converse, socialize and interact with kids at their same developmental level."

The language intervention trial was also supported by a grant from the National Institute of Child Health and Human Development (NICHD) to the Kansas Mental Retardation and Developmental Disabilities Research Center (KIDDRC) at the University of Kansas.

Section 23.3

Autism Spectrum Disorders and Stuttering

This section contains text excerpted from the following sources:
Text in this section begins with excerpts from "Neurodevelopmental
Disorders," U.S. Environmental Protection Agency (EPA), October
2015. Reviewed October 2018; Text beginning with the heading
"What Is Stuttering?" is excerpted from "Stuttering," National
Institute on Deafness and Other Communication
Disorders (NIDCD), March 6, 2017.

Autism spectrum disorders (ASDs) are a group of developmental
disabilities defined by significant social, communication, and behavioral impairments. The term "spectrum disorders" refers to the fact
that although people with ASDs share some common symptoms,
ASDs affect different people in different ways, with some experiencing very mild symptoms and others experiencing severe symptoms.
ASDs encompass autistic disorder and the generally less severe forms,
Asperger syndrome (AS) and pervasive developmental disorder-not
otherwise specified (PDD-NOS). Children with ASDs may lack interest
in other people, have trouble showing or talking about feelings, and
avoid or resist physical contact. A range of communication problems
are seen in children with ASDs: some speak very well, while many children with an ASD do not speak at all. Another hallmark characteristic
of ASDs is the demonstration of restrictive or repetitive interests or
behaviors, such as lining up toys, flapping hands, rocking his or her
body, or spinning in circles.

What Is Stuttering?

Stuttering is a speech disorder characterized by repetition of sounds,
syllables, or words; prolongation of sounds; and interruptions in speech
known as blocks. An individual who stutters exactly knows what she or
he would like to say but has trouble producing a normal flow of speech.
These speech disruptions may be accompanied by struggle behaviors,
such as rapid eye blinks or tremors of the lips. Stuttering can make
it difficult to communicate with other people, which often affects a
person's quality of life and interpersonal relationships. Stuttering
can also negatively influence job performance and opportunities, and
treatment can come at a high financial cost.

Symptoms of stuttering can vary significantly throughout a person's
day. In general, speaking before a group or talking on the telephone

may make a person's stuttering more severe, while singing, reading, or speaking in unison may temporarily reduce stuttering.

Stuttering is sometimes referred to as stammering and by a broader term, disfluent speech.

Who Stutters?

Roughly 3 million Americans stutter. Stuttering affects people of all ages. It occurs most often in children between the ages of 2 and 6 as they are developing their language skills. Approximately 5 to 10 percent of all children will stutter for some period in their life, lasting from a few weeks to several years. Boys are 2 to 3 times as likely to stutter as girls and as they get older this gender difference increases; the number of boys who continue to stutter is three to four times larger than the number of girls. Most children outgrow stuttering. Approximately 75 percent of children recover from stuttering. For the remaining 25 percent who continue to stutter, stuttering can persist as a lifelong communication disorder.

How Is Speech Normally Produced?

We make speech sounds through a series of precisely coordinated muscle movements involving breathing, phonation (voice production), and articulation (movement of the throat, palate, tongue, and lips). Muscle movements are controlled by the brain and monitored through our senses of hearing and touch.

What Are the Causes and Types of Stuttering?

The precise mechanisms that cause stuttering are not understood. Stuttering is commonly grouped into two types termed developmental and neurogenic.

Developmental Stuttering

Developmental stuttering occurs in young children while they are still learning speech and language skills. It is the most common form of stuttering. Some scientists and clinicians believe that developmental stuttering occurs when children's speech and language abilities are unable to meet the child's verbal demands. Most scientists and clinicians believe that developmental stuttering stems from complex interactions of multiple factors. Brain imaging studies have shown consistent differences in those who stutter compared to nonstuttering peers. Developmental stuttering may also run in families and research has shown that genetic factors contribute to this type of stuttering. Starting in 2010, researchers at the National Institute on Deafness and Other Communication Disorders (NIDCD) have identified four different genes in which mutations are associated with stuttering.

Neurogenic Stuttering

Neurogenic stuttering may occur after a stroke, head trauma, or other type of brain injury. With neurogenic stuttering, the brain has difficulty coordinating the different brain regions involved in speaking, resulting in problems in the production of clear, fluent speech.

At one time, all stuttering was believed to be psychogenic, caused by emotional trauma, but today we know that psychogenic stuttering is rare.

How Is Stuttering Diagnosed?

Stuttering is usually diagnosed by a speech-language pathologist (SLP), a health professional who is trained to test and treat individuals with voice, speech, and language disorders. The speech-language pathologist will consider a variety of factors, including the child's case history (such as when the stuttering was first noticed and under what circumstances), an analysis of the child's stuttering behaviors, and an evaluation of the child's speech and language abilities and the impact of stuttering on his or her life.

When evaluating a young child for stuttering, a speech-language pathologist will try to determine if the child is likely to continue his or her stuttering behavior or outgrow it. To determine this difference, the speech-language pathologist will consider such factors as the family's history of stuttering, whether the child's stuttering has lasted six months or longer, and whether the child exhibits other speech or language problems.

How Is Stuttering Treated?

Although there is currently no cure for stuttering, there are a variety of treatments available. The nature of the treatment will differ, based upon a person's age, communication goals, and other factors. If you or your child stutters, it is important to work with a speech-language pathologist to determine the best treatment options.

Therapy for Children

For very young children, early treatment may prevent developmental stuttering from becoming a lifelong problem. Certain strategies can help children learn to improve their speech fluency while developing positive attitudes toward communication. Health professionals generally recommend that a child be evaluated if she or he has stuttered for three to six months, exhibits struggle behaviors associated with stuttering, or has a family history of stuttering or related communication disorders. Some researchers recommend that a child be evaluated every three months to determine if the stuttering is increasing or decreasing. Treatment often involves teaching parents about ways to support their child's production of fluent speech. Parents may be encouraged to:

- Provide a relaxed home environment that allows many opportunities for the child to speak. This includes setting aside time to talk to one another, especially when the child is excited and has a lot to say.

- Listen attentively when the child speaks and focus on the content of the message, rather than responding to how it is said or interrupting the child.

- Speak in a slightly slowed and relaxed manner. This can help reduce time pressures the child may be experiencing.

- Listen attentively when the child speaks and wait for him or her to say the intended word. Don't try to complete the child's sentences. Also, help the child learn that a person can communicate successfully even when stuttering occurs.

- Talk openly and honestly to the child about stuttering if she or he brings up the subject. Let the child know that it is okay for some disruptions to occur.

Stuttering Therapy

Many of the current therapies for teens and adults who stutter focus on helping them learn ways to minimize stuttering when they speak, such as by speaking more slowly, regulating their breathing, or gradually progressing from single-syllable responses to longer words and more complex sentences. Most of these therapies also help address the anxiety a person who stutters may feel in certain speaking situations.

Drug Therapy

The U.S. Food and Drug Administration (FDA) has not approved any drug for the treatment of stuttering. However, some drugs that are approved to treat other health problems—such as epilepsy, anxiety, or depression—have been used to treat stuttering. These drugs often have side effects that make them difficult to use over a long period of time.

Electronic Devices

Some people who stutter use electronic devices to help control fluency. For example, one type of device fits into the ear canal, much like a hearing aid, and digitally replays a slightly altered version of the wearer's voice into the ear so that it sounds as if she or he is speaking in unison with another person. In some people, electronic devices may help improve fluency in a relatively short period of time. Additional research is needed to determine how long such effects may last and whether people are able to easily use and benefit from these devices in real-world situations. For these reasons, researchers are continuing to study the long-term effectiveness of these devices.

Self-Help Groups

Many people find that they achieve their greatest success through a combination of self-study and therapy. Self-help groups (SHGs) provide a way for people who stutter to find resources and support as they face the challenges of stuttering.

Chapter 24

ASD, Seizures, and Epilepsy

What Are the Epilepsies?

The epilepsies are chronic neurological disorders in which clusters of nerve cells, or neurons, in the brain sometimes signal abnormally and cause seizures. Neurons normally generate electrical and chemical signals that act on other neurons, glands, and muscles to produce human thoughts, feelings, and actions. During a seizure, many neurons fire (signal) at the same time—as many as 500 times a second, much faster than normal. This surge of excessive electrical activity happening at the same time causes involuntary movements, sensations, emotions, and behaviors and the temporary disturbance of normal neuronal activity may cause a loss of awareness.

Epilepsy can be considered a spectrum disorder because of its different causes, different seizure types, its ability to vary in severity and impact from person to person, and its range of coexisting conditions. Some people may have convulsions (sudden onset of repetitive general contraction of muscles) and lose consciousness. Others may simply stop what they are doing, have a brief lapse of awareness, and stare into space for a short period. Some people have seizures very infrequently, while other people may experience hundreds of seizures each day. There also are many different types of epilepsy, resulting

This chapter includes text excerpted from "The Epilepsies and Seizures: Hope through Research," National Institute of Neurological Disorders and Stroke (NINDS), August 8, 2018.

from a variety of causes. Recent adoption of the term "the epilepsies" underscores the diversity of types and causes.

In general, a person is not considered to have epilepsy until she or he has had two or more unprovoked seizures separated by at least 24 hours. In contrast, a provoked seizure is one caused by a known precipitating factor such as a high fever, nervous system infections, acute traumatic brain injury, or fluctuations in blood sugar or electrolyte levels.

Anyone can develop epilepsy. About 2.3 million adults and more than 450,000 children and adolescents in the United States currently live with epilepsy. Each year, an estimated 150,000 people are diagnosed with epilepsy. Epilepsy affects both males and females of all races, ethnic backgrounds, and ages. In the United States alone, the annual costs associated with the epilepsies are estimated to be $15.5 billion in direct medical expenses and lost or reduced earnings and productivity.

The majority of those diagnosed with epilepsy have seizures that can be controlled with drug therapies and surgery. However, as much as 30–40 percent of people with epilepsy continue to have seizures because available treatments do not completely control their seizures (called intractable or medication-resistant epilepsy).

While many forms of epilepsy require lifelong treatment to control the seizures, for some people the seizures eventually go away. The odds of becoming seizure-free are not as good for adults or for children with severe epilepsy syndromes, but it is possible that seizures may decrease or even stop over time. This is more likely if the epilepsy starts in childhood, has been well-controlled by medication, or if the person has had surgery to remove the brain focus of the abnormal cell firing.

Many people with epilepsy lead productive lives, but some will be severely impacted by their epilepsy. Medical and research advances in the past two decades have led to a better understanding of the epilepsies and seizures. More than 20 different medications and a variety of dietary treatments and surgical techniques (including two devices) are now available and may provide good control of seizures. Devices can modulate brain activity to decrease seizure frequency. Advance neuroimaging can identify brain abnormalities that give rise to seizures which can be cured by neurosurgery. Even dietary changes can effectively treat certain types of epilepsy. Research on the underlying causes of the epilepsies, including identification of genes for some forms of epilepsy, has led to a greatly improved understanding of these disorders that may lead to more effective treatments or even to new ways of preventing epilepsy in the future.

What Causes the Epilepsies?

The epilepsies have many possible causes, but for up to half of people with epilepsy a cause is not known. In other cases, the epilepsies are clearly linked to genetic factors, developmental brain abnormalities, infection, traumatic brain injury, stroke, brain tumors, or other identifiable problems. Anything that disturbs the normal pattern of neuronal activity—from illness to brain damage to abnormal brain development—can lead to seizures.

The epilepsies may develop because of an abnormality in brain wiring, an imbalance of nerve signaling in the brain (in which some cells either over-excite or over-inhibit other brain cells from sending messages), or some combination of these factors. In some pediatric conditions, abnormal brain wiring causes other problems such as intellectual impairment.

In other persons, the brain's attempts to repair itself after a head injury, stroke, or other problem may inadvertently generate abnormal nerve connections that lead to epilepsy. Brain malformations and abnormalities in brain wiring that occur during brain development also may disturb neuronal activity and lead to epilepsy.

Genetics

Genetic mutations may play a key role in the development of certain epilepsies. Many types of epilepsy affect multiple blood-related family members, pointing to a strong inherited genetic component. In other cases, gene mutations may occur spontaneously and contribute to development of epilepsy in people with no family history of the disorder (called "de novo" mutations). Overall, researchers estimate that hundreds of genes could play a role in the disorders.

Several types of epilepsy have been linked to mutations in genes that provide instructions for ion channels, the "gates" that control the flow of ions in and out of cells to help regulate neuronal signaling. For example, most infants with Dravet syndrome, a type of epilepsy associated with seizures that begin before the age of one year, carry a mutation in the SCN1A gene that causes seizures by affecting sodium ion channels.

Genetic mutations also have been linked to disorders known as the progressive myoclonic epilepsies (PMEs), which are characterized by ultra-quick muscle contractions (myoclonus) and seizures over time. For example, Lafora disease (LD), a severe, progressive form of myoclonic epilepsy that begins in childhood, has been linked to a gene that helps to break down carbohydrates in brain cells.

169

Mutations in genes that control neuronal migration—a critical step in brain development—can lead to areas of misplaced or abnormally formed neurons, called cortical dysplasia, in the brain that can cause these miswired neurons to misfire and lead to epilepsy.

Other genetic mutations may not cause epilepsy, but may influence the disorder in other ways. For example, one study showed that many people with certain forms of epilepsy have an abnormally active version of a gene that results in resistance to antiseizure drugs. Genes also may control a person's susceptibility to seizures, or seizure threshold, by affecting brain development.

Other Disorders

Epilepsies may develop as a result of brain damage associated with many types of conditions that disrupt normal brain activity. Seizures may stop once these conditions are treated and resolved. However, the chances of becoming seizure-free after the primary disorder is treated are uncertain and vary depending on the type of disorder, the brain region that is affected, and how much brain damage occurred prior to treatment. Examples of conditions that can lead to epilepsy include:

- Brain tumors, including those associated with neurofibromatosis or tuberous sclerosis complex (TSC), two inherited conditions that cause benign tumors called hamartomas to grow in the brain

- Head trauma

- Alcoholism or alcohol withdrawal

- Alzheimer disease (AD)

- Strokes, heart attacks, and other conditions that deprive the brain of oxygen (a significant portion of new-onset epilepsy in elderly people is due to stroke or other cerebrovascular disease)

- Abnormal blood vessel formation (arteriovenous malformations) or bleeding in the brain (hemorrhage)

- Inflammation of the brain

- Infections such as meningitis, human immunodeficiency virus (HIV), and viral encephalitis

Cerebral palsy (CP) or other developmental neurological abnormalities may also be associated with epilepsy. About 20 percent of seizures in children can be attributed to developmental neurological conditions. Epilepsies often co-occur in people with abnormalities of brain development or other neurodevelopmental disorders. Seizures are more common, for example, among individuals with autism spectrum disorder or intellectual impairment. In one study, fully a third of children with autism spectrum disorder had treatment-resistant epilepsy.

Seizure Triggers

Seizure triggers do not cause epilepsy but can provoke first seizures in those who are susceptible or can cause seizures in people with epilepsy who otherwise experience good seizure control with their medication. Seizure triggers include alcohol consumption or alcohol withdrawal, dehydration or missing meals, stress, and hormonal changes associated with the menstrual cycle. In surveys of people with epilepsy, stress is the most commonly reported seizure trigger. Exposure to toxins or poisons such as lead or carbon monoxide, street drugs, or even excessively large doses of antidepressants or other prescribed medications also can trigger seizures.

Sleep deprivation is a powerful trigger of seizures. Sleep disorders are common among people with the epilepsies and appropriate treatment of coexisting sleep disorders can often lead to improved control of seizures. Certain types of seizures tend to occur during sleep, while others are more common during times of wakefulness, suggesting to physicians how to best adjust a person's medication.

For some people, visual stimulation can trigger seizures in a condition known as photosensitive epilepsy (PSE). Stimulation can include such things as flashing lights or moving patterns.

How Are the Epilepsies Diagnosed?

A number of tests are used to determine whether a person has a form of epilepsy and, if so, what kind of seizures the person has.

Imaging and Monitoring

An electroencephalogram, or EEG, can assess whether there are any detectable abnormalities in the person's brain waves and may help to determine if antiseizure drugs would be of benefit. This most common diagnostic test for epilepsy records electrical activity detected by electrodes placed on the scalp. Some people who are diagnosed with a specific syndrome may have abnormalities in brain activity, even when they are not experiencing a seizure. However, some people continue to show normal electrical activity patterns even after they have experienced a seizure. These occur if the abnormal activity is generated deep in the brain where the EEG is unable to detect it. Many people who do not have epilepsy also show some unusual brain activity on an EEG. Whenever possible, an EEG should be performed within 24 hours of an individual's first seizure. Ideally, EEGs should be performed while the person is drowsy as well as when she or he is awake because brain activity during sleep and drowsiness is often more revealing of activity resembling epilepsy. Video monitoring may be used in conjunction with EEG to determine the nature of a person's seizures and to rule out other disorders such as psychogenic nonepileptic seizures, cardiac arrhythmia, or narcolepsy that may look like epilepsy.

A magnetoencephalogram (MEG) detects the magnetic signals generated by neurons to help detect surface abnormalities in brain activity. MEG can be used in planning a surgical strategy to remove focal areas involved in seizures while minimizing interference with brain function.

The most commonly used brain scans include CT (computed tomography), PET (positron emission tomography) and MRI (magnetic resonance imaging). CT and MRI scans reveal structural abnormalities of the brain such as tumors and cysts, which may cause seizures. A type of MRI called functional magnetic resonance imaging (fMRI) can be used to localize normal brain activity and detect abnormalities in functioning. SPECT (single photon emission computed tomography) is sometimes used to locate seizure foci in the brain. A modification of SPECT, called ictal SPECT, can be very helpful in localizing the brain area generating seizures. In a person admitted to the hospital for epilepsy monitoring, the SPECT blood flow tracer is injected within 30 seconds of a seizure, then the images of brain blood flow at the time of the seizure are compared with blood flow images taken in between seizures. The seizure onset area shows a high blood flow region on the scan. PET scans can be used to identify brain regions with lower than normal metabolism, a feature of the epileptic focus after the seizure has stopped.

Medical History

Taking a detailed medical history, including symptoms and duration of the seizures, is still one of the best methods available to determine what kind of seizures a person has had and to determine any form of epilepsy. The medical history should include details about any past illnesses or other symptoms a person may have had, as well as any family history of seizures. Since people who have suffered a seizure often do not remember what happened, caregiver or other accounts of seizures are vital to this evaluation. The person who experienced the seizure is asked about any warning experiences. The observers will be asked to provide a detailed description of events in the timeline they occurred.

Blood Tests

Blood samples may be taken to screen for metabolic or genetic disorders that may be associated with the seizures. They also may be used to check for underlying health conditions such as infections, lead poisoning, anemia, and diabetes that may be causing or triggering the seizures. In the emergency department, it is standard procedure to screen for exposure to recreational drugs in anyone with a first seizure.

Developmental, Neurological, and Behavioral Tests

Tests devised to measure motor abilities, behavior, and intellectual ability are often used as a way to determine how epilepsy is affecting an individual. These tests also can provide clues about what kind of epilepsy the person has.

How Can Epilepsy Be Treated?

Accurate diagnosis of the type of epilepsy a person has is crucial for finding an effective treatment. There are many different ways to successfully control seizures. Doctors who treat the epilepsies come from many different fields of medicine and include neurologists, pediatricians, pediatric neurologists, internists, and family physicians, as well as neurosurgeons. An epileptologist is someone who has completed advanced training and specializes in treating the epilepsies.

Once epilepsy is diagnosed, it is important to begin treatment as soon as possible. Research suggests that medication and other treatments may be less successful once seizures and their consequences become established. There are several treatment approaches that can be used depending on the individual and the type of epilepsy. If seizures are not controlled quickly, referral to an epileptologist at a specialized epilepsy center should be considered, so that careful consideration of treatment options, including dietary approaches, medication, devices, and surgery, can be performed in order to gain optimal seizure treatment.

Medications

The most common approach to treating the epilepsies is to prescribe antiseizure drugs. More than 20 different antiseizure medications are available, all with different benefits and side effects. Most seizures can be controlled with one drug (called monotherapy). Deciding on which drug to prescribe, and at what dosage, depends on many different factors, including seizure type, lifestyle and age, seizure frequency, drug side effects, medicines for other conditions, and, for a woman, whether she is pregnant or will become pregnant. It may take several months to determine the best drug and dosage. If one treatment is unsuccessful, another may work better.

Seizure medications include:

Table 24.1. Seizure Medication Drugs

Generic	Brand Name (United States)
Carbamazepine	Carbatrol, Tegretol
Clobazam	Frisium, Onfi
Clonazepam	Klonopin
Diazepam	Diastat, Diazepam, Valium
Divalproex Sodium	Depakote, Depakote ER
Eslicarbazepine Acetate	Aptiom
Ezogabine	Potiga
Felbamate	Felbatol
Gabapentin	Neurontin
Lacosamide	Vimpat
Lamotrigine	Lamictal
Levetiracetam	Keppra, Keppra XR
Lorazepam	Ativan
Oxcarbazepine	Oxtellar, Oxtellar XR, Trileptal
Perampanel	Fycompa
Phenobarbital	
Phenytoin	Dilantin, Phenytek,
Pregabalin	Lyrica
Primidone	Mysoline
Rufinamide	Banzel
Tiagabine Hydrochloride	Gabitril
Topiramate	Topamax, Topamax XR
Valproic Acid	Depakene
Vigabatrin	Sabril

In June 2018 the U.S. Food and Drug Administration (FDA) approved cannabidiol (Epidiolex, derived from marijuana) for the treatment of seizures associated with Lennox-Gastaut syndrome (LGS) and Dravet syndrome (DS) for children age 2 and older. The drug contains only a small amount of the psychoactive element in marijuana and does not induce euphoria associated with the drug.

For many people with epilepsy, seizures can be controlled with monotherapy at the optimal dosage. Combining medications may amplify side effects such as fatigue and dizziness, so doctors usually prescribe just one drug whenever possible. Combinations of drugs, however, are still sometimes necessary for some forms of epilepsy that do not respond to monotherapy.

When starting any new antiseizure medication, a low dosage will usually be prescribed initially followed by incrementally higher dosages, sometimes with blood-level monitoring, to determine when the optimal dosage has been reached. It may take time for the dosage to achieve optimal seizure control while minimizing side effects. The latter are usually worse when first starting a new medicine.

Most side effects of antiseizure drugs are relatively minor, such as fatigue, dizziness, or weight gain. Antiseizure medications have different effects on mood: some may worsen depression, where others may improve depression or stabilize mood. However, severe and life-threatening reactions such as allergic reactions or damage to the liver or bone marrow can occur. Antiseizure medications can interact with many other drugs in potentially harmful ways. Some antiseizure drugs can cause the liver to speed the metabolism of other drugs and make the other drugs less effective, as may be the case with oral contraceptives. Since people can become more sensitive to medications as they age, blood levels of medication may need to be checked occasionally to see if dosage adjustments are necessary. The effectiveness of a medication can diminish over time, which can increase the risk of seizures. Some citrus fruit and products, in particular grapefruit juice, may interfere with the breakdown of many drugs, including antiseizure medications—causing them to build up in the body, which can worsen side effects.

Some people with epilepsy may be advised to discontinue their antiseizure drugs after two to three years have passed without a seizure. Others may be advised to wait for four to five years. Discontinuing medication should always be done with supervision of a healthcare professional. It is very important to continue taking antiseizure medication for as long as it is prescribed. Discontinuing medication too early is one of the major reasons people who have been seizure-free start having new seizures and can lead to status epilepticus. Some evidence also suggests that uncontrolled seizures may trigger changes in the brain that will make it more difficult to treat the seizures in the future.

The chance that a person will eventually be able to discontinue medication varies depending on the person's age and his or her type of epilepsy. More than half of children who go into remission with medication can eventually stop their medication without having new seizures. One study showed that 68 percent of adults who had been seizure-free for 2 years before stopping medication were able to do so without having more seizures and 75 percent could successfully discontinue medication if they had been seizure-free for 3 years. However, the odds of successfully stopping medication are not as good for people with a family history of epilepsy, those who need multiple medications, those with focal seizures, and those who continue to have abnormal EEG results while on medication.

There are specific syndromes in which certain antiseizure medications should not be used because they may make the seizures worse. For example, carbamazepine can worsen epilepsy in children diagnosed with Dravet syndrome.

Diet

Dietary approaches and other treatments may be more appropriate depending on the age of the individual and the type of epilepsy. A high-fat, very low carbohydrate ketogenic diet is often used to treat medication-resistant epilepsies. The diet induces a state known as ketosis, which means that the body shifts to breaking down fats instead of carbohydrates to survive. A ketogenic diet effectively reduces seizures for some people, especially children with certain forms of epilepsy. Studies have shown that more than 50 percent of people who try the ketogenic diet have a greater than 50 percent improvement in seizure control and 10 percent experience seizure freedom. Some children are able to discontinue the ketogenic diet after several years and remain seizure-free, but this is done with strict supervision and monitoring by a physician.

The ketogenic diet is not easy to maintain, as it requires strict adherence to a limited range of foods. Possible side effects include impaired growth due to nutritional deficiency and a buildup of uric acid in the blood, which can lead to kidney stones.

Researchers are looking at modified versions of and alternatives to the ketogenic diet. For example, studies show promising results for a modified Atkins diet and for a low-glycemic-index treatment, both of which are less restrictive and easier to follow than the ketogenic diet, but well-controlled randomized controlled trials have yet to assess these approaches.

Surgery

Evaluation of persons for surgery is generally recommended only after focal seizures persist despite the person having tried at least two appropriately chosen and well-tolerated medications, or if there is an identifiable brain lesion (a dysfunctional part of the brain) believed to cause the seizures. When someone is considered to be a good candidate for surgery experts generally agree that it should be performed as early as possible.

Surgical evaluation takes into account the seizure type, the brain region involved, and the importance of the area of the brain where seizures originate (called the focus) for everyday behavior. Prior to surgery, individuals with epilepsy are monitored intensively in order to pinpoint the exact location in the brain where seizures begin. Implanted electrodes may be used to record activity from the surface of the brain, which yields more detailed information than an external scalp EEG. Surgeons usually avoid operating in areas of the brain that are necessary for speech, movement, sensation, memory and thinking, or other important abilities. fMRI can be used to locate such "eloquent" brain areas involved in an individual.

While surgery can significantly reduce or even halt seizures for many people, any kind of surgery involves some level of risk. Surgery for epilepsy does not always successfully reduce seizures and it can result in cognitive or personality changes as well as physical disability, even in people who are excellent candidates for it. Nonetheless, when medications fail, several studies have shown that surgery is much more likely to make someone seizure-free compared to attempts to use other medications. Anyone thinking about surgery for epilepsy should be assessed at an epilepsy center experienced in surgical techniques and should discuss with the epilepsy specialists the balance between the risks of surgery and desire to become seizure-free.

Even when surgery completely ends a person's seizures, it is important to continue taking antiseizure medication for some time. Doctors generally recommend continuing medication for at least two years after a successful operation to avoid recurrence of seizures.

Surgical procedures for treating epilepsy disorders include:

- Surgery to remove a seizure focus involves removing the defined area of the brain where seizures originate. It is the most common type of surgery for epilepsy, which doctors may refer to as a lobectomy or lesionectomy, and is appropriate only for focal seizures that originate in just one area of the brain. In general, people have a better chance of becoming seizure-free after surgery if they have a small, well-defined seizure focus. The most common type of lobectomy is a temporal lobe resection, which is performed for people with medial temporal lobe epilepsy. In such individuals, one hippocampus (there are two, one on each side of the brain) is seen to be shrunken and scarred on an MRI scan.

- Multiple subpial transection (MST) may be performed when seizures originate in part of the brain that cannot be removed. It involves making a series of cuts that are designed to prevent seizures from spreading into other parts of the brain while leaving the person's normal abilities intact.

- Corpus callosotomy (CC), or severing the network of neural connections between the right and left halves (hemispheres) of the brain, is done primarily in children with severe seizures that start in one half of the brain and spread to the other side. Corpus callosotomy can end drop attacks and other generalized seizures. However, the procedure does not stop seizures in the side of the brain where they originate, and these focal seizures may even worsen after surgery.

- Hemispherectomy and hemispherotomy involve removing half of the brain's cortex, or outer layer. These procedures are used predominantly in children who have seizures that do not respond to medication because of damage that involves only half the brain, as occurs with conditions such as Rasmussen encephalitis (RE). While this type of surgery is very excessive and is performed only when other therapies have failed, with intense rehabilitation, children can recover many abilities.

Devices

Electrical stimulation of the brain remains a therapeutic strategy of interest for people with medication-resistant forms of epilepsy who are not candidates for surgery.

The vagus nerve stimulation device for the treatment of epilepsy was approved by the FDA in 1997. The vagus nerve stimulator is surgically implanted under the skin of the chest and is attached to the vagus nerve in the lower neck. The device delivers short bursts of electrical energy to the brain via the vagus nerve. On average, this stimulation reduces seizures by about 20 to 40 percent. Individuals usually cannot stop taking epilepsy medication because of the stimulator, but they often experience fewer seizures and they may be able to reduce the dosage of their medication.

Responsive stimulation involves the use of an implanted device that analyzes brain activity patterns to detect a forthcoming seizure. Once detected, the device administers an intervention, such as electrical stimulation or a fast-acting drug to prevent the seizure from occurring. These devices also are known as closed-loop systems. NeuroPace, one of the first responsive stimulation, closed-loop devices, received pre-market approval by the FDA in late 2013 and is available for adults with refractory epilepsy (hard to treat epilepsy that does not respond well to trials of at least two medicines).

Experimental devices: not approved by the FDA for use in the United States

- Deep brain stimulation (DBS) using mild electrical impulses has been tried as a treatment for epilepsy in several different brain regions. It involves surgically implanting an electrode connected to an implanted pulse generator—similar to a heart pacemaker—to deliver electrical stimulation to specific areas in the brain to regulate electrical signals in neural circuits. Stimulation of an area called the anterior thalamic nucleus has been particularly helpful in providing at least partial relief from seizures in people who had medication-resistant forms of the disorder.

- A report on trigeminal nerve stimulation (TNS) (using electrical signals to stimulate parts of the trigeminal nerve and affected brain regions) showed efficacy rates similar to those for vagal nerve stimulation, with responder rates hovering around 50 percent. (A responder is defined as someone having greater than a 50% reduction in seizure frequency.) Freedom from seizures, although reported, remains rare for both methods. At the time of this writing, a trigeminal nerve stimulation device was available for use in Europe, but it had not yet been approved in the United States.

- Transcutaneous magnetic stimulation (TMS) involves a device being placed outside the head to produce a magnetic field to induce an electrical current in nearby areas of the brain. It has been shown to reduce cortical activity associated with specific epilepsy syndromes.

Chapter 25

Nonverbal Learning Disability and Asperger Syndrome

Nonverbal learning disability (NLD) is a brain-based learning disability that causes individuals to experience difficulty with abstract thinking, spatial relationships, and identifying and interpreting concepts and patterns. Nonverbal learning disability occurs in 0.1 to 1.0 percent of the general population and is sometimes called a nonverbal learning disorder (NVLD) or right-hemisphere learning disorder.

People use the spoken word in many ways. Sometimes they say exactly what they mean. Sometimes they expect the listener to pick up another meaning from their facial expressions or the tone of their voices. Sometimes they expect the listener to fill in information from past experiences or other sources of information. For example, "I love rainy days" may be a simple declaration of truth. But, if the same phrase is accompanied by a frown or eye roll and is said in a growly tone, then the speaker is communicating sarcastically and is really conveying a dislike of rainy days to the listener. Finally, if the speaker says, "You know how I feel about rainy days," then the listener is expected to fill in some previously learned information.

A person with a nonverbal learning disability is unable to interpret these facial expressions and tones of voice, and thus accepts such untrue statements as literal truth. Nor can these listeners draw on existing patterns of previously learned information, and thus are unable to accurately interpret what the speaker is communicating.

Signs of Nonverbal Learning Disability

Children with NLD tend to be very smart. They develop large vocabularies in comparison to other children of their age, memorize facts, talk freely, and read earlier than their peers. Intelligence tests indicate high verbal IQ (intelligence quotient) levels, but low performance IQ levels attributable to visual–spatial difficulties.

Five main characteristic areas of weakness are prevalent in people with NLD. However, the population may not exhibit these weaknesses in all five areas, nor may they exhibit them all at once. The weaknesses tend to become more obvious as children progress in school and are required to rely more on identifying patterns and less on memorized facts.

The five main areas of weakness are:

1. **Visual/Spatial Awareness.** Children with NLD may have problems estimating distance, size, and/or the shape of objects. They may be clumsy, spill drinks, bump into people or objects, or be unable to catch a ball. They may also have a poor sense of direction and be unable to distinguish left from right.

2. **Motor Skills.** Children with NLD may have trouble mastering basic motor skills. both large—such as dressing themselves, running, or riding a bike—or small—such as writing or using scissors.

3. **Abstract Thinking.** Children with NLD may have difficulty seeing or understanding the big picture. They can read a story and relate the details, but cannot answer questions about how the details fit together.

4. **Conceptual Skills.** Children with NLD may have trouble grasping the larger concept of a situation. For example, they may be unable to determine how pieces of a puzzle fit together or how to identify the steps required to solve a problem. This contributes to specific problems with math.

5. **Social Skills.** Children with NLD may have trouble making friends or socializing in a group setting. They may interrupt

others or behave inappropriately in social situations. These children use previously learned skills to cope with new social situations, whether appropriate or not.

Because NLD occurs in the right side of the brain, children with NLD also may have a distorted sense of touch or feel, and exhibit poor coordination on the left side of their bodies.

These areas of weakness are often masked in preschool and the early elementary years, when students are learning basic (rote) skills such as reading and arithmetic. By the fourth or fifth grade, however, students are required to process what they read or remember patterns from previous examples. This is when the weaknesses are likely to become evident. At the same time, these very smart children may begin to exhibit behavioral problems brought on by frustration with not "getting it" or feelings of being socially inept.

Diagnosis of Nonverbal Learning Disability

The diagnosis of NLD is controversial. NLD is not listed in the fifth edition of the American Psychiatric Association's (APA) *Diagnostic and Statistical Manual of Mental Disorders* (DSM) manual, which is used by doctors and therapists to diagnose learning disabilities. Nor is NLD recognized as a disability covered by the Individuals with Disabilities Education Act (IDEA). Nonetheless, if a child is exhibiting signs of NLD, then there are steps that parents should take to identify and address the symptoms.

- **A medical examination.** A thorough physical examination and discussion about the child's learning problems will help a medical doctor rule out any physical causes for the learning challenges.

- **A mental-health consultation.** Most likely the family doctor will refer the child to a neurologist or other specialist. The specialist will discuss the learning challenges with the parents and child, and may administer a variety of motor skills, speech and language, and visual–spatial relationships tests. The results, coupled with information from the parents and child, will help the specialist analyze the strengths and weaknesses associated with NLD and make a final diagnosis.

As with many learning disorders, the symptoms of NLD can vary from child to child, Thus, a comprehensive assessment is needed to determine an individual child's needs. With input and support from

183

learning professionals and therapists, as well as from the family, a student facing these challenges can be helped.

Help for Nonverbal Learning Disability

It is important to work with the child's school specialists to develop accommodations for the child's NLD. Formal accommodations may be developed through an Individualized Education Program (IEP) or 504 plan. If the child does not qualify for either plan, informal accommodations may be made in the classroom. Classroom accommodations may include modifying homework assignments and tests for time and content, presenting lectures with PowerPoint slides so that the student can see as well as hear the material being covered, and/or working with a reading specialist to read a passage aloud and then extracting key terms and ideas from the content.

Parents can help their child in various ways that will make things easier for both the student and the family. They can:

- Establish structure and routine

- Offer clear instructions

- Keep a chart of the day's social and academic activities

- Make transitions easier by providing logical, step-by-step explanations of what is going to happen. (We are going to a restaurant for dinner. We need to leave in one hour.).

- Break tasks into small steps that follow a logical sequence.

- Play games with the child to have them identify specific emotions from facial expressions or voice tone.

- Avoid sarcasm—or if it happens, use the experience to help the child identify the signs of sarcasm.

- Set up one-on-one play dates with another child who shares an interest with yours. Playdates should be structured, monitored, and time bound.

- Avoid situations that may overwhelm the child with too much sensory input–noise, smells, activity, and so on.

Other sources of help are available for parents and students. Social skills groups can help the student in social situations. Parent behavioral training can help parents learn how to collaborate with teachers. Occupational and physical therapy may help the child improve movement and writing skills as well as build tolerance for outside experiences. Cognitive therapy can help the child deal with anxiety, depression, and other mental-health issues.

Although NLD presents many challenges for both the student and the family, help is available—and, with patience and effort, there will be improvements.

Asperger Syndrome and NVLD

Asperger syndrome is one kind of autism. People diagnosed with Asperger syndrome hear, see, and feel the things around them differently. Some of the signs of Asperger syndrome include language and speech issues, social symptoms, cognitive behavioral symptoms, and physical symptoms.

Asperger syndrome and NVLD are different conditions that share many similarities. Research has proven that most children diagnosed with Asperger syndrome also have NVLD, but children diagnosed with NVLD do not necessarily have Asperger syndrome. Children with either diagnosis face challenges with learning social skills, though.

Problems with motor skills and physical space: People with NVLD most often struggle with understanding the physical space around them as they move through it. They may not be able to understand where they are standing or sitting, and this makes them prone to accidents. They may also have a problem with motor skills and have difficulty processing things they do with their hands. People diagnosed with Asperger syndrome also struggle to perform motor skills.

Problems with understanding body language: NVLD-affected people have problems differentiating the shapes of different objects, and find it difficult to process the differences in people's body language. People with Asperger syndrome may be aware of another person's body language, but are typically unable to understand the meaning of the body language.

References

1. Epstein, Varda. "Nonverbal Learning Disorder: Is This What Your Child Has?" Kars4Kids, July 1, 2015.

2. Miller, Caroline. "What Is Nonverbal Learning Disorder?" Child Mind Institute, 2016.

3. Patino, Erica. "Understanding Nonverbal Learning Disabilities," Understood, May 21, 2014.

4. "Quick Facts on Nonverbal Learning Disorder," Child Mind Institute, 2016.

5. Thompson, Sue. "Nonverbal Learning Disorders," LDonline, 1996.

6. Griffin, J. Mark. "Are Nonverbal Learning Disabilities the Same as Asperger's Syndrome?" Understood.org, August 31, 2014.

7. Olsen, Lisa Linnell. "Non-Verbal Learning Disability vs. Asperger's," Verywell Family, June 30, 2018.

8. Marks, Julie. "Asperger's Syndrome: What Are the Signs and Symptoms of the Disorder?" Everyday Health, March 22, 2018.

Chapter 26

Co-Occurring Genetic Disorders in People with Autism Spectrum Disorders

Chapter Contents

Section 26.1

Angelman Syndrome

This section includes text excerpted from "Angelman
Syndrome Information Page," National Institute of Neurological
Disorders and Stroke (NINDS), August 30, 2018.

Angelman syndrome (AS) is a genetic disorder that causes neurological and psychological problems including seizures, difficult behaviors, movement disorders, and sleep problems. Gastrointestinal, orthopedic, and eye problems also are often present. Infants with AS appear normal at birth but often have feeding problems in the first months of life and exhibit noticeable developmental delays by 6–12 months. Seizures often begin between 2–3 years of age and occur in 80–85 percent of those with AS. Features that help define the syndrome include very happy demeanor with frequent laughter, poor balance, tremor, and minimal to no speech. The disorder results from the absence of the *UBE3A* gene inherited from the mother. The gene provides instructions for a protein that plays a critical role in the normal development and function of the nervous system.

Types of Angelman Syndrome

There are four types of Angelman syndrome, involving problems with chromosomes or mutations in the *UBE3A* gene. Other children may have a genetic syndrome that looks like AS but is caused by a different gene. Dr. Harry Angelman first reported the syndrome in 1965, when he described three children in his practice with similar symptoms.

Treatment for Angelman Syndrome

There is no specific therapy for Angelman syndrome at this time. The best treatment is to minimize seizures, anxiety, and gastrointestinal (GI) issues and maximize sleep. Seizures are treated with medications and dietary therapies, while sleep issues are treated with medications and sleep training. It is also important to test for and treat any problems with vision, hearing, and mobility. Intensive therapies such as physical, occupational, and speech therapies are critical to begin early and continue as long as necessary. Applied behavior analysis and/or behavior therapy also are important for many individuals.

Prognosis of Angelman Syndrome

Most individuals with Angelman syndrome will have significant developmental delays, speech limitations, and motor difficulties, but they understand much of what is said and often learn to communicate nonverbally and by using communication devices. Those with deletions are more severely affected, whereas those with nondeletions typically make more developmental progress with better communications skills. Individuals with AS appear to have normal lifespans and generally do not show developmental regression as they age.

As individuals move into adolescence and adulthood, seizures improve or resolve for most people, sleep tends to improve but is still an issue for many, and gastrointestinal symptoms do not change much over time. Anxiety tends to worsen after puberty and can lead to difficult behaviors. Many teens and adults with AS also have frequent twitching in their hands, called myoclonus, which can spread to their arms and the rest of the body. Myoclonus is not seizure activity but can interfere with quality of life and may be treated with medication.

Section 26.2

Fragile X Syndrome

This section includes text excerpted from "Fragile X Syndrome," National Institute of Mental Health (NIMH), September 18, 2015. Reviewed October 2018.

The products of mutated genes in syndromic forms of autism indicate a link between disrupted synaptic function and the regulation of protein synthesis. There are two such neurodevelopmental disorders: Fragile X syndrome (FXS) and tuberous sclerosis complex (TSC).

FXS is the most common inherited form of cognitive disability in males with an estimated frequency of 1/4000. FXS is usually caused by the expansion of a CGG repeat sequence in the fragile X mental retardation gene (*FMR1*) on the X chromosome. Normally, the CGG

189

repeat sequence has 4–54 repeats. The fragile X premutation is characterized by a CGG repeat sequence length of 55–200. In this range, the repeat sequence is unstable and tends to expand in succeeding generations. When the sequence length expands to greater than 200 repeats, *FMR1* is silenced, and, as a consequence, its protein product, fragile X mental retardation protein (FMRP) is absent. This is known as FXS or the full mutation.

Normally, FMRP suppresses protein synthesis, hence in its absence (as in FXS), protein synthesis may be elevated. The studies address increased rates of cerebral protein synthesis as a core phenotype of FXS in both a mouse model of the disease (*Fmr1* KO) and young adult human subjects with the full FXS mutation. In the mouse model, the effects of proposed treatments on protein synthesis are examined. The rates of protein synthesis in FXS subjects and healthy Volunteers are also being measured to ascertain whether the phenotype seen in the mouse model can be detected in the human disease. The goal is to establish rates of protein synthesis as a biomarker for FXS, and use this method to test efficacy of potential treatments.

Section 26.3

Landau-Kleffner Syndrome

This section includes text excerpted from "Landau-Kleffner Syndrome Information Page," National Institute of Neurological Disorders and Stroke (NINDS), August 27, 2018.

Landau-Kleffner syndrome (LKS) is a rare, childhood neurological disorder characterized by the sudden or gradual development of aphasia (the inability to understand or express language) and an abnormal electroencephalogram (EEG). Specifically, the EEG typically shows an increase to nearly continuous abnormal brain activity firing (spikes) during sleep that scientists believe impair memory formation. LKS affects the parts of the brain that control comprehension and speech, typically affecting understanding rather than expression.

The disorder usually occurs in children between the ages of five and seven years. Typically, children with LKS develop normally but then lose their language skills for no apparent reason. While many of the affected individuals have seizures, some do not.

Diagnosis of Landau-Kleffner Syndrome

The disorder can be difficult to diagnose and may be misdiagnosed and should be recognized as different from the more common causes of autism, pervasive developmental disorder (PDD), hearing impairment, learning disability, auditory/verbal processing disorder, attention deficit disorder (ADD), childhood schizophrenia, or emotional/behavioral problems.

Treatment for Landau-Kleffner Syndrome

Treatment for LKS usually consists of antiseizure medications and corticosteroids, and speech therapy, which should be started early. A controversial treatment option involves a surgical technique called multiple subpial transection (MST) in which the pathways of abnormal electrical brain activity are severed.

Prognosis of Landau-Kleffner Syndrome

The prognosis for children with LKS varies. Some affected children may have a permanent severe language disorder, while others may regain much of their language abilities (although it may take months or years). In some cases, remission and relapse may occur. The prognosis is improved when the onset of the disorder is after age six and when speech therapy is started early. Seizures generally disappear by adulthood, and the distinctive epilepsy activity on EEG also tends to improve by that time.

Section 26.4

Mitochondrial Disease

This section includes text excerpted from "Mitochondrial Disease—Frequently Asked Questions," Centers for Disease Control and Prevention (CDC), April 26, 2018.

What Are Mitochondrial Diseases or Disorders?

Mitochondria are tiny parts of almost every cell in your body. Mitochondria are like the powerhouse of the cells. They turn sugar and oxygen into energy that the cells need to work. In mitochondrial diseases, the mitochondria cannot efficiently turn sugar and oxygen into energy, so the cells do not work correctly.

There are many types of mitochondrial disease, and they can affect different parts of the body: the brain, kidneys, muscles, heart, eyes, ears, and others. Mitochondrial diseases can affect one part of the body or can affect many parts. They can affect those part(s) mildly or very seriously.

Not everyone with a mitochondrial disease will show symptoms. However, when discussing the group of mitochondrial diseases that tend to affect children, symptoms usually appear in the toddler and preschool years.

Mitochondrial diseases and disorders are the same things.

Is There a Relationship between Mitochondrial Disease and Autism?

A child with a mitochondrial disease:

- may also have an autism spectrum disorder,
- may have some of the symptoms/signs of autism, or
- may not have any signs or symptoms related to autism.

A child with autism may or may not have a mitochondrial disease. When a child has both autism and a mitochondrial disease, they sometimes have other problems as well, including epilepsy, problems with muscle tone, and/or movement disorders.

More research is needed to find out how common it is for people to have autism and a mitochondrial disorder. Right now, it seems rare. In general, more research about mitochondrial disease and autism is needed.

What Is Regressive Encephalopathy?

Encephalopathy is a medical term for a disease or disorder of the brain. It usually means a slowing down of brain function. Regression happens when a person loses skills that they used to have like walking or talking or even being social. Regressive encephalopathy means there is a disease or disorder in the brain that makes a person lose skills they once had.

We know that sometimes children with mitochondrial diseases seem to be developing as they should, but around toddler or preschool age, they regress. The disease was there all the time, but something happens that "sets it off." This could be something like malnutrition, an illness such as flu, a high fever, dehydration, or it could be something else.

Is There a Relationship between Autism and Encephalopathy?

Most children with an autism spectrum disorder do not and have not had an encephalopathy. Some children with an autism spectrum disorder have had regression and some have had a regressive encephalopathy.

What Do We Know about the Relationship between Mitochondrial Disease and Other Disorders Related to the Brain?

Different parts of the brain have different functions. The area of the brain that is damaged by a mitochondrial disease determines how the person is impacted. This means that a person could have seizures; trouble talking or interacting with people; difficulty eating; muscle weakness, or other problems. They could have one issue or several.

Do Vaccines Cause or Worsen Mitochondrial Diseases?

As of now, there are no scientific studies that say vaccines cause or worsen mitochondrial diseases. We do know that certain illnesses that can be prevented by vaccines, such as the flu, can trigger the regression that is related to a mitochondrial disease. More research is needed to determine if there are rare cases where underlying mitochondrial disorders are triggered by anything related to vaccines. However, we know that for most children, vaccines are a safe and important way to prevent them from getting life-threatening diseases.

Are All Children Routinely Tested for Mitochondrial Diseases? What about Children with Autism?

Children are not routinely tested for mitochondrial diseases. This includes children with autism and other developmental delays.

Testing is not easy and may involve getting multiple samples of blood, and often samples of muscle. Doctors decide whether testing for mitochondrial diseases should be done based on a child's signs and symptoms.

Should I Have My Child Tested for a Mitochondrial Disease?

If you are worried that your child might have a mitochondrial disease, talk to your child's doctor.

Section 26.5

Moebius Syndrome

This section includes text excerpted from "Moebius Syndrome Information Page," National Institute of Neurological Disorders and Stroke (NINDS), June 15, 2018.

Moebius syndrome is a rare birth defect caused by the absence or underdevelopment of the 6th and 7th cranial nerves, which control eye movements and facial expression. Many of the other cranial nerves may also be affected, including the 3rd, 5th, 8th, 9th, 11th, and 12th.

Symptoms of Moebius Syndrome

The first symptom, present at birth, is an inability to suck. Other symptoms can include: feeding, swallowing, and choking problems; excessive drooling; crossed eyes; lack of facial expression; inability to smile; eye sensitivity; motor delays; high or cleft palate; hearing problems and speech difficulties. Children with Moebius syndrome are unable to move their eyes back and forth. Decreased numbers of muscle fibers have been reported. Deformities of the tongue, jaw, and limbs, such as clubfoot and missing or webbed fingers, may also occur. As children get older, lack of facial expression and inability to smile become the dominant visible symptoms. Approximately 30 to 40 percent of children with Moebius syndrome have some degree of autism.

Categories of Moebius Syndrome

There are four recognized categories of Moebius syndrome:

- Group I, characterized by small or absent brainstem nuclei that control the cranial nerves;

- Group II, characterized by loss and degeneration of neurons in the facial peripheral nerve;

- Group III, characterized by loss and degeneration of neurons and other brain cells, microscopic areas of damage, and hardened tissue in the brainstem nuclei, and,

- Group IV, characterized by muscular symptoms in spite of a lack of lesions in the cranial nerve.

Treatment for Moebius Syndrome

There is no specific course of treatment for Moebius syndrome. Treatment is supportive and in accordance with symptoms. Infants may require feeding tubes or special bottles to maintain sufficient nutrition. Surgery may correct crossed eyes and improve limb and jaw deformities. Physical and speech therapy often improves motor skills and coordination, and leads to better control of speaking and eating abilities. Plastic reconstructive surgery may be beneficial in some individuals. Nerve and muscle transfers to the corners of the mouth have been performed to provide limited ability to smile.

Prognosis of Moebius Syndrome

There is no cure for Moebius syndrome. In spite of the impairments that characterize the disorder, proper care and treatment give many individuals a normal life expectancy.

Section 26.6

Prader-Willi Syndrome

This section includes text excerpted from "Prader-Willi Syndrome (PWS): Condition Information," *Eunice Kennedy Shriver* National Institute of Child Health and Human Development (NICHD), December 1, 2016.

The term Prader-Willi syndrome (PWS) refers to a genetic disorder that affects many parts of the body. Genetic testing can successfully diagnose nearly all infants with PWS.

The syndrome usually results from deletions or partial deletions on chromosome 15 that affect the regulation of gene expression, or how genes turn on and off. Andrea Prader and Heinrich Willi first described the syndrome in the 1950s.

One of the main symptoms of PWS is the inability to control eating. In fact, PWS is the leading genetic cause of life-threatening obesity. Other symptoms include low muscle tone and poor feeding as an infant, delays in intellectual development, and difficulty controlling emotions.

There is no cure for PWS, but people with the disorder can benefit from a variety of treatments to improve their symptoms. These treatments depend on the individual's needs, but they often include strict dietary supervision, physical therapy, behavioral therapy, and treatment with growth hormone, among others. As adults, people with PWS usually do best in special group homes for people with this disorder. Some can work in sheltered environments.

Scientists do not know what increases the risk for Prader-Willi syndrome. The genetic error that leads to Prader-Willi syndrome occurs randomly, usually very early in fetal development. The syndrome is usually not hereditary.

Section 26.7

Smith-Lemli-Opitz Syndrome

This section includes text excerpted from "Smith-Lemli-Opitz Syndrome," Genetics Home Reference (GHR), National Institutes of Health (NIH), October 16, 2018.

Smith-Lemli-Opitz syndrome (SLOS) is a developmental disorder that affects many parts of the body. This condition is characterized by distinctive facial features, small head size (microcephaly), intellectual disability (ID) or learning problems, and behavioral problems. Many affected children have the characteristic features of autism, a developmental condition that affects communication and social interaction. Malformations of the heart, lungs, kidneys, gastrointestinal (GI) tract, and genitalia are also common. Infants with Smith-Lemli-Opitz syndrome have weak muscle tone (hypotonia), experience feeding difficulties, and tend to grow more slowly than other infants. Most affected individuals have fused second and third toes (syndactyly), and some have extra fingers or toes (polydactyly).

Causes of Smith-Lemli-Opitz Syndrome

Mutations in the *DHCR7* gene cause Smith-Lemli-Opitz syndrome. The *DHCR7* gene provides instructions for making an enzyme called 7-dehydrocholesterol reductase. This enzyme is responsible for the final step in the production of cholesterol. Cholesterol is a waxy, fat-like substance that is produced in the body and obtained from foods that come from animals (particularly egg yolks, meat, poultry, fish, and dairy products). Cholesterol is necessary for normal embryonic development and has important functions both before and after birth. It is a structural component of cell membranes and the protective substance covering nerve cells (myelin). Additionally, cholesterol plays a role in the production of certain hormones and digestive acids.

Mutations in the *DHCR7* gene reduce or eliminate the activity of 7-dehydrocholesterol reductase, preventing cells from producing enough cholesterol. A lack of this enzyme also allows potentially toxic byproducts of cholesterol production to build up in the blood, nervous system, and other tissues. The combination of low cholesterol levels and an accumulation of other substances likely disrupts the growth and development of many body systems. It is not known, however, how this disturbance in cholesterol production leads to the specific features of Smith-Lemli-Opitz syndrome.

Inheritance Pattern

This condition is inherited in an autosomal recessive pattern, which means both copies of the gene in each cell have mutations. The parents of an individual with an autosomal recessive condition each carry one copy of the mutated gene, but they typically do not show signs and symptoms of the condition.

Signs and Symptoms of Smith-Lemli-Opitz Syndrome

The signs and symptoms of Smith-Lemli-Opitz syndrome vary widely. Mildly affected individuals may have only minor physical abnormalities with learning and behavioral problems. Severe cases can be life-threatening and involve profound intellectual disability and major physical abnormalities.

Frequency of Smith-Lemli-Opitz Syndrome

Smith-Lemli-Opitz syndrome affects an estimated 1 in 20,000–60,000 newborns. This condition is most common in whites of European ancestry, particularly people from Central European countries such as Slovakia and the Czech Republic. It is very rare among African and Asian populations.

Section 26.8

Tourette Syndrome

This section includes text excerpted from "Tourette Syndrome Fact Sheet," National Institute of Neurological Disorders and Stroke (NINDS), June 7, 2018.

What Is Tourette Syndrome?

Tourette syndrome (TS) is a neurological disorder characterized by repetitive, stereotyped, involuntary movements and vocalizations called tics. The disorder is named for Dr. Georges Gilles de la Tourette, the pioneering French neurologist who in 1885 first described the condition in an 86-year-old French noblewoman.

The early symptoms of TS are typically noticed first in childhood, with the average onset between the ages of 3 and 9 years. TS occurs in people from all ethnic groups; males are affected about three to four times more often than females. It is estimated that 200,000 Americans have the most severe form of TS, and as many as one in 100 exhibits milder and less complex symptoms such as chronic motor or vocal tics. Although TS can be a chronic condition with symptoms lasting a lifetime, most people with the condition experience their worst tic symptoms in their early teens, with improvement occurring in the late teens and continuing into adulthood.

What Are the Symptoms?

Tics are classified as either simple or complex. Simple motor tics are sudden, brief, repetitive movements that involve a limited number of muscle groups. Some of the more common simple tics include eye blinking and other eye movements, facial grimacing, shoulder shrugging, and head or shoulder jerking. Simple vocalizations might include repetitive throat-clearing, sniffing, or grunting sounds. Complex tics are distinct, coordinated patterns of movements involving several muscle groups. Complex motor tics might include facial grimacing combined with a head twist and a shoulder shrug. Other complex motor tics may actually appear purposeful, including sniffing or touching objects, hopping, jumping, bending, or twisting. Simple vocal tics may include throat-clearing, sniffing/snorting, grunting, or barking. More complex vocal tics include words or phrases. Perhaps the most dramatic and disabling tics include motor movements that result in self-harm such as punching oneself in the face or vocal tics including coprolalia (uttering socially inappropriate words such as swearing) or echolalia (repeating the words or phrases of others). However, coprolalia is only present in a small number (10–15%) of individuals with TS. Some tics are preceded by an urge or sensation in the affected muscle group, commonly called a premonitory urge. Some with TS will describe a need to complete a tic in a certain way or a certain number of times in order to relieve the urge or decrease the sensation.

Tics are often worse with excitement or anxiety and better during calm, focused activities. Certain physical experiences can trigger or worsen tics, for example, tight collars may trigger neck tics, or hearing another person sniff or throat-clear may trigger similar sounds. Tics do not go away during sleep but are often significantly diminished.

What Is the Course of Tourette Syndrome?

Tics come and go over time, varying in type, frequency, location, and severity. The first symptoms usually occur in the head and neck area and may progress to include muscles of the trunk and extremities. Motor tics generally precede the development of vocal tics and simple tics often precede complex tics. Most patients experience peak tic severity before the mid-teen years with improvement for the majority of patients in the late teen years and early adulthood. Approximately 10 to 15 percent of those affected have a progressive or disabling course that lasts into adulthood.

Can People with Tourette Syndrome Control Their Tics?

Although the symptoms of TS are involuntary, some people can sometimes suppress, camouflage, or otherwise manage their tics in an effort to minimize their impact on functioning. However, people with TS often report a substantial buildup in tension when suppressing their tics to the point where they feel that the tic must be expressed (against their will). Tics in response to an environmental trigger can appear to be voluntary or purposeful but are not.

What Causes Tourette Syndrome?

Although the cause of TS is unknown, current research points to abnormalities in certain brain regions (including the basal ganglia, frontal lobes, and cortex), the circuits that interconnect these regions, and the neurotransmitters (dopamine, serotonin, and norepinephrine) responsible for communication among nerve cells. Given the often complex presentation of TS, the cause of the disorder is likely to be equally complex.

What Disorders Are Associated with Tourette Syndrome?

Many individuals with TS experience additional neurobehavioral problems that often cause more impairment than the tics themselves. These include inattention, hyperactivity and impulsivity (attention deficit hyperactivity disorder (ADHD)); problems with reading, writing, and arithmetic; and obsessive-compulsive symptoms such as intrusive thoughts/worries and repetitive behaviors. For example, worries about dirt and germs may be associated with repetitive hand-washing, and concerns about bad things happening may be associated with ritualistic behaviors such as counting, repeating, or ordering and arranging.

People with TS have also reported problems with depression or anxiety disorders, as well as other difficulties with living, that may or may not be directly related to TS. In addition, although most individuals with TS experience a significant decline in motor and vocal tics in late adolescence and early adulthood, the associated neurobehavioral conditions may persist. Given the range of potential complications, people with TS are best served by receiving medical care that provides a comprehensive treatment plan.

How Is Tourette Syndrome Diagnosed?

TS is a diagnosis that doctors make after verifying that the patient has had both motor and vocal tics for at least one year. The existence of other neurological or psychiatric conditions can also help doctors arrive at a diagnosis. Common tics are not often misdiagnosed by knowledgeable clinicians. However, atypical symptoms or atypical presentations (for example, onset of symptoms in adulthood) may require specific specialty expertise for diagnosis. There are no blood, laboratory, or imaging tests needed for diagnosis. In rare cases, neuroimaging studies, such as magnetic resonance imaging (MRI) or computerized tomography (CT), electroencephalogram (EEG) studies, or certain blood tests may be used to rule out other conditions that might be confused with TS when the history or clinical examination is atypical.

It is not uncommon for patients to obtain a formal diagnosis of TS only after symptoms have been present for some time. The reasons for this are many. For families and physicians unfamiliar with TS, mild and even moderate tic symptoms may be considered inconsequential, part of a developmental phase, or the result of another condition. For example, parents may think that eye blinking is related to vision problems or that sniffing is related to seasonal allergies. Many patients are self-diagnosed after they, their parents, other relatives, or friends read or hear about TS from others.

How Is Tourette Syndrome Treated?

Because tic symptoms often do not cause impairment, the majority of people with TS require no medication for tic suppression. However, effective medications are available for those whose symptoms interfere with functioning. Neuroleptics (drugs that may be used to treat psychotic and nonpsychotic disorders) are the most consistently useful medications for tic suppression; a number are available but some are more effective than others (for example, haloperidol and pimozide).

201

Unfortunately, there is no one medication that is helpful to all people with TS, nor does any medication completely eliminate symptoms. In addition, all medications have side effects. Many neuroleptic side effects can be managed by initiating treatment slowly and reducing the dose when side effects occur. The most common side effects of neuroleptics include sedation, weight gain, and cognitive dulling. Neurological side effects such as tremor, dystonic reactions (twisting movements or postures), parkinsonian-like symptoms, and other dyskinetic (involuntary) movements are less common and are readily managed with dose reduction.

Discontinuing neuroleptics after long-term use must be done slowly to avoid rebound increases in tics and withdrawal dyskinesias. One form of dyskinesia called tardive dyskinesia (TD) is a movement disorder distinct from TS that may result from the chronic use of neuroleptics. The risk of this side effect can be reduced by using lower doses of neuroleptics for shorter periods of time.

Other medications may also be useful for reducing tic severity, but most have not been as extensively studied or shown to be as consistently useful as neuroleptics. Additional medications with demonstrated efficacy include alpha-adrenergic agonists such as clonidine and guanfacine. These medications are used primarily for hypertension but are also used in the treatment of tics. The most common side effect from these medications that precludes their use is sedation. However, given the lower side effect risk associated with these medications, they are often used as first-line agents before proceeding to treatment with neuroleptics.

Effective medications are also available to treat some of the associated neurobehavioral disorders that can occur in patients with TS. Research shows that stimulant medications such as methylphenidate and dextroamphetamine can lessen ADHD symptoms in people with TS without causing tics to become more severe. However, the product labeling for stimulants currently contraindicates the use of these drugs in children with tics/TS and those with a family history of tics. Scientists hope that future studies will include a thorough discussion of the risks and benefits of stimulants in those with TS or a family history of TS and will clarify this issue. For obsessive-compulsive symptoms that significantly disrupt daily functioning, the serotonin reuptake inhibitors (SRIs) (clomipramine, fluoxetine, fluvoxamine, paroxetine, and sertraline) have been proven effective in some patients.)

Behavioral treatments such as awareness training and competing response training can also be used to reduce tics. A National Institutes of Health (NIH)-funded, multicenter randomized control trial called Cognitive Behavioral Intervention for Tics, or CBIT, showed that training to voluntarily move in response to a premonitory urge can reduce tic symptoms. Other behavioral therapies, such as biofeedback or supportive therapy, have not been shown to reduce tic symptoms. However, supportive therapy can help a person with TS better cope with the disorder and deal with the secondary social and emotional problems that sometimes occur.

Is Tourette Syndrome Inherited?

Evidence from twin and family studies suggests that TS is an inherited disorder. Although early family studies suggested an autosomal dominant mode of inheritance (an autosomal dominant disorder is one in which only one copy of the defective gene, inherited from one parent, is necessary to produce the disorder), more studies suggest that the pattern of inheritance is much more complex. Although there may be a few genes with substantial effects, it is also possible that many genes with smaller effects and environmental factors may play a role in the development of TS.

Genetic studies also suggest that some forms of ADHD and obsessive-compulsive disorder (OCD) are genetically related to TS, but there is less evidence for a genetic relationship between TS and other neurobehavioral problems that commonly co-occur with TS. It is important for families to understand that genetic predisposition may not necessarily result in full-blown TS; instead, it may express itself as a milder tic disorder or as obsessive-compulsive behaviors. It is also possible that the gene-carrying offspring will not develop any TS symptoms.

The gender of the person also plays an important role in TS gene expression. At-risk males are more likely to have tics and at-risk females are more likely to have obsessive-compulsive symptoms.

Genetic counseling of individuals with TS should include a full review of all potentially hereditary conditions in the family.

What Is the Prognosis?

Although there is no cure for TS, the condition in many individuals improves in the late teens and early twenties. As a result, some may actually become symptom-free or no longer need medication for tic suppression. Although the disorder is generally lifelong and chronic, it is not a degenerative condition. Individuals with TS have a normal life expectancy. TS does not impair intelligence. Although tic symptoms tend to decrease with age, it is possible that neurobehavioral disorders such as ADHD, OCD, depression, generalized anxiety, panic attacks, and mood swings can persist and cause impairment in adult life.

What Is the Best Educational Setting for Children with Tourette Syndrome?

Although students with TS often function well in the regular classroom, ADHD, learning disabilities, obsessive-compulsive symptoms, and frequent tics can greatly interfere with academic performance or social adjustment. After a comprehensive assessment, students should be placed in an educational setting that meets their individual needs. Students may require tutoring, smaller or special classes, and in some cases special schools.

All students with TS need a tolerant and compassionate setting that both encourages them to work to their full potential and is flexible enough to accommodate their special needs. This setting may include a private study area, exams outside the regular classroom, or even oral exams when the child's symptoms interfere with his or her ability to write. Untimed testing reduces stress for students with TS.

Section 26.9

Tuberous Sclerosis

This section includes text excerpted from "Tuberous Sclerosis Fact Sheet," National Institute of Neurological Disorders and Stroke (NINDS), June 7, 2018.

What Is Tuberous Sclerosis?

Tuberous sclerosis—also called tuberous sclerosis complex (TSC)—is a rare, multi-system genetic disease that causes benign tumors to grow in the brain and on other vital organs such as the kidneys, heart, eyes, lungs, and skin. It usually affects the central nervous system and results in a combination of symptoms including seizures, developmental delay, behavioral problems, skin abnormalities, and kidney disease.

The disorder affects as many as 25,000–40,000 individuals in the United States and about 1–2 million individuals worldwide, with an estimated prevalence of one in 6,000 newborns. TSC occurs in all races and ethnic groups, and in both genders.

The name tuberous sclerosis comes from the characteristic tuber or potato-like nodules in the brain, which calcify with age and become hard or sclerotic. The disorder—once known as epiloia or Bourneville disease—was first identified by a French physician more than 100 years ago.

Many TSC patients show evidence of the disorder in the first year of life. However, clinical features can be subtle initially, and many signs and symptoms take years to develop. As a result, TSC can be unrecognized or misdiagnosed for years.

What Causes Tuberous Sclerosis?

TSC is caused by defects, or mutations, on two genes—*TSC1* and *TSC2*. Only one of the genes needs to be affected for TSC to be present. The *TSC1* gene, discovered in 1997, is on chromosome 9 and produces a protein called hamartin. The *TSC2* gene, discovered in 1993, is on chromosome 16 and produces the protein tuberin. Scientists believe these proteins act in a complex as growth suppressors by inhibiting the activation of a master, evolutionarily conserved kinase called mTOR. Loss of regulation of mTOR occurs in cells lacking either hamartin or tuberin, and this leads to abnormal differentiation and development, and to the generation of enlarged cells, as are seen in TSC brain lesions.

Is TSC Inherited?

Although some individuals inherit the disorder from a parent with TSC, most cases occur as sporadic cases due to new, spontaneous mutations in *TSC1* or *TSC2*. In this situation, neither parent has the disorder or the faulty gene(s). Instead, a faulty gene first occurs in the affected individual.

In familial cases, TSC is an autosomal dominant disorder, which means that the disorder can be transmitted directly from parent to child. In those cases, only one parent needs to have the faulty gene in order to pass it on to a child. If a parent has TSC, each offspring has a 50 percent chance of developing the disorder. Children who inherit TSC may not have the same symptoms as their parent and they may have either a milder or a more severe form of the disorder.

Rarely, individuals acquire TSC through a process called gonadal mosaicism. These patients have parents with no apparent defects in the two genes that cause the disorder. Yet these parents can have a child with TSC because a portion of one of the parent's reproductive cells (sperm or eggs) can contain the genetic mutation without the other cells of the body being involved. In cases of gonadal mosaicism, genetic testing of a blood sample might not reveal the potential for passing the disease to offspring.

What Are the Signs and Symptoms of TSC?

TSC can affect many different systems of the body, causing a variety of signs and symptoms. Signs of the disorder vary depending on which system and which organs are involved. The natural course of TSC varies from individual to individual, with symptoms ranging from very mild to quite severe. In addition to the benign tumors that frequently occur in TSC, other common symptoms include seizures, cognitive impairment, behavior problems, and skin abnormalities. Tumors can grow in nearly any organ, but they most commonly occur in the brain, kidneys, heart, lungs, and skin. Malignant tumors are rare in TSC. Those that do occur primarily affect the kidneys.

Brain involvement in TSC: Three types of brain lesions are seen in TSC: cortical tubers, for which the disease is named, generally form on the surface of the brain but may also appear in the deep areas of the brain: subependymal nodules (SEN), which form in the walls of the ventricles—the fluid-filled cavities of the brain; and subependymal giant-cell astrocytomas (SEGA), which develop from SEN and grow such that they may block the flow of fluid within the brain, causing a buildup of fluid and pressure and leading to headaches and blurred vision.

TSC usually causes the greatest problems for those affected and their family members through effects on brain function. Most individuals with TSC will have seizures at some point during their life. Seizures of all types may occur, including infantile spasms; tonic-clonic seizures (also known as grand mal seizures); or tonic, akinetic, atypical absence, myoclonic, complex partial or generalized squires. Infantile spasms can occur as soon as the day of birth and are often difficult to recognize. Seizures can also be difficult to control by medication, and sometimes surgery or other measures are used.

About one-half to two-thirds of individuals with TSC have developmental delays ranging from mild learning disabilities to severe impairment. Behavior problems, including aggression, sudden rage, attention deficit hyperactivity disorder, acting out, obsessive-compulsive disorder, and repetitive, destructive, or self-harming behavior occur in children with TSC and can be difficult to manage. About one-third of children with TSC meet criteria for autism spectrum disorder.

Kidney problems such as cysts and angiomyolipomas occur in an estimated 70–80 percent of individuals with TSC, usually occurring between ages 15 and 30. Cysts are usually small, appear in limited numbers, and cause no serious problems. Approximately 2 percent of individuals with TSC develop large numbers of cysts in a pattern similar to polycystic kidney disease during childhood. In these cases, kidney function is compromised and kidney failure occurs. In rare instances, the cysts may bleed, leading to blood loss and anemia.

Angiomyolipomas-benign growths consisting of fatty tissue and muscle cells are the most common kidney lesions in TSC. These growths are seen in the majority of individuals with TSC, but are also found in about one of every 300 people without TSC. Angiomyolipomas caused by TSC are usually found in both kidneys and in most cases they produce no symptoms. However, they can sometimes grow so large that they cause pain or kidney failure. Bleeding from angiomyolipomas may also occur, causing both pain and weakness. If severe bleeding does not stop naturally, there may severe blood loss, resulting in profound anemia and a life-threatening drop in blood pressure, warranting urgent medical attention.

Other rare kidney problems include renal cell carcinoma (RCC), developing from an angiomyolipoma, and oncocytomas, benign tumors unique to individuals with TSC.

Tumors called cardiac rhabdomyomas are often found in the hearts of infants and young children with TSC, and they are often seen on prenatal fetus ultrasound exams. If the tumors are large or there are multiple tumors, they can block circulation and cause death. However, if they do not cause problems at birth-when in most cases they are at their largest size-they usually become smaller with time and do not affect the individual in later life.

Benign tumors called phakomas are sometimes found in the eyes of individuals with TSC, appearing as white patches on the retina. Generally they do not cause vision loss or other vision problems, but they can be used to help diagnose the disease.

Additional tumors and cysts may be found in other areas of the body, including the liver, lung, and pancreas. Bone cysts, rectal polyps, gum fibromas, and dental pits may also occur.

A wide variety of skin abnormalities may occur in individuals with TSC. Most cause no problems but are helpful in diagnosis. Some cases may cause disfigurement, necessitating treatment. The most common skin abnormalities include:

- Hypomelanotic macules ("ash leaf spots"), which are white or lighter patches of skin that may appear anywhere on the body and are caused by a lack of skin pigment or melanin-the substance that gives skin its color.

- Reddish spots or bumps called facial angiofibromas (also called adenoma sebaceum), which appear on the face (sometimes resembling acne) and consist of blood vessels and fibrous tissue.

- Raised, discolored areas on the forehead called forehead plaques, which are common and unique to TSC and may help doctors diagnose the disorder.

- Areas of thick leathery, pebbly skin called shagreen patches, usually found on the lower back or nape of the neck.

- Small fleshy tumors called ungual or subungual fibromas that grow around and under the toenails or fingernails and may need to be surgically removed if they enlarge or cause bleeding. These usually appear later in life, ages 20 to 50.

- Other skin features that are not unique to individuals with TSC, including molluscum fibrosum or skin tags, which typically occur across the back of the neck and shoulders, café au lait spots or flat brown marks, and poliosis, a tuft or patch of white hair that may appear on the scalp or eyelids.

Lung lesions are present in about one-third of adult women with TSC and are much less commonly seen in men. Lung lesions include lymphangioleiomyomatosis (LAM) and multinodular multifocal pneumocyte hyperplasia (MMPH). LAM is a tumor-like disorder in which cells proliferate in the lungs, and there is lung destruction with cyst formation. There is a range of symptoms with LAM, with many TSC individuals having no symptoms, while others suffer with breathlessness, which can progress and be severe. MMPH is a more benign tumor that occurs in men and women equally.

How Is TSC Diagnosed?

The diagnosis of TSC is based upon clinical criteria. In many cases the first clue to recognizing TSC is the presence of seizures or delayed development. In other cases, the first sign may be white patches on the skin (hypomelanotic macules) or the identification of cardiac tumor rhabdomyoma.

Diagnosis of the disorder is based on a careful clinical exam in combination with computed tomography (CT) or magnetic resonance imaging (MRI) of the brain, which may show tubers in the brain, and an ultrasound of the heart, liver, and kidneys, which may show tumors in those organs. Doctors should carefully examine the skin for the wide variety of skin features, the fingernails and toenails for ungual fibromas, the teeth and gums for dental pits and/or gum fibromas, and the eyes for retinal lesions. A Wood's lamp or ultraviolet light may be used to locate the hypomelanotic macules which are sometimes hard to see on infants and individuals with pale or fair skin. Because of the wide variety of signs of TSC, it is best if a doctor experienced in the diagnosis of TSC evaluates a potential patient.

In infants TSC may be suspected if the child has cardiac rhabdomyomas or seizures (infantile spasms) at birth. With a careful examination of the skin and brain, it may be possible to diagnose TSC in a very young infant. However, many children are not diagnosed until later in life when their seizures begin and other symptoms such as facial angiofibromas appear.

How Is TSC Treated?

There is no cure for TSC, although treatment is available for a number of the symptoms. Antiepileptic drugs may be used to control seizures. Vigabatrin is a particularly useful medication in TSC, and has been approved by the U.S. Food and Drug Administration (FDA) for treatment of infantile spasms in TSC, although it has significant side effects. The FDA has approved the drug everolimus (Afinitor®) to treat subependymal giant cell astrocytomas (SEGA brain tumors) and angiomyolipoma kidney tumors. Specific medications may be prescribed for behavior problems. Intervention programs including special schooling and occupational therapy may benefit individuals with special needs and developmental issues. Surgery may be needed in case of complications connected to tubers, SEN or SEGA, as well as in risk of hemorrhage from kidney tumors. Respiratory insufficiency due to LAM can be treated with supplemental oxygen therapy or lung transplantation if severe.

Because TSC is a lifelong condition, individuals need to be regularly monitored by a doctor to make sure they are receiving the best possible treatments. Due to the many varied symptoms of TSC, care by a clinician experienced with the disorder is recommended.

Basic laboratory studies have revealed insight into the function of the TSC genes and has led to recent use of rapamycin and related drugs for treating some manifestations of TSC. Rapamycin has been shown to be effective in treating SEGA, the brain tumor seen in TSC. However, its benefit for a variety of other aspects of and tumors seen in people with TSC is less certain, and clinical trials looking at the benefit carefully are continuing. Rapamycin and related drugs are not yet approved by the FDA for any purpose in individuals with TSC.

What Is the Prognosis?

The prognosis for individuals with TSC is highly variable and depends on the severity of symptoms. Those individuals with mild symptoms usually do well and have a normal life expectancy, while paying attention to TSC-specific issues. Individuals who are severely affected can suffer from severe mental retardation and persistent epilepsy.

All individuals with TSC are at risk for life-threatening conditions related to the brain tumors, kidney lesions, or LAM. Continued monitoring by a physician experienced with TSC is important. With appropriate medical care, most individuals with the disorder can look forward to normal life expectancy.

Chapter 27

Autism Affects Functioning of Entire Brain

A study provides evidence that autism affects the functioning of virtually the entire brain, and is not limited to the brain areas involved with social interactions, communication behaviors, and reasoning abilities, as had been previously thought. The study, conducted by scientists in a research network supported by the National Institutes of Health (NIH), found that autism also affects a broad array of skills and abilities, including those involved with sensory perception, movement, and memory.

The findings, appearing in the *August Child Neuropsychology,* strongly suggest that autism is a disorder in which the various parts of the brain have difficulty working together to accomplish complex tasks.

The study was conducted by researchers in the Collaborative Program of Excellence in Autism (CPEA), a research network funded by two components of the NIH, the *Eunice Kennedy Shriver* National Institute of Child Health and Human Development (NICHD) and the National Institute on Deafness and Other Communication Disorders (NIDCD).

"These findings suggest that further understanding of autism will likely come not from the study of factors affecting one brain area or

This chapter includes text excerpted from "Study Provides Evidence That Autism Affects Functioning of Entire Brain," National Institutes of Health (NIH), August 16, 2006. Reviewed October 2018.

system, but from studying factors affecting many systems," said the director of NICHD, Duane Alexander, M.D.

People with autism tend to display three characteristic behaviors, which are the basis of the diagnosis of autism, explained the study's senior author, Nancy Minshew, M.D., Professor of Psychiatry and Neurology at the University of Pittsburgh School of Medicine (UPSOM). These behaviors involve difficulty interacting socially, problems with verbal and nonverbal communications, and repetitive behaviors or narrow, obsessive interests. Traditionally, Dr. Minshew said, researchers studying autism have concentrated on these behavioral areas.

Within the last 20 years, however, researchers began studying other aspects of thinking and brain functioning in autism, discovering that people with autism have difficulty in many other areas, including balance, movement, memory, and visual perception skills.

In the study, Dr. Minshew and her colleagues administered a comprehensive array of neuropsychological tests to a group of children with autism. The researchers tested 56 autistic children, and compared their responses to those of 56 children who did not have autism. The children with autism were classified as having higher functioning autism—an I.Q. of 80 or above, and the ability to speak, read, and write. All of the children in the study ranged in age from 8 to 15 years. The purpose of the test array, Dr. Minshew said, was to determine whether there were any patterns in mental functioning unique to autism.

"We set out to find commonalities across a broad range of measures, so that we could make inferences about what's going on in the brain," Dr. Minshew said.

The researchers found that, across the entire series of tests, the children with autism performed as well as—and in some instances even better than—the other children on measures of basic functioning. Uniformly, however, they had trouble with complex tasks.

For example, regarding visual and spatial skills, the children with autism were very good at finding small objects in a cluttered visual field, on tasks like finding Waldo in the "Where's Waldo" picture books series. However, when asked to perform a complex task, like telling the difference between the faces of similar looking people, they had great difficulty.

Although their memory for the detail in a story was phenomenal, the children with autism had great difficulty comprehending the story. Many were highly proficient at spelling and had a good command of grammar, but had difficulty understanding complex figures of speech, like idioms and metaphors.

"We see this with our patients," Dr. Minshew said. "If you use an expression like 'hop to it,' a child with autism may literally hop."

Other complex tasks were also difficult for them. The children with autism either had poor handwriting, or wrote very slowly. Many had difficulty tying their shoes and with using scissors.

"These findings show that you can't compartmentalize autism under three basic areas," Dr. Minshew said. "It's much more complex than that."

Dr. Minshew explained that the major implication of the finding is that when seeking to understand autism, researchers need to look for a cause or causes that affect multiple brain areas, rather than limiting their search to brain areas dealing with the three characteristic behaviors involving social interactions, communication, and repetitive behaviors or obsessive interests.

"Our paper strongly suggests that autism is not primarily a disorder of social interaction, but a global disorder affecting how the brain processes the information it receives—especially when the information becomes complicated."

In previous research with an imaging technology known as functional magnetic resonance imaging, or fMRI, Dr. Minshew and her coworkers determined that adults with autism have abnormalities in the neurological wiring through which brain areas communicate. In those studies, the researchers found that people with autism had difficulty performing certain complex tasks that involved brain areas working together.

Dr. Minshew said that such abnormalities in brain circuitry provide the most likely explanation for why the children with autism in the study have difficulty with complex tasks that require coordination among brain regions but do well on tasks that require only one region of the brain at a time.

The researchers undertook the study as a follow up to an earlier study they did of adults with autism. The researchers studied children to determine if the features of autism were consistent throughout life, or changed as people with autism grow older. For the most part, the study revealed that both adults and children with autism experience the same kinds of difficulties with complex tasks.

One difference is that adults with autism appear to score higher on tests involving sensory interpretation than do children with autism. Such tests would involve identifying a number traced on a fingertip, or identifying an object placed in one's hand without looking at it. Dr. Minshew said that as people with autism grow older, they may have less sensory difficulty than they did as children.

Still, adults with autism fare much worse on tests of complex language and reasoning than do other adults. This gap in complex language and reasoning ability between the two groups is not as pronounced when children with autism are compared to other children. This is because children's brains have not yet developed these skills, Dr. Minshew said. However, the gap widens with time. As typical children get older, they develop these higher order language and reasoning skills while adolescents and adults with autism do not.

Chapter 28

Other Conditions That May Accompany Autism Spectrum Disorders

Chapter Contents

Section 28.1

Thin Bones and Autism Spectrum Disorder

This section contains text excerpted from the following sources:
Text in this section begins with excerpts from "Thin Bones
Seen in Boys with Autism and Autism Spectrum Disorder,"
Eunice Kennedy Shriver National Institute of Child Health and
Human Development (NICHD), January 29, 2008. Reviewed
October 2018; Text under the heading "Good Nutrition Is
Important" is excerpted from "Nutritional Therapy for Autism,"
Eunice Kennedy Shriver National Institute of Child Health and
Human Development (NICHD), January 31, 2017.

Results of an early study suggest that dairy-free diets and unconventional food preferences could put boys with autism and autism spectrum disorder (ASD) at higher than normal risk for thinner, less dense bones when compared to a group of boys the same age who do not have autism.

The study, by researchers from the National Institutes of Health (NIH) and the Cincinnati Children's Hospital Medical Center (CCHMC), was published online in the *Journal of Autism and Developmental Disorders*.

The researchers believe that boys with autism and ASD are at risk for poor bone development for a number of reasons. These factors are lack of exercise, a reluctance to eat a varied diet, lack of vitamin D, digestive problems, and diets that exclude casein, a protein found in milk and milk products. Dairy products provide a significant source of calcium and vitamin D. Casein-free diets are a controversial treatment thought by some to lessen the symptoms of autism.

Funding for the study was provided by the NIH's *Eunice Kennedy Shriver* National Institute of Child Health and Human Development (NICHD) and National Center for Research Resources (NCRR). The research team that conducted the study was led by Mary L. Hediger, Ph.D., a biological anthropologist in NICHD's Division of Epidemiology, Statistics, and Prevention Research (DESPR).

"Our results suggest that children with autism and autism spectrum disorder may be at risk for calcium and vitamin D deficiencies," Dr. Hediger said. "Parents of these children may wish to include a dietitian in their children's healthcare team, to ensure that they receive a balanced diet."

Dr. Hediger stressed that the study results need to be confirmed by larger studies. Until definitive information is available, however, it would be prudent for parents of children with autism and ASD to include a dietitian in their care, particularly if the children's diets do not include dairy products or they are not otherwise eating a balanced diet, she said. Because girls are much less likely to have autism or ASD than are boys, the researchers were unable to enroll a sufficient number of girls within the short time frame of the study to allow them to draw firm conclusions. Dr. Hediger added that if a girl with autism or ASD is not eating dairy products or eating a balanced diet, it would be prudent for a dietitian to be included in her healthcare team.

Autism is a complex brain disorder involving communication and social difficulties as well as repetitive behavior or narrow interests. Autism is often grouped with similar disorders, which are often referred to collectively as autism spectrum disorders. The underlying causes of autism and ASD are unclear. There is no cure for the disorders and treatments are limited.

When the boys were enrolled in the study, the researchers asked the boys' parents if the boys were taking over-the-counter (OTC) or prescription medications, were taking any vitamin or mineral supplements, or were on a restricted diet.

During the study, researchers X-rayed the hands of 75 boys between the ages of 4 and 8 years old who had been diagnosed with autism or ASD. The researchers then measured the thickness of the bone located between the knuckle of the index finger and the wrist and compared its development to a standardized reference based on a group of boys without autism.

Dr. Hediger said that the research team measured cortical bone thickness. She added that this procedure was done as a substitute for a conventional bone scan, which measures bone density. Bone density is an indication of bones' mineral content. Less dense bones may indicate a risk of bone fracture.

The researchers used the measure of bone thickness because many of the boys were unable to remain still long enough for the conventional scan, which requires individuals to lie immobile for an extended period of time. To successfully complete the bone scan, many of the boys would have required sedation—a step the researchers were reluctant to take for an early study.

The hand X-ray, Dr. Hediger explained, offers an approximate indication of bone density. She added, however, that because the researchers were unable to use a conventional bone scan, the results of the study should be confirmed by additional studies using conventional bone scans.

The investigators found that the bones of the boys with autism were growing longer but were not thickening at a normal rate. During normal bone development, material from inside the bone is transferred to the outside of the bone, increasing thickness, while at the same time, the bones are also growing longer.

At five or six years of age, the bones of the autistic boys were significantly thinner than the bones of boys without autism and the difference in bone thickness became even greater at ages seven and eight.

The bone thinning was particularly notable because the boys with autism and ASD were heavier than average and would, therefore, be expected to have thicker bones.

The researchers do not know for certain why the boys had thinner than normal bones. A possible explanation is the lack of calcium and vitamin D in their diets. Dr. Hediger explained that a deficiency of these important nutrients in the boys' diets could result from a variety of causes. Many children with autism, she said, have aversions to certain foods. Some will insist on eating the same foods nearly every day, to the exclusion of other foods. So while they may consume enough calories to meet their needs—or even more calories than they need—they may lack certain nutrients, like calcium and vitamin D.

Other children with autism may have digestive problems which interfere with the absorption of nutrients. Moreover, many children with autism remain indoors because they require supervision during outdoor activity. Lack of exercise hinders proper bone development, she said. Similarly, if children remain indoors and are not exposed to sunlight, they may not make enough vitamin D, which is needed to process calcium into bones. The boys in the study who were on a casein-free diet had the thinnest bones. In fact, the 9 boys who were on a casein-free diet had bones that were 20 percent thinner than normal for children their age. Boys who were not on a casein-free diet showed a 10 percent decrease in bone thickness when compared to boys with normal bone development.

The study authors wrote that bone development of children on casein-free diets should be monitored very carefully. They noted that studies of casein-free diets had not proven the diets to be effective in treating the symptoms of autism or ASD.

Only nine boys on casein-free diets were available to participate in the study, Dr. Hediger said. When conducting a scientific study, it's easier to obtain statistically valid results by studying a larger number of individuals than with a smaller number of individuals. However, the dramatic difference in the boys' bone thickness when they were either on a casein-free diet or an unrestricted diet and when compared to normally developing bones strongly suggest that the bone thinning the researchers observed was statistically valid.

The researchers recommended that larger studies be conducted to confirm their results.

Until those studies can be conducted, Dr. Hediger offered the following advice: "Our study shows that it couldn't hurt—and would probably help—if parents of children with autism or autism spectrum disorder consulted with a dietitian during their children's routine medical care to make sure that their diets are balanced."

Good Nutrition Is Important

Research shows that children with autism tend to have thinner bones than children without autism. Restricting access to bone-building foods, such as dairy products, can make it even harder for their bones to grow strong. Working with a healthcare provider can help ensure that children who are on special diets still get the bone-building and other nutrients they need.

Section 28.2

High Growth Hormones in Boys with Autism Spectrum Disorder

This section includes text excerpted from "Boys with Autism, Related Disorders, Have High Levels of Growth Hormones," National Institutes of Health (NIH), June 22, 2007. Reviewed October 2018.

Boys with autism and autism spectrum disorder had higher levels of hormones involved with growth in comparison to boys who do not have autism, reported researchers from the National Institutes of Health (NIH), the Centers for Disease Control and Prevention (CDC), the Cincinnati Children's Hospital (CCH) and the University of Cincinnati College of Medicine (UCCOM).

The researchers believe that the higher hormone levels might explain the greater head circumference seen in many children with autism. Earlier studies had reported that many children with autism have very rapid head growth in early life, leading to a proportionately larger head circumference than children who do not have autism.

The researchers found that, in addition to a larger head circumference, the boys with autism and autism spectrum disorder who took part in the study were heavier than boys without these conditions.

"The study authors have uncovered a promising new lead in the quest to understand autism," said Duane Alexander, M.D., Director of the *Eunice Kennedy Shriver* National Institute of Child Health and Human Development, the NIH institute that funded the study. "Future research will determine whether the higher hormone levels the researchers observed are related to abnormal head growth as well as to other features of autism."

Autism is a complex developmental disorder that includes problems with social interaction and communication. The term autism spectrum disorder (ASD) refers to individuals who have a less severe form of autism.

The study was published online in *Clinical Endocrinology.*

The researchers compared the height, weight, head circumference and levels of growth-related hormones to growth and maturation in 71 boys with autism and with ASD to a group of 59 boys who did not have these conditions.

The investigators found that the boys with autism had higher levels of two hormones that directly regulate growth (insulin-like growth factors 1 and 2). These growth-related hormones stimulate cellular growth. The researchers did not measure the boys' levels of human growth hormone, which for technical reasons is difficult to evaluate.

The boys with autism also had higher levels of other hormones related to growth, such as insulin-like growth factor binding protein and growth hormone binding protein.

In addition to greater head circumference, the boys with autism and those with autism spectrum disorders weighed more and had a higher body mass index (BMI). BMI is a ratio of a person's weight and height. A higher BMI often indicates that a person is overweight or obese. The boys' higher BMI may be related to their higher hormone levels, said the study's principal investigator, NICHD's James L. Mills, M.D., a senior investigator in the Division of Epidemiology, Statistics and Prevention Research's (DESPR) Epidemiology Branch. Dr. Mills and his coworkers also found that there was no difference in height between the two groups of boys.

The levels of growth-related hormones were significantly higher in the boys with autism even after the researchers compensated for the fact that higher levels of these hormones would be expected in children with a greater BMI.

"The higher growth-related hormone levels are not a result of the boys with autism simply being heavier," said Dr. Mills.

While it has long been noted that many children with autism have a larger head circumference than other children, few studies have investigated whether these children are also taller and heavier, Dr. Mills added.

Researchers analyzed medical records and blood samples from 71 boys diagnosed with autism and ASD who were patients at Cincinnati Children's Hospital Medical Center (CCHMC) from March 2002 to February 2004. The researchers compared the information on the boys with autism and autism spectrum disorders to other boys treated for other conditions at the hospital and who do not have autism. Children with conditions that may have affected their growth—such as being born severely premature, long-term illness, or the genetic condition fragile X were not included in the study. Girls are much less likely to develop autism than are boys, and the researchers were unable to recruit a sufficient number of girls with autism to participate in the study.

Dr. Mills explained that the bone age of the boys with autism—the bone development assessed by taking X-rays* and comparing the size and shape of the bones to similarly-aged children—were not more advanced in the group of boys with autism. For this reason, Dr. Mills and his coworkers ruled out the possibility that they were merely maturing more rapidly than were the other boys.

X-ray: A type of high-energy radiation. In low doses, X-rays are used to diagnose diseases by making pictures of the inside of the body.

Dr. Mills said that future studies could investigate whether the higher levels of growth hormones seen in children with autism could be directly related to the development of the condition itself.

Section 28.3

Unhealthy Weight in the U.S. Adolescents with Autism

This section includes text excerpted from "Key Findings: Prevalence and Impact of Unhealthy Weight in a National Sample of U.S. Adolescents with Autism and Other Learning and Behavioral Disorders," Centers for Disease Control and Prevention (CDC), April 26, 2018.

The *Maternal and Child Health Journal* has published a study that focuses on unhealthy weight among adolescents with developmental disabilities. Researchers from the Centers for Disease Control and Prevention (CDC) and the Health Resources and Services Administration (HRSA) found that obesity is high among adolescents with learning and behavioral developmental disabilities and highest among children with autism compared to adolescents without these conditions. This puts these already vulnerable adolescents at risk for lifelong health conditions related to being obese. There are no specific recommendations for preventing obesity among children or adolescents with developmental disabilities. Obesity prevention and management approaches for this at-risk group need further consideration.

Main Findings from This Study

Adolescents with learning and behavioral developmental disabilities were about 1.5 times more likely to be obese than adolescents without developmental disabilities.

Adolescents with autism were about two times more likely to be obese than adolescents without developmental disabilities.

Among adolescents with either attention deficit hyperactivity disorder (ADHD) or learning disorder/other developmental delay, those who were not taking prescription medications were more likely to be obese than adolescents without developmental disabilities.

About 5.6 percent of adolescents with learning and behavioral developmental disabilities were underweight, compared with 3.5 percent of adolescents without developmental disabilities. This means that adolescents with learning and behavioral developmental disabilities were about 1.5 times more likely to be underweight.

Adolescents with intellectual disability were four times more likely to be underweight than adolescents without developmental disabilities.

However, this likelihood decreased when taking into account whether the adolescent was born too small (less than 5.5 lbs).

Both obese adolescents (with or without developmental disabilities) and adolescents with developmental disabilities (with or without obesity) were more likely to have health conditions, such as asthma, eczema, and migraine headaches in comparison to nonobese adolescents without developmental disabilities.

Adolescents with both obesity and developmental disabilities had the highest number of these same health conditions.

Table 28.1. Percentage of Adolescents Who Are Obese

With any Learning Behavioral Developmental Disability	20.40%
With Autism	31.80%
With Intellectual Disability	19.80%
With ADHD	17.60%
With Learning Disorder/Other Developmental Delay	20.30%

About This Study

This study looked at parent-reported information collected as part of the National Health Interview Survey (NHIS). Specifically, researchers analyzed data on over 9,600 adolescents who were 12 to 17 years old in 2008–2010. Parents of over 1,400 of these adolescents identified their adolescents as having autism, ADHD, intellectual disability, and/ or learning disability or other developmental delay.

Section 28.4

Childhood Vision Impairment, Hearing Loss, and Co-Occurring Autism Spectrum Disorder

This section includes text excerpted from "Key Findings: Childhood Vision Impairment, Hearing Loss and Co-Occurring Autism Spectrum Disorder," Centers for Disease Control and Prevention (CDC), April 9, 2018.

The *Disability and Health Journal* has published a new study: "Childhood vision impairment, hearing loss, and co-occurring autism spectrum disorder." This study is based on information from the Metropolitan Atlanta Developmental Disabilities Surveillance Program (MADDSP). The study found that autism spectrum disorder was more common among children who also have vision impairment or hearing loss compared with the overall population of eight-year-old children with an autism spectrum disorder in metro Atlanta. More needs to be done to ensure that all children with autism spectrum disorder are identified as early as possible so that they can get the help they need.

Main Findings
Vision Impairment

- About 1 in 830 children in metro Atlanta has vision impairment.

- Approximately seven percent of the children with vision impairment also had autism spectrum disorder compared with about one percent of children in metro Atlanta with autism spectrum disorder overall.

- Compared to children with vision impairment without an autism spectrum disorder, the children with vision impairment and autism spectrum disorder were significantly more likely to:

  - Be born too early

  - Be born too small

  - Have intellectual disability

- The children with vision impairment and autism spectrum disorder were first evaluated by a community provider at about the same age as children without vision impairment. However, children with vision impairment were diagnosed with autism spectrum disorder later than those without vision impairment (6 years and 7 months compared to 4 years and 8 months).

Hearing Loss

- About 1 in 770 children in metro Atlanta has hearing loss.

- About six percent of the children with hearing loss also had autism spectrum disorder compared with about one percent of children in metro Atlanta with autism spectrum disorder overall.

- Compared to children with hearing loss without an autism spectrum disorder, the children with hearing loss and autism spectrum disorder were more likely to:

  - Be boys

  - Have intellectual disability and/or cerebral palsy (CP)

- The children with hearing loss and autism spectrum disorder were first evaluated by a community provider earlier than children without hearing loss (three years and four months compared with four years and two months, respectively). However, both groups were diagnosed with autism spectrum disorder at about the same age (four years and seven months).

What Is the Take-Home Message?

This study highlights the need for:

- Greater awareness of the signs and symptoms of autism spectrum disorder among doctors and other providers serving children with vision impairment or hearing loss;

- More tools that can be used to diagnose autism spectrum disorder among children with vision impairment or hearing loss; and

- Early treatment and improved services to address autism spectrum disorder among children with vision impairment or hearing loss.

This study found that certain factors, such as being born too early, increase the chance of a child having both autism spectrum disorder and either vision impairment or hearing loss. These findings could help guide future research.

225

Part Five

Interventions and Treatments for Autism Spectrum Disorders

Chapter 29

What Are Autism Spectrum Disorder Interventions?

Interventions—also known as procedures, programs, services, strategies, supports, or treatments—are designed to help people with autism spectrum disorders (ASDs) and their families negotiate the challenges associated with ASD and achieve positive outcomes. There are many different types of ASD interventions, and they vary in terms of goals, purpose, scope, intensity, timing, duration, and methodology. Some interventions focus on improving communication skills, encouraging social interaction, promoting independence, or increasing educational achievement. Other interventions aim to address challenging or inappropriate behaviors, treat sensory-processing issues, or develop adaptive skills. All interventions are intended to help people with ASD capitalize on their strengths, improve upon their deficits, and maximize their growth and development. Most individuals with ASD receive a combination of interventions from multiple providers, such as psychologists, behavior specialists, speech pathologists, physical therapists, and special education teachers.

Autism is a complex disorder that affects each person differently, so the key is to develop the right combination of interventions and therapies to meet an individual's unique needs. In general, though, research has shown that early intervention is a critical factor in terms of improving social skills and behavior for children with ASD. The biological processes underlying brain systems and functions are most

---

"ASD Interventions," © 2016 Omnigraphics. Reviewed October 2018.

responsive to outside influences during the first few years of life, so the likelihood of interventions leading to significant breakthroughs is highest at that time. Appropriate interventions can still produce positive results for older children, teenagers, and adults with ASD, however. Studies have shown that interventions can reduce ASD symptoms and lead to improvements in health, independence, and quality of life for people with ASD.

Effective ASD interventions typically include a predictable schedule, structured activities, and positive reinforcement of behavior. Outcomes are also enhanced when treatment programs break tasks down into simple steps, engage the person's attention and build on their interests, and promote self-esteem and independence. Successful interventions require the involvement of parents and caregivers because they play such a prominent role in shaping the experiences and environment of the person with ASD. The professional who leads the intervention must have the necessary skills and experience in working with people with autism, as well as a style that is a good fit with the patient. Finally, the process works best when professionals work collaboratively and coordinate their efforts across different types of interventions.

The Intervention Process

ASD intervention can be viewed as part of a process. The process begins with screening children for symptoms of autism, diagnosing ASD, and conducting assessments of skills, abilities, challenges, and deficits in functioning. Once an individual's unique needs have been identified through assessments, the next step is planning interventions to help the individual reach his or her goals. After the intervention plan has been developed and implemented, the final step in the process involves monitoring progress and revising the plan as needed.

Assessment

Assessment for intervention planning is typically conducted by a multidisciplinary team of professionals. A thorough assessment of an individual's symptoms, behavior, communication, social competence, and psychological functioning is required to determine what interventions will be most effective. The information gathered in the assessments guides the development of an individualized intervention plan.

Intervention Planning

Once the assessment results have identified the strengths and needs of the person with ASD, the individual and her or his parents and caregivers work with a team of professionals to review and select interventions to meet their goals. Interventions chosen should be supported by evidence-based research findings, reflect the values and preferences of the individual and his or her family, and be accessible given family and community resources. The final part of the intervention plan involves determining procedures to be used for monitoring progress toward meeting objectives.

Monitoring Progress

Once the intervention plan is put in place, data is collected and compared to the initial assessment results to monitor the individual's progress in response to the interventions. This data helps families and professionals determine whether the interventions are working as intended and whether the desired changes or improvements are occurring. If not, adjustments and revisions can be made to the intervention plan.

Types of Interventions

There are many different types of interventions available to address many different aspects of ASD. A few of the more common interventions include:

- Social skills training to help children with ASD express thoughts and feelings appropriately and interact with others in social situations

- Speech-language therapy to help children with ASD communicate better and interpret the verbal and nonverbal signals of others

- Sensory integration therapy to help children with ASD develop their motor skills, gain control over their senses, or improve their responses to sensory stimuli

- Cognitive behavior therapy (CBT) to help people with ASD manage their emotions, fears, and anxieties in order to reduce challenging behaviors and respond more appropriately in various situations

- Applied behavioral analysis (ABA)—a highly structured method of breaking down skills into small steps and providing positive reinforcement for achieving the desired result—to teach people with ASD communication, social, academic, adaptive, and other skills, as well as to reduce challenging behaviors

- Parent education and training to enable caregivers to incorporate aspects of treatment programs into the daily home life of a child with ASD. Interventions such as social skills and behavior training tend to be more successful when they are reinforced consistently in multiple settings.

References

1. "Autism Spectrum Disorders: Guide to Evidence-Based Interventions," Missouri Autism Guidelines Initiative (MAGI), 2012.

2. "Interventions and Treatment Options," Autism Speaks, 2016.

Chapter 30

Evidence for ASD Interventions

Based on that studies included five randomized controlled trials (RCTs) of good quality, six of fair quality, and one of poor quality. Individual studies using intensive University of California, Los Angeles (UCLA)/Lovaas-based interventions, the Early Start Denver Model (ESDM), the Learning Experiences and Alternate Program for Preschoolers and their Parents (LEAP) program, and eclectic variants reported improvements in outcomes for young children. Improvements were most often seen in cognitive abilities and language acquisition, with less robust and consistent improvements seen in adaptive skills, core autism spectrum disorder (ASD) symptom severity, and social functioning.

Young children receiving high-intensity applied behavior analysis (ABA)-based interventions over extended time frames (i.e., eight months to two years) displayed improvement in cognitive functioning and language skills relative to community controls. However, the magnitude of these effects varied across studies. This variation may reflect subgroups showing differential responses to particular interventions. Intervention response is likely moderated by both treatment and child factors, but exactly how these moderators function is not clear. Despite multiple studies of early intensive treatments, intervention approaches

This chapter includes text excerpted from "Therapies for Children with Autism Spectrum Disorder: Behavioral Interventions Update," Effective Health Care Program, Agency for Healthcare Research and Quality (AHRQ), August 2014. Reviewed October 2018.

still vary substantially, which makes it difficult to tease apart what these unique treatment and child factors may be. Further, the long-term impact of these early skill improvements is not yet clear, and many studies did not follow children beyond late preschool or early school years.

Studies of high-intensity early intervention services also demonstrated improvements in children's early adaptive behavior skills, but these improvements were more variable than those found for early cognitive and language skills. Treatment effects were not consistently maintained over follow-up assessments across studies. Many studies measured different adaptive behavior domains (creating within-scale variability), and some evidence suggests that adaptive behavior changes may be contingent on baseline child characteristics, such as cognitive/language skills and ASD severity.

Evidence for the impact of early intensive intervention on core ASD symptoms is limited and mixed. Children's symptom severity often decreased during treatment, but these improvements often did not differ from those of children in control groups. Better quality studies reported positive effects of intervention on symptom severity, but multiple lower quality studies did not.

Since the Evidence-based Practice Center's (EPC) previous review, there have been substantially more studies of well-controlled low-intensity interventions that provide parent training in bolstering social communication skills. Although parent training programs modified parenting behaviors during interactions, data were more limited about their ability to improve broad developmental skills (such as cognition, adaptive behavior, and ASD symptom severity) beyond language gains for some children. Children receiving low-intensity interventions have not demonstrated the same substantial gains in cognitive skills seen in the early intensive intervention paradigms.

Social Skills Studies

The EPC located 13 studies addressing interventions targeting social skills, including 11 RCTs. The overall quality of studies improved in comparison with the previous review, with 2 good quality and 10 fair-quality studies. Social skills interventions varied widely in terms of scope and intensity. A few studies replicated interventions using the Skillstreaming model, which uses a published treatment manual (i.e., is manualized) to promote a consistent approach. Other studies incorporated peer-mediated and/or group-based approaches, and still others described interventions that focused on emotion identification and Theory of Mind (ToM) training. The studies also varied in intensity, with most interventions consisting of 1–2 hour sessions/week lasting approximately 4–5 weeks. However, some of the group-based approaches lasted 15–16 weeks.

Most studies reported short-term gains in either parent-rated social skills or directly tested emotion recognition. However, EPC's confidence (strength of evidence) in that effect is low. Although it now has higher quality studies of social skills interventions that demonstrate positive effects, the ability to determine effectiveness continues to be limited by the diversity of the intervention protocols and measurement tools (i.e., no consistent outcome measures used across studies). Studies also included only participants considered "high functioning" and/or with intelligence quotient (IQ) test scores >70, thus limiting generalization of results to children with more significant impairments. Maintenance and generalization of these skills beyond the intervention setting are also inconsistent, with parent and clinician raters noting variability in performance across environments.

Play-/Interaction-Focused Studies

Since EPC's previous review, more studies of well-controlled joint attention interventions across a range of intervention settings (e.g., clinician, parent, teacher delivered) have been published. This growing evidence base includes 11 RCTs of good and fair quality and suggests that joint attention interventions may be associated with positive outcomes for toddler and preschool children with ASD, particularly when targeting joint attention skills themselves as well as related social communication and language skills. Although joint attention intervention studies demonstrated changes within this theoretically important domain, data are more limited about their ability to improve broad developmental skills (such as cognition, adaptive behavior, and ASD symptom severity) beyond direct measures of joint attention and related communication and language gains over time.

Specific training that used naturalistic approaches to promote imitation (e.g., Reciprocal Imitation Training (RIT)) was associated with some improvements, not only in imitation skills, but also potentially in other social communication skills (such as joint attention). Additionally, parent training in a variety of play-based interventions was associated with enhanced early social communication skills (e.g., joint attention, engagement, play interactions), play skills, and early-language skills.

235

Studies of Interventions Targeting Conditions Commonly Associated with Autism Spectrum Disorder

Six RCTs (five good and one fair quality) of interventions addressing conditions commonly associated with ASD measured anxiety symptoms as a primary outcome. Five of these studies reported significantly greater improvements in anxiety symptoms in the intervention group compared with controls. Two found positive effects of cognitive behavioral therapy (CBT) on the core ASD symptom of socialization, and one reported improvements in executive function in the treatment group. The one RCT that did not find a significant benefit of CBT compared it with social recreational therapy rather than with treatment as usual or a wait-listed control group.

The studies examining the effects of CBT on anxiety had largely consistent methodologies. Six studies provided follow-up data reflecting treatment effects that lasted beyond the period of direct intervention. Two common factors limit the applicability of the results, however. Due to the nature of CBT, which is often language intensive and requires a certain level of reasoning skills to make abstract connections between concepts, most studies included only children with IQs much greater than 70. These studies report positive results regarding the use of CBT to treat anxiety in children with ASD. They also report some positive results in socialization, executive function, and communication; however, these results were less robust, and it is unclear in some studies if these improvements exceeded improvements related to the impact of ameliorated anxiety itself.

Additional data in the review relate to parent training to address challenging behavior. Specifically, one fair-quality study combined a parent-training approach with risperidone. This combination significantly reduced irritability, stereotypical behaviors, and hyperactivity, and improved socialization and communication skills. However, these effects were not maintained at one year after treatment.

Other Behavioral Studies

Two RCTs (one fair and one poor quality) examined neurofeedback and found some improvements on parent-rated measures of communication and tests of executive function. Three fair-quality RCTs reported on sleep-focused interventions, with little positive effect of a sleep education pamphlet for parents in one, improvements in sleep quality in treatment arms (melatonin alone, melatonin + CBT) in another, and some improvements in time to fall asleep in one short-term RCT of sleep education programs for parents. One poor-quality study of parent education to mitigate feeding problems reported no significant effects.

Modifiers of Treatment Effects

Among the potential modifiers or moderators of early intensive ABA-based interventions, younger age at intake was associated with better outcomes for children in a limited number of studies. Greater baseline cognitive skills and higher adaptive behavior scores were associated with better outcomes across behavioral interventions, but again, these associations were not consistent. In general, children with lower symptom severity or less severe diagnoses improved more than participants with greater impairments. Many studies (e.g., social skills, CBT) restricted the range of participants' impairment at baseline (e.g., recruiting only participants with IQs >70), limiting understanding of intervention impact on broader populations. Studies assessing parental responsiveness to children's communication typically reported better outcomes in children whose parents were more aligned with the child's communication versus those who attempted to redirect or were less synchronized. Regarding intervention-related factors, duration of treatment had an inconsistent effect. Some studies reported improved outcomes with more intervention time and others reported no association. Overall, most studies were not adequately designed or controlled to identify true moderators of treatment response.

Treatment Phase Changes That Predict Outcomes

The reviewed literature offers little information about what specific early changes from baseline measurements of child characteristics might predict long-term outcome and response.

Treatment Effects That Predict Long-Term Outcomes

Few studies assess end-of-treatment effects that may predict outcomes. Several early intensive behavioral and developmental interventions are associated with changes in outcome measures over the course of very lengthy treatments, but such outcomes usually have not been assessed beyond treatment windows. One family of studies attempted to follow young children receiving early joint attention intervention until they were school aged, but this study failed to include adequate followup of control conditions. It also involved children who were receiving many hours of uncontrolled interventions during the course of study.

Generalization of Treatment Effects

The majority of the social skills and behavioral intervention studies targeting associated conditions attempted to collect outcomes based on parent, self, teacher, and peer report of targeted symptoms (e.g., anxiety, externalizing behaviors, social skills, peer relations) at home, at school, and in the community. Although such ratings outside of the clinical setting may be suggestive of generalization in that they improve outcomes in the daily context/life of the child, in most cases, these outcomes are parent-reported and not confirmed with direct observation. Behavioral intervention studies rarely measured outcomes beyond the intervention period, and therefore, cannot assume that effects were maintained over time.

Treatment Components That Drive Outcomes

EPC did not identify any studies meeting the inclusion criteria that addressed this question.

Treatment Approaches for Children under Age Two at Risk for Diagnosis of Autism Spectrum Disorder

In the studies addressing interventions for younger children, children who received behavioral interventions seemed to improve regardless of intervention type (including the comparator interventions, which were also behavioral). None of the fair- or good-quality studies compared treatment groups with a no-treatment control group. Potential modifiers of treatment efficacy include baseline levels of object interest. Most outcome measures of adaptive functioning were based on parent report, and the effect of parental perception of treatment efficacy on perception (and report) of child functioning was generally not explored.

Chapter 31

Early Intervention for Children with Developmental Delays

Chapter Contents

Section 31.1

Overview of Early Intervention

This section includes text excerpted from "Early Intervention for Autism," *Eunice Kennedy Shriver* National Institute of Child Health and Human Development (NICHD), January 31, 2017.

Research shows that early diagnosis of and interventions for autism are more likely to have major long-term positive effects on symptoms and later skills. Autism spectrum disorder (ASD) can sometimes be diagnosed in children before they are two years of age. Some children with ASD whose development seems normal up to that point begin to regress just before or sometime during their second year.

Early interventions occur at or before preschool age, as early as two or three years of age. In this period, a young child's brain is still forming, meaning it is more "plastic" or changeable than at older ages. Because of this plasticity, treatments have a better chance of being effective in the longer term. Early interventions not only give children the best start possible, but also the best chance of developing to their full potential. The sooner a child gets help, the greater the chance for learning and progress. In fact, guidelines suggest starting an integrated developmental and behavioral intervention as soon as ASD is diagnosed or seriously suspected.

With early intervention, some children with autism make so much progress that they are no longer on the autism spectrum when they are older. Many of the children who later go off the spectrum have some things in common:

- Diagnosis and treatment at younger ages

- A higher intelligence quotient (IQ, a measure of thinking ability) than the average child with autism

- Better language and motor skills

Goals of Early Intervention

Early intervention programs help children gain the basic skills that they usually learn in the first two years of life, such as:

- Physical skills

- Thinking skills

- Communication skills
- Social skills
- Emotional skills

State-Run Programs

Each state has its own early intervention program for children from birth to age two years who are diagnosed with developmental delays or disabilities, including ASD. These programs are specified by Part C of Public Law 108-77: Individuals with Disabilities Education Improvement Act (2004) (idea.ed.gov/part-c/search/new.html), sometimes called "IDEA." Some states also provide services for children who are at risk for developmental delays and disabilities.

Section 31.2

Diagnoses of Autism Spectrum Disorder Made at Earlier Ages

This section includes text excerpted from "CDC's 'Learn the Signs. Act Early.' Program," Centers for Disease Control and Prevention (CDC), May 1, 2011. Reviewed October 2018.

The Importance of Early Identification of Developmental Delay and Disability

- The Centers for Disease Control and Prevention (CDC) estimates that 1 in 88 children has been identified with an autism spectrum disorder and about 1 in 6 children aged 3 to 17 has a developmental disability.

- Many children with a developmental disability are not identified until after entering school.

- Early intervention (before school age) can have a significant impact on a child's ability to learn new skills as well as reduce the need for costly interventions over time.

Improving Early Identification of Developmental Delay and Disability

The CDC's "Learn the Signs. Act Early." program aims to improve early identification of children with autism and other developmental disabilities so children and families can get the services and support they need as early as possible.

The program is made up of three components:

- Health education campaign promotes awareness of

  - Healthy developmental milestones in early childhood

  - The importance of tracking each child's development

  - The importance of acting early if there are concerns

- Act Early Initiative works with state, territorial, and national partners to improve early childhood systems by

  - Enhancing collaborative efforts to improve screening and referral to early intervention services

  - Supporting the work of Act Early Ambassadors to promote "Learn the Signs. Act Early." messages and tools and improve early identification efforts in their state

- Research and evaluation improve campaign materials and implementation activities and increases the understanding of the factors that influence early identification and referral.

The CDC works with the Health Resources and Services Administration (HRSA), the Association of University Centers on Disabilities (AUCD), the Association of Maternal and Child Health Programs (AMCHP) and other partners in the delivery of this program.

"Learn the Signs. Act Early." aims to change perceptions about the importance of identifying developmental concerns early and gives parents and professionals the tools to help.

The CDC offers parent-friendly materials that are research-based, free, easily accessible and customizable.

- Materials are available for parents, early educators, and healthcare providers.

- Milestone checklists, tips for parents, early warning signs, fact sheets, and other materials can be downloaded or ordered for free.

- All materials are available in English and Spanish; some are available in other languages.

- Find materials at www.cdc.gov/actearly.

National, state, and local programs that serve parents of young children can add "Learn the Signs." materials to their resources for parents.

- The CDC's materials help programs address the need for child development resources.

- Programs can customize the CDC's materials with their own contact information and distribute them to the populations they serve.

Research and evaluation projects advance the understanding of how to improve early identification of children with autism and other developmental disabilities in population groups with health disparities.

African American children and Hispanic children are less likely than white children to be identified as having an autism spectrum disorder.

- Research projects address information needs of parents, healthcare providers, and early educators to improve early identification in populations with health disparities.

- Evaluation and feasibility studies address how to reach special populations with campaign messages and how to improve systems that identify and serve children with developmental delays.

Section 31.3

Early Services for Autism Spectrum Disorder

This section includes text excerpted from "Autism Spectrum Disorder (ASD)—Treatment," Centers for Disease Control and Prevention (CDC), April 26, 2018.

There are no medications that can cure autism spectrum disorder (ASD) or treat the core symptoms. However, there are medications that can help some people with ASD function better. For example, medication might help manage high energy levels, inability to focus, depression, or seizures.

Medications might not affect all children in the same way. It is important to work with a healthcare professional who has experience in treating children with ASD. Parents and healthcare professionals must closely monitor a child's progress and reactions while she or he is taking a medication to be sure that any negative side effects of the treatment do not outweigh the benefits.

It is also important to remember that children with ASD can get sick or injured just like children without ASD. Regular medical and dental exams should be part of a child's treatment plan. Often it is hard to tell if a child's behavior is related to the ASD or is caused by a separate health condition. For instance, head banging could be a symptom of the ASD, or it could be a sign that the child is having headaches. In those cases, a thorough physical exam is needed. Monitoring healthy development means not only paying attention to symptoms related to ASD, but also to the child's physical and mental health, as well.

Early Intervention Services

Research shows that early intervention treatment services can greatly improve a child's development. Early intervention services help children from birth to 3 years old (36 months) learn important skills. Services include therapy to help the child talk, walk, and interact with others. Therefore, it is important to talk to your child's doctor as soon as possible if you think your child has an ASD or other developmental problem.

Even if your child has not been diagnosed with an ASD, she or he may be eligible for early intervention treatment services. The Individuals with Disabilities Education Act (IDEA) (sites.ed.gov/idea) says that children under the age of 3 years (36 months) who are at risk of having developmental delays may be eligible for services. These services are provided through an early intervention system in your state. Through this system, you can ask for an evaluation.

In addition, treatment for particular symptoms, such as speech therapy for language delays, often does not need to wait for a formal ASD diagnosis. While early intervention is extremely important, intervention at any age can be helpful.

Types of Treatments

There are many different types of treatments available. For example, auditory training, discrete trial training, vitamin therapy, anti-yeast therapy, facilitated communication, music therapy, occupational therapy, physical therapy, and sensory integration.

The different types of treatments can generally be broken down into the following categories:

- Behavior and Communication Approaches

- Dietary Approaches

- Medication

- Complementary and Alternative Medicine

Behavior and Communication Approaches

According to reports by the American Academy of Pediatrics (AAP) and the National Research Council (NRC), behavior and communication approaches that help children with ASD are those that provide structure, direction, and organization for the child in addition to family participation.

Applied Behavior Analysis

A notable treatment approach for people with an ASD is called applied behavior analysis (ABA). ABA has become widely accepted among healthcare professionals and used in many schools and treatment clinics. ABA encourages positive behaviors and discourages negative behaviors in order to improve a variety of skills. The child's progress is tracked and measured.

There are different types of ABA. Following are some examples:

- **Discrete Trial Training (DTT).** DTT is a style of teaching that uses a series of trials to teach each step of a desired behavior or response. Lessons are broken down into their simplest parts and positive reinforcement is used to reward correct answers and behaviors. Incorrect answers are ignored.

- **Early Intensive Behavioral Intervention (EIBI).** This is a type of ABA for very young children with an ASD, usually younger than five, and often younger than three.

- **Pivotal Response Training (PRT).** PRT aims to increase a child's motivation to learn, monitor his own behavior, and initiate communication with others. Positive changes in these behaviors should have widespread effects on other behaviors.

- **Verbal Behavior Intervention (VBI).** VBI is a type of ABA that focuses on teaching verbal skills.

Other therapies that can be part of a complete treatment program for a child with an ASD include:

- **Developmental, Individual Differences, Relationship-Based Approach (DIR; also called "Floortime").** Floortime focuses on emotional and relational development (feelings, relationships with caregivers). It also focuses on how the child deals with sights, sounds, and smells.

- **Treatment and Education of Autistic and Related Communication-Handicapped Children (TEACCH)** (teacch. com). TEAACH uses visual cues to teach skills. For example, picture cards can help teach a child how to get dressed by breaking information down into small steps.

- **Occupational Therapy.** It teaches skills that help the person live as independently as possible. Skills might include dressing, eating, bathing, and relating to people.

- **Sensory Integration Therapy.** It helps the person deal with sensory information, like sights, sounds, and smells. Sensory integration therapy could help a child who is bothered by certain sounds or does not like to be touched.

- **Speech Therapy.** It helps to improve the person's communication skills. Some people are able to learn verbal communication skills. For others, using gestures or picture boards is more realistic.

- **The Picture Exchange Communication System (PECS).** PECS uses picture symbols to teach communication skills. The person is taught to use picture symbols to ask and answer questions and have a conversation.

Dietary Approaches

Some dietary treatments have been developed by reliable therapists. But many of these treatments do not have the scientific support needed for widespread recommendation. An unproven treatment might help one child, but may not help another.

Many biomedical interventions call for changes in diet. Such changes include removing certain types of foods from a child's diet and using vitamin or mineral supplements. Dietary treatments are based on the idea that food allergies or lack of vitamins and minerals cause symptoms of ASD. Some parents feel that dietary changes make a difference in how their child acts or feels.

If you are thinking about changing your child's diet, talk to the doctor first. Or talk with a nutritionist to be sure your child is getting important vitamins and minerals.

Medication

There are no medications that can cure ASD or even treat the main symptoms. But there are medications that can help some people with related symptoms. For example, medication might help manage high energy levels, inability to focus, depression, or seizures.

Complementary and Alternative Treatments

To relieve the symptoms of ASD, some parents and healthcare professionals use treatments that are outside of what is typically recommended by the pediatrician. These types of treatments are known as complementary and alternative treatments. They might include special diets, chelation (a treatment to remove heavy metals such as lead from the body), biologicals (e.g., secretin), or body-based systems (like deep pressure).

These types of treatments are very controversial. Research shows that as many as one third of parents of children with an ASD may have tried complementary or alternative medicine treatments, and up to 10 percent may be using a potentially dangerous treatment. Before starting such a treatment, check it out carefully, and talk to your child's doctor.

Section 31.4

Autism Intervention for Toddlers Improves Developmental Outcomes

This section includes text excerpted from "Towards Interventions across the Autism Spectrum," National Institute of Mental Health (NIMH), April 26, 2017.

Improving Outcomes: The Earlier the Better

Although the Centers for Disease Control and Prevention (CDC) says that it is possible to diagnose autism spectrum disorder (ASD) in children at age two, the median age of diagnosis is older than four. Moreover, research suggests that identifying early signs and symptoms of the disorder could help diagnose children even sooner. And this is really important, since children do better when interventions are started earlier.

First things first: It is challenging to develop effective interventions for ASD due to the variability in the condition. There is great variability within and across these domains of functioning, and interventions are needed that address individual needs.

There are therapies that help improve outcomes, enabling many children with ASD to learn skills that help them function better. Among these are comprehensive therapies, targeting a range of ASD-related deficits. An example is the Early Start Denver Model (ESDM), in which a trained therapist works with a child and his or her parents in an approach that makes use of everyday activities to help children improve across the domains affected in ASD. Children at ages 13–30 months receiving ESDM in a clinical trial improved in communication, motor, and daily living skills. Follow-up studies found that children receiving this early intervention showed patterns of brain activity, measured by electroencephalogram (EEG), closer to typically developing children when compared with children receiving more usual treatment. Two years following the end of the intensive treatment, the children's gains in terms of core symptoms were still evident.

Another approach, parent-mediated social communication therapy (PACT), involves a therapist working with a parent and child in a way that emphasizes the parent's role, enhancing the parent's sensitivity to the child's communication and using play and verbal strategies to encourage communication skills. Six years following the end of treatment, children continued to have reduced symptoms relative to children who received treatment as usual. In another trial, a parent-supported social communication intervention delivered to children between 9 and 14 months of age with a sibling with ASD, but who have not otherwise been identified as being other than typically developing, resulted in improvement in autism prodromal symptoms, sustained two years following the intervention.

To maximize the efficacy of these treatments, we need to be able to identify children with ASD early, and to ensure access to evidence-based interventions and services. To enhance early identification, the National Institute of Mental Health (NIMH) funded the ASD Pediatric, Early Detection, Engagement, and Services Research (PEDS) Network, which comprises of five separate but coordinated studies to test a range of strategies for universal screening and early engagement in treatment. The various study sites have agreed to collect common data elements, pool their resources, and share their data in a truly collaborative effort that will enhance the reliability and impact of their findings. These studies are expected to be completed in 2019.

The NIMH participates in other research efforts aimed at developing novel treatments and enhancing implementation of existing ones. For example, it partnered with four other institutes—the *Eunice Kennedy Shriver* National Institute of Child Health and Human Development (NICHD), the National Institute on Deafness and Other Communication Disorders (NIDCD), the National Institute of Neurological Disorders and Stroke (NINDS), and the National Institute of Environmental Health Sciences (NIEHS)—to establish 11 Autism Centers of Excellence (ACE) across the country. These centers focus on causes and improved treatment, as well as studies of specific populations affected by ASD, including females and African Americans. In a partnership with the Simons Foundation for Autism Research Initiative (SFARI) (sfari.org), NICHD, and NINDS, the NIMH supports a multiyear project to develop and improve clinical research tools for studying ASD. Part of the Biomarkers Consortium, this project will test and refine clinical measures of social impairment in ASD to better evaluate potential behavioral and drug therapies.

Treatment across the Lifespan

While continued research on interventions and services for young children with ASD is crucial, research on the needs of transition-age youth and adults with ASD is equally important. Despite this clear need, relatively little about how best to support individuals with

ASD as they transition to adulthood is known. Postsecondary education and vocational training, supported employment, appropriate residential opportunities, continued development of social skills, and access to services and supports, including psychosocial interventions and technological supports, are all thought to be helpful to transition-age youth and adults. Nonetheless, the evidence base in support of these approaches is lacking, and precisely how best to meet the needs of transition-age youth and adults this need is unclear.

The NIMH is investing in research to remedy this lack of information. The ServASD initiative is funding efforts to develop and test the effectiveness of community-based interventions that can be delivered across a variety of service systems to improve functional and health outcomes of individuals with ASD throughout the lifespan, including the transition from youth to adulthood. These strategies take into account the structure and staffing of the service setting, such as educational, vocational, healthcare, and independent living programs, to ensure that, should the interventions prove effective, they can be delivered consistently and sustainably. Projects funded are aimed at developing and testing models for the delivery of needed services, including screening services, early intervention, transition services, and services for adults that target employment, social relationships, housing, and independent living.

Section 31.5

Challenging Behaviors

This section includes text excerpted from "Why Act Early If You're Concerned about Development?" Centers for Disease Control and Prevention (CDC), April 30, 2018.

Act early on developmental concerns to make a real difference for your child and you! If you're concerned about your child's development, don't wait. You know your child best.

Early intervention helps children improve their abilities and learn new skills. Take these steps to help your child today:

- Tell your child's doctor or nurse if you notice any signs of possible developmental delay and ask for a developmental screening.

If you or the doctor still feel worried,

- Ask for a referral to a specialist; and
- Call your state or territory's early intervention program to find out if your child can get services to help.

What Is Early Intervention?

Early intervention:

- Is the term used to describe services and support that help babies and toddlers (from birth to three years of age in most states/territories) with developmental delays or disabilities and their families
- May include speech therapy, physical therapy, and other types of services based on the needs of the child and family
- Can have a significant impact on a child's ability to learn new skills and increase their success in school and life
- Programs are available in every state and territory. These services are provided for free or at a reduced cost for any child who meets the state's criteria for developmental delay.

Why Early Intervention Is Important

Earlier Is Better!

Intervention is likely to be more effective when it is provided earlier in life rather than later.

"If it's autism, waiting for a child to 'catch up' on his or her own just won't work. Acting early can help a child communicate, play, and learn from the world now and for the future. It can also prevent frustration—so common in children with communication difficulties— from turning into more difficult behaviors." (Pennsylvania clinical psychologist)

The connections in a baby's brain are most adaptable in the first three years of life. These connections, also called neural circuits, are the foundation for learning, behavior, and health. Over time, these connections become harder to change.

251

"The earlier developmental delays are detected and intervention begins, the greater the chance a young child has of achieving his or her best potential." (Georgia pediatrician)

Intervention Works!

Early intervention services can change a child's developmental path and improve outcomes for children, families, and communities.

"Acting early gives your child a chance to receive the appropriate therapy, giving him or her the best chance for a good outcome in the future. I believe that early intervention is the reason my high-functioning son is now able to blend in with his peers and attend kindergarten in a regular classroom with no supports." (Kansas mom)

Help Your Child, Help Your Family!

Families benefit from early intervention by being able to better meet their children's needs from an early age and throughout their lives.

"Action replaced fear and empowered me with the knowledge to help my son. He has overcome most of his symptoms and is headed to college next year." (Florida mom)

Chapter 32

Therapies for Children with Autism Spectrum Disorder

What Is Autism Spectrum Disorder?

Autism spectrum disorder (ASD) includes a range of behavioral symptoms.

The two core features of ASD are:

- Difficulty with social interactions and communication
- Repetitive behaviors, interests, and activities

How Common Is Autism Spectrum Disorder?

About one in every 68 children in the United States has ASD. It is about four times more common in boys than girls. It can affect children of all races and social classes wherever they live. Researchers are not sure what causes ASD.

No Two Children with ASD Are Alike

ASD is called a "wide-spectrum disorder" because the symptoms are different for each child. Symptoms can range from mild to severe,

This chapter includes text excerpted from "Therapies for Children with Autism Spectrum Disorder," Effective Health Care Program, Agency for Healthcare Research and Quality (AHRQ), September 23, 2014. Reviewed October 2018.

and can change as the child grows. No two children with ASD are alike. This makes understanding ASD and finding the best therapies difficult.

How Do I Make Sense of All the Different Treatments?

Treatments for ASD can be grouped into different categories. Each category focuses on a type of treatment.

Figure 32.1. *Categories of ASD Treatment*

Because children with ASD may show different symptoms, a family will need to choose from the available treatments, therapies, and programs based on their child's needs. The treatment plan for your child may have some treatments from each of these categories.

What Can the Research Tell Me?

There is a lot of research being done on how to treat the symptoms of ASD in children or to help children overcome the challenges of ASD. But to decide whether something helps or not (or works better than something else), researchers need to look at the results from many studies rather than just one. One study may find that something helped, while another study may find that it did not. The information in this section will tell you about each type of treatment and what researchers found when they looked at all the studies at once.

Behavior Programs

These programs address social skills, attention, sleep, play, anxiety, parent interaction, and challenging behaviors. Some programs also help with children's overall development.

Many of these programs use specially trained providers who work with parents and children for up to 25 hours every week. The programs can last as long as 12 weeks to 3 years. They are held in homes, schools, and clinics.

Early intensive behavioral intervention, cognitive behavioral therapy (CBT), and social skills training are types of behavior programs. Early intensive behavioral interventions target children's overall development. Programs such as the Lovaas Model and Early Start Denver Model mostly focus on working with children. Other programs, such as Pivotal response training (PRT) and Hanen More Than Words, focus on teaching parents how to help their children.

Programs that use cognitive behavioral therapy help children manage anxiety. Coping Cat and Facing Your Fears are examples of this type of program.

Social skills programs address social skills, attention, and play. Programs such as Skillstreaming help older children with their social skills. Programs such as Joint Attention Symbolic Play Engagement and Regulation (JASPER) aim to help younger children with issues such as trouble with cooperative play.

The behavior programs in your area may be based on these or other models. However, they might be called by different names.

Do They Help?

- Early intensive behavioral interventions that focus on helping children with their overall development may improve a young child's reasoning and communication skills. Research is not clear about whether they improve social skills, daily-living skills, or the severity of ASD symptoms.

- Programs that focus on teaching parents how to help their children show promise, but researchers do not yet know if they work.

- Cognitive behavioral therapy reduces anxiety in some older children with ASD who do not have other developmental delays and have average reasoning and language skills.

- Social skills programs may help school-age children without other developmental or language delays for short periods of time. More research is needed to know whether children remember and use these skills after the end of the program.

255

- Programs that address how children play may improve children's social interactions, but more research is needed to know for sure.

What Are the Costs?

The costs of behavior programs vary by state. Providers have different fees. Insurance may not cover some costs. You should check with your insurance plan to find out about coverage. Other assistance may be available. Ask your doctor.

What Else Should I Think About?

Because of the amount of time involved, you may need to change your family's schedule or routine to participate in some programs.

Education and Learning Programs

These programs are offered in schools or other learning centers. They focus on learning and reasoning skills and "whole life" approaches. Schools may have different names for their programs, but many of these programs are based on the Treatment and Education of Autistic and Communication related handicapped CHildren (TEACCH) approach. Programs like TEACCH use visual tools and arrange the classroom in ways that are easier to manage for a child with ASD. Other programs are classroom- or center-based and use "applied behavior analysis" (commonly known as ABA) strategies like positive reinforcement.

Do They Help?

- Some children in the TEACCH program showed improvement in motor skills (the ability to walk, run, hold items, or sit up straight), eye–hand coordination, and thinking and reasoning. There were not enough studies for researchers to say for sure, however, whether TEACCH was effective.

- Other education programs have not been studied enough to know if they work.

What Are the Costs?

Usually, these services are included in the cost of the school or learning center, so there may not be any other costs to you if you are a resident of the school district or community.

What Else Should I Think About?

Your school district or learning center may have other names for these educational approaches, so you may want to ask about the exact types of strategies they use. Schools or other public agencies may be able to help pay for these programs if there are costs.

Medications
What Medicines Are Used to Treat ASD Symptoms?

- Antipsychotics
  - Risperidone (brand name: Risperdal®)
  - Aripiprazole (brand name: Abilify®)
- Serotonin-reuptake inhibitors or "SRIs" (antidepressants)
  - Examples include Prozac®, Sarafem®, Celexa ®, and Cipramil®
- Stimulants and other hyperactivity medicines
  - Examples include Ritalin®, Adderall®, and Tenex®
- Secretin. This medicine is used for digestion problems but some researchers thought it might help children with ASD symptoms as well.
- Chelation. This therapy uses substances to remove heavy metals from the body, which some people think causes autism.

Do They Help?

- Research found that two antipsychotic drugs—risperidone (Risperdal®) and aripiprazole (Abilify®)—can help reduce emotional distress, aggression, hyperactivity, and self-injury. Many people who take risperidone and aripiprazole report side effects such as weight gain, sleepiness, tremors, and abnormal movements. Because of these side effects, these medicines may be best only for children who have more severe symptoms or have symptoms that might increase their risk of hurting themselves.
- SRIs and a hyperactivity medicine called methylphenidate (Ritalin®) have not been studied enough to know if they help treat ASD symptoms.
- Research showed that secretin is not effective in improving autistic symptoms.

- According to the U.S. Food and Drug Administration (FDA), there are serious safety issues associated with chelation products. Even when used under the care of a doctor, these products can cause serious harm, including dehydration, kidney failure, and death. Research does not support the use of chelation for ASD.

What Are the Costs?

The cost to you for each type of medicine will depend on your health insurance, the amount (dose) your child needs to take, and whether a generic form of the medicine is available.

Other Treatments and Therapies

You may have heard or read of other types of treatments or therapies that have been used for children with ASD, such as:

- Speech and language therapy
- Music therapy
- Occupational therapy
- Acupuncture
- Vitamins and mineral supplements
- Massage therapy
- The Picture Exchange Communication System (PECS)
- Responsive Prelinguistic Milieu Teaching (PMT)
- Neurofeedback
- Sleep education and training

Do They Help?

These other therapies have not been studied enough to know if they help or have any side effects. This does not mean that they do not work or are not safe. It just means that researchers do not have enough information to know for sure.

What Else Should I Think About?

Because little is known about how well these treatments or therapies work, talking about them with your doctor, other healthcare or education professionals, your family, and other people that you trust may help you decide whether to try them.

Why Is There so Little Known about ASD and These Treatments?

The research reviewed for this guide showed that some treatments can make specific improvements in the way a child thinks or acts. But researchers do not have enough information to know whether one type of treatment works better than any other. For most treatments, researchers also do not know which treatments will work best for specific children. For example, research does not show whether a program usually works best for older or younger children, or for children with severe or less severe ASD.

This does not mean that a treatment, therapy, or program will not be helpful for your child. It only means that researchers do not have enough information to say so with strong confidence.

Researchers are still studying these treatments and therapies. Check with your doctor or a support group to find out about new research on the programs and treatments in this chapter and about new options.

Making a Decision

There are many things for you to consider when choosing therapies or programs for your child. There are many people you should talk to, including your doctor, social worker, school administrator, and health insurance representative. Here are some questions to ask:

What Plan Is Best for My Child?

- Do you think an early intensive intervention would help my child?

- What other types of programs might be helpful?

- Do you think my child would benefit from taking medicine?

What Is Available in My Community?

- Are there any early intensive intervention programs in this community?

- Do the schools in this district have programs for children with ASD?

- What support groups are available?

What Are the Costs?

- How much will it cost for us to participate in these programs?
- Is help available from the schools or other public agencies?
- Does my health insurance plan cover any costs?

What Changes to Our Work Schedules and Life Will We Need to Make?

- How much time does each option take?
- What are the ways that other families have fit these programs into their lives?
- What else can we do to help our child?

Which Medicine, If Any, Is Best for My Child?

- What symptoms will the medicines help?
- How soon should I see changes in my child's symptoms?
- What are the warning signs that my child may be having a harmful side effect?
- What else is available if my child needs different medicine?

Chapter 33

Treatments for Autism Spectrum Disorder

There is currently no one standard treatment for autism spectrum disorder (ASD). But there are many ways to help minimize the symptoms and maximize abilities. People who have ASD have the best chance of using all of their abilities and skills if they receive appropriate therapies and interventions. The most effective therapies and interventions are often different for each person. However, most people with ASD respond best to highly structured and specialized programs. In some cases, treatment can help people with autism to function at near-normal levels.

Research shows that early diagnosis and interventions, such as during preschool or before, are more likely to have major positive effects on symptoms and later skills.

Because there can be overlap in symptoms between ASD and other disorders, such as attention deficit hyperactivity disorder (ADHD), it's important that treatment focus on a person's specific needs, rather than the diagnostic label.

Behavioral Management Therapy for Autism

Behavior management therapy tries to reinforce wanted behaviors and reduce unwanted behaviors. It also suggests what caregivers can do before, during, after, and between episodes of problem behaviors.

This chapter includes text excerpted from "What Are the Treatments for Autism?" *Eunice Kennedy Shriver* National Institute of Child Health and Human Development (NICHD), January 31, 2017.

Behavioral therapy is often based on applied behavior analysis (ABA), a widely accepted approach that tracks a child's progress in improving his or her skills.

Different types of ABA commonly used to treat autism spectrum disorder (ASD) include:

- **Positive Behavioral and Support (PBS).** PBS aims to figure out why a child does a particular problem behavior. It works to change the environment, teach skills, and make other changes that make a correct behavior more positive for the child. This encourages the child to behave in a less problematic manner.

- **Pivotal Response Training (PRT).** PRT takes place in the child's everyday environment. Its goal is to improve a few "pivotal" skills, such as motivation and taking initiative to communicate. These help the child to learn many other skills and deal with many situations.

- **Early Intensive Behavioral Intervention (EIBI).** EIBI provides individualized behavioral instruction to very young children with ASD. It requires a large time commitment and provides one-on-one or small-group instruction.

- **Discrete Trial Teaching (DTT).** DTT teaches skills in a controlled, step-by-step way. The teacher uses positive feedback to encourage the child to use new skills.

Keep in mind that other behavioral therapies, beyond ABA, may also be effective for people with ASD. Talk to your healthcare provider about the best options for your child.

Cognitive Behavior Therapy for Autism

Cognitive behavior therapy (CBT) focuses on the connection between thoughts, feelings, and behaviors.

Together, the therapist, the person with autism spectrum disorder (ASD), and/or the parents come up with specific goals for the course of therapy. Throughout the sessions, the person with autism learns to identify and change thoughts that lead to problem feelings or behaviors in particular situations.

Cognitive behavior therapy is structured into specific phases of treatment. However, it is also individualized to patients' strengths and weaknesses. Research shows that this therapy helps people with some types of ASD deal with anxiety. It can also help some people with autism cope with social situations and better recognize emotions.

Educational and School-Based Therapies for Autism

Children with autism are guaranteed free, appropriate public education under the federal laws of Public Law 108-177: Individuals with Disabilities Education Improvement Act (2004), sometimes called "IDEA."

IDEA ensures that children diagnosed with certain disabilities or conditions, including autism spectrum disorder (ASD), get free educational services and educational devices to help them to learn as much as they can.

Eunice Kennedy Shriver National Institute of Child Health and Human Development (NICHD)-funded researchers have also incorporated communications interventions for children with ASD within the classroom setting, with successful outcomes. Although the specific interventions used in the study are not a guaranteed part of IDEA, components from the program could provide an important evidence-based foundation for future school-based therapies.

IDEA Covers Children and Young Adults

In most states, each child is entitled to these services from age 3 years through high school, or until age 21, whichever comes first. Some states now offer these types of services beyond age 21. You can find the specific rules of IDEA for each state at the National Early Childhood Technical Assistance Center (NECTAC) website (ectacenter.org/sec619/stateregs.asp).

Educational Environment

IDEA states that children must be taught in the "least restrictive environment, appropriate for that individual child." This means the teaching environment should:

- Be designed to meet a child's specific needs and skills
- Minimize restrictions on the child's access to typical learning experiences and interactions

Educating people with autism often includes a combination of one-on-one, small group, and regular classroom instruction.

Individualized Education Program

The special education team in your child's school will work with you to design an individualized education program (IEP) for your child. An IEP is a written document that:

- Lists individualized goals for your child

- Specifies the plan for services your child will receive

- Lists the developmental specialists who will work with your child

Qualifying for Special Education

To qualify for access to special-education services, the child must be evaluated by the school system and meet specific criteria as outlined by federal and state guidelines. To learn how to have your child assessed for special services, you can:

- Contact a local school principal or special-education coordinator

- Visit the Center for Parent Information and Resources (CPIR) (www.parentcenterhub.org)

Consult a parents' organization to get information on therapeutic and educational services and how to get these services for a child.

Joint Attention Therapy for Autism

Research shows that many people with autism have difficulty with joint attention, which is the ability to share focus on an object or area with another person. Examples of joint attention skills include following someone else's gaze or pointed finger to look at something.

Joint attention is important to communication and language learning. Joint attention therapy focuses on improving specific skills related to shared attention, such as:

- Pointing

- Showing

- Coordinating looks between a person and an object

Improvements from such treatments can last for years.

Medication Treatment for Autism

There is no medication that can cure autism spectrum disorder (ASD) or all of its symptoms. But some medications can help treat certain symptoms associated with ASD, especially certain behaviors.

The NICHD does not endorse or support the use of any medications not approved by the U.S. Food and Drug Administration (FDA) for treating symptoms of autism or other conditions.

Healthcare providers often use medications to deal with a specific behavior, such as to reduce self-injury or aggression. Minimizing a symptom so that it is no longer a problem allows the person with autism to focus on other things, including learning and communication. Research shows that medication is most effective when used in combination with behavioral therapies.

In 2006, the FDA approved the drug risperidone for treating irritability in children with autism who are between 5 years and 16 years of age. Risperidone is the only FDA-approved drug for the treatment of specific autism symptoms.

Other drugs are often used to help improve symptoms of autism, but they are not approved by the FDA for this specific purpose. Some medications on this list are not approved for those younger than 18 years of age. Please consult with the FDA for complete information on the medications listed below.

All medications carry risks, some of them serious. Families should work closely with their children's healthcare providers to ensure safe use of any medication.

- **Selective serotonin reuptake inhibitors (SSRIs)**

  - This group of antidepressants treats some problems that result from imbalances in the body's chemical systems.

  - SSRIs might reduce the frequency and intensity of repetitive behaviors; decrease anxiety, irritability, tantrums, and aggressive behavior; and improve eye contact.

- **Tricyclics**

  - These medications are another type of antidepressant used to treat depression and obsessive-compulsive behaviors.

  - These drugs seem to cause more minor side effects than do SSRIs. They are sometimes more effective than SSRIs for treating certain people and certain symptoms.

- **Psychoactive or antipsychotic medications**

  - These types of medications affect the brain of the person taking them. The antipsychotic drug risperidone is approved for reducing irritability in 5-to-16-year-olds with autism.

- These medications can decrease hyperactivity, reduce stereotyped behaviors, and minimize withdrawal and aggression among people with autism.

- **Stimulants**
  - This group of medications can help to increase focus and decrease hyperactivity in people with autism. They are particularly helpful for those with mild ASD symptoms.

- **Antianxiety medications**
  - This group of medications can help relieve anxiety and panic disorders, which are often associated with ASD.

- **Anticonvulsants**

  - These medications treat seizures and seizure disorders, such as epilepsy. (Seizures are attacks of jerking or staring and seeming frozen.)

  - Almost one-third of people with autism symptoms have seizures or seizure disorders.

  - Autism Speaks, one of the leading autism science and family-support organizations in the United States, offers a tool to help parents and caregivers make informed decisions about medication.

Creating a Medication Plan

Healthcare providers usually prescribe a medication on a trial basis to see if it helps. Some medications may make symptoms worse at first or take several weeks to work. Your child's healthcare provider may have to try different dosages or different combinations of medications to find the most effective plan.

Families, caregivers, and healthcare providers need to work together to make sure that the medication plan is safe and that all medications have some benefit.

Nutritional Therapy for Autism

For a variety of reasons, children with ASD may not get the nutrition they need for healthy growth and development. Some children with autism will only eat certain foods because of how the foods feel in their mouths. Other times, they might avoid eating foods because they associate them with stomach pain or discomfort. Some children are put on limited diets in hopes of reducing autism symptoms.

It is important that parents and caregivers work with a nutrition specialist—such as a registered dietitian—or healthcare provider to design a meal plan for a person with autism, especially if they want to try a limited diet. Such providers can help to make sure the child is still getting all the nutrients she or he needs to grow into a healthy adult, even while on the special diet.

For example, many children with ASD are on gluten-free or casein-free diets. (Gluten and casein are types of proteins found in wheat and milk products, respectively.) Available research data do not support the use of a casein-free diet, a gluten-free diet, or a combined gluten-free, casein-free diet as a primary treatment for individuals with ASD.

Good Nutrition Is Important

Research shows that children with autism tend to have thinner bones than children without autism. Restricting access to bone-building foods, such as dairy products, can make it even harder for their bones to grow strong. Working with a healthcare provider can help ensure that children who are on special diets still get the bone-building and other nutrients they need.

Digestive Problems in Autism Spectrum Disorder

Some people with autism also have digestive problems, such as constipation, abdominal (belly) pain, or vomiting. Some research suggests that digestive problems occur more often in people with autism than in people without autism, but research is still being done on this topic. Working with a healthcare provider can help ensure that a diet does not make digestive problems worse.

Occupational Therapy for Autism

Occupational therapy helps people with ASD do everyday tasks by finding ways to work within and make the most of their needs, abilities, and interests.

An occupational therapist might:

- Find a specially designed computer mouse and keyboard to ease communication

- Teach personal care skills such as getting dressed and eating

- Do many of the same types of activities that physical therapists do

The American Occupational Therapy Association (AOTA) offers several resources related to occupational therapy and autism.

Parent-Mediated Therapy in Autism

In parent-mediated therapy, parents learn therapy techniques from professionals and provide specific therapies to their own child. This approach gives children with ASD consistent reinforcement and training throughout the day. Parents can also conduct some therapies with children who are at risk of autism but are too young to be diagnosed.

Several types of therapies can be parent-mediated activities, including:

- Joint attention therapy

- Social communication therapy

- Behavioral therapy

Studies suggest that parent-mediated therapies might be able to improve the child's communication skills and interactions with others. Researchers are still collecting evidence on parent-mediated therapies.

Physical Therapy for Autism

Physical therapy includes activities and exercises that build motor skills and improve strength, posture, and balance. For example, this type of therapy aims to help a child build muscle control and strength so that she or he can play more easily with other children.

Problems with movement are common in ASD, and many children with autism receive physical therapy. However, there is not yet solid evidence that particular therapies can improve movement skills in those with autism.

Social Skills Training for Autism

Social skills training teaches children the skills they need to interact with others. It includes repeating and reinforcing certain desired behaviors.

The Children's Friendship Training (CFT) intervention, for instance, helps elementary school-age children improve several social skills:

- Conversation

- Handling teasing

- Being a good sport

- Showing good host behavior during playdates

Speech-Language Therapy for Autism

Speech-language therapy can help people with ASD improve their abilities to communicate and interact with others.

Verbal Skills

This type of therapy can help some people improve their spoken or verbal skills, such as:

- Correctly naming people and things

- Better explaining feelings and emotions

- Using words and sentences better

- Improving the rate and rhythm of speech

Nonverbal Communication

Speech-language therapy can also teach nonverbal communication skills, such as:

- Using hand signals or sign language

- Using picture symbols to communicate (Picture Exchange Communication System (PECS))

Speech-language therapy activities can also include social skills and normal social behaviors. For example, a child might learn how to make eye contact or stand at a comfortable distance from another person. These skills make it a little easier to interact with others.

If you have a question about treatment, talk to a healthcare provider who specializes in caring for people with ASD.

Chapter 34

Communication Therapies for Autism Spectrum Disorder

Chapter Contents

Section 34.1

Language Instruction for Children with Autism: Learning Words

This section includes text excerpted from "Language and Speech Disorders," Centers for Disease Control and Prevention (CDC), May 23, 2018.

Children are born ready to learn a language, but they need to learn the language or languages that their family and environment use. Learning a language takes time, and children vary in how quickly they master milestones in language and speech development. Typically developing children may have trouble with some sounds, words, and sentences while they are learning. However, most children can use language easily around five years of age.

Helping Children Learn Language

Parents and caregivers are the most important teachers during a child's early years. Children learn language by listening to others speak and by practicing. Even young babies notice when others repeat and respond to the noises and sounds they make. Children's language and brain skills get stronger if they hear many different words. Parents can help their child learn in many different ways, such as:

- Responding to the first sounds, gurgles, and gestures a baby makes

- Repeating what the child says and adding to it

- Talking about the things that a child sees

- Asking questions and listening to the answers

- Looking at or reading books

- Telling stories

- Singing songs and sharing rhymes

This can happen both during playtime and during daily routines. Parents can also observe the following:

- How their child hears and talks and compare it with typical milestones for communication skills

- How their child reacts to sounds and have their hearing tested if they have concerns

What to Do If There Are Concerns

Some children struggle with understanding and speaking and they need help. They may not master the language milestones at the same time as other children, and it may be a sign of a language or speech delay or disorder.

Language development has different parts, and children might have problems with one or more of the following:

- Understanding what others say (receptive language). This could be due to:

  - Not hearing the words (hearing loss)

  - Not understanding the meaning of the words

- Communicating thoughts using language (expressive language). This could be due to:

  - Not knowing the words to use

  - Not knowing how to put words together

  - Knowing the words to use but not being able to express them

Language and speech disorders can exist together or by themselves. Examples of problems with language and speech development include the following:

- Speech disorders

  - Difficulty with forming specific words or sounds correctly

  - Difficulty with making words or sentences flow smoothly, like stuttering or stammering

- Language delay—the ability to understand and speak develops more slowly than is typical

- Language disorders

  - Aphasia (difficulty understanding or speaking parts of language due to a brain injury or how the brain works)

  - Auditory processing disorder (APD) (difficulty understanding the meaning of the sounds that the ear sends to the brain)

Language or speech disorders can occur with other learning disorders that affect reading and writing. Children with language disorders may feel frustrated that they cannot understand others or make themselves understood, and they may act out, act helpless, or withdraw. Language or speech disorders can also be present with emotional or behavioral disorders, such as attention deficit hyperactivity disorder (ADHD) or anxiety. Children with developmental disabilities including autism spectrum disorder may also have difficulties with speech and language. The combination of challenges can make it particularly hard for a child to succeed in school. Properly diagnosing a child's disorder is crucial so that each child can get the right kind of help.

Detecting Problems with Language or Speech

If a child has a problem with language or speech development, talk to a healthcare provider about an evaluation. An important first step is to find out if the child may have a hearing loss. Hearing loss may be difficult to notice particularly if a child has hearing loss only in one ear or has partial hearing loss, which means they can hear some sounds but not others.

A language development specialist such as a speech-language pathologist (SLP) will conduct a careful assessment to determine what type of problem with language or speech the child may have.

Overall, learning more than one language does not cause language disorders, but children may not follow exactly the same developmental milestones as those who learn only one language. Developing the ability to understand and speak in two languages depends on how much practice the child has using both languages, and the kind of practice. If a child who is learning more than one language has difficulty with language development, careful assessment by a specialist who understands development of skills in more than one language may be needed.

Treatment for Language or Speech Disorders and Delays

Children with language problems often need extra help and special instruction. Speech-language pathologists can work directly with children and their parents, caregivers, and teachers.

Having a language or speech delay or disorder can qualify a child for early intervention (for children up to three years of age) and special education services (for children aged three years and older). Schools can do their own testing for language or speech disorders to see if a child needs intervention. An evaluation by a healthcare professional is needed if there are other concerns about the child's hearing, behavior, or emotions. Parents, healthcare providers, and the school can work together to find the right referrals and treatment.

What Every Parent Should Know

Children with specific learning disabilities, including language or speech disorders, are eligible for special education services or accommodations at school under the Individuals with Disabilities in Education Act (IDEA) and Section 504, an antidiscrimination law.

The Role of Healthcare Providers

Healthcare providers can play an important part in collaborating with schools to help a child with speech or language disorders and delay or other disabilities get the special services they need. The American Academy of Pediatrics (AAP) has created a report that describes the roles that healthcare providers can have in helping children with disabilities, including language or speech disorders.

Section 34.2

Augmentative and Alternative Communication

"Augmentative and Alternative Communication," © 2019 Omnigraphics. Reviewed October 2018.

A specialized area of assistive technology called "augmentative and alternative communication" (AAC) aids adults and children whose communications are limited by language and speech barriers. AAC allows people to express their ideas, hopes, and needs and to connect with family and friends, access education, and better understand what is happening around them. AAC provides promising new methods through which people can communicate without speaking. People whose communications are limited by language and speech barriers are now able to use AAC as a part of their daily lives.

Importance of Augmentative and Alternative Communication

ACC is important because it provides new and enhanced means of meaningful communicative expression. Person who struggle to speak can now use different forms of AAC instead. The communication can be through actions, gestures, or written communication. AAC has gone through several stages of developmental, the latest being technological methods of communication that have benefited this population greatly.

Types of Augmentative and Alternative Communication

The two main types of AAC are:

1. Unaided system

2. Aided system

Unaided Augmentative and Alternative Communication System

This form of AAC relies on body language rather than assistive devices for communication purposes. People using the unaided AAC system strategically uses their own bodies as a means of communication, and employ sign language, eye contact, facial expression, and body gestures to convey meaning and information. Some forms of unaided system include:

- Touch cues include body contact that allows a caregiver or other person to understand what the other speechless person is trying to communicate.

- Key word signing includes hand signs and gestures that help caregivers and others understand what a hearing speechless person is trying to communicate.

- Body signs convey information primarily to people who are blind or visually impaired and allow this population to better understand what is happening around them.

Aided Augmentative and Alternative Communication System

This AAC system uses assistive devices or external aids to help people with limited or no speech to communicate. There are two basic types of aided systems:

- **Basic/Low Technology:** This system uses basic tools such as a pen and paper, pointing to pictures or words, drawing, communication boards, visual strategies, access boards, and many others.

- **High Technology:** The high-end technology used in this system includes such things such as speech-generating devices (SGD), voice amplifiers, communication apps and software, and touching pictures or words on a computer screen that then voices out the content based on the high-end aided system.

Working with Your Healthcare Provider

A speech-language pathologist (SLP) will help a person with limited or no speech or language identify the kind of AAC system that best suits their needs. Some people will need an AAC for only a short period of time—people who are recovering from a stroke or mouth surgery, for example—while others may rely on them for extended periods of time. Healthcare providers recognize that not every AAC device or method will work for everybody, and work with individuals to identify the right AAC device or form of AAC for them.

What to Consider When Identifying an AAC

Some of the key things to watch out while exploring an AAC include:

- **Cost:** Buying any high-end equipment is expensive, and the cost needs to be calculated and understood before any purchase is made. This cost should include ongoing maintenance and repair charges as well as associated replacement costs. Funding for high-end AAC equipment is sometimes available.

- **Consultation with a speech pathologist:** It is vital that people consult with a speech pathologist before purchasing any kind of specialized equipment. A speech pathologist has specialized knowledge and will be able to assist the person in both identifying the right device for them and in learning how to use the device.

Other things to consider include training and support from suppliers, wear and tear on equipment, and how to optimally operate the equipment.

References

1. "What Is 'Augmentative and Alternative Communication?'" Novita Tech, May 24, 2018.

2. "Augmentative and Alternative Communication (AAC)," American Speech Language Hearing Association (ASHA), November 13, 2017.

3. "Augmentative and Alternative Communication (AAC)," Acquired Brain Injury Outreach Service (ABIOS), August 2017.

4. "Augmentative and Alternative Communication (AAC)," Department of Human Services, Government of South Australia, September 2018.

Section 34.3

Assistive Devices for People with Hearing, Voice, Speech, or Language Disorders

This section includes text excerpted from "Assistive Devices for People with Hearing, Voice, Speech, or Language Disorders," National Institute on Deafness and Other Communication Disorders (NIDCD), March 6, 2017.

What Are Assistive Devices?

The terms "assistive device" or "assistive technology" can refer to any device that helps a person with hearing loss or a voice, speech, or language disorder to communicate. These terms often refer to devices that help a person to hear and understand what is being said more clearly or to express thoughts more easily. With the development of digital and wireless technologies, more and more devices are becoming available to help people with hearing, voice, speech, and language disorders communicate more meaningfully and participate more fully in their daily lives.

What Types of Assistive Devices Are Available?

Health professionals use a variety of names to describe assistive devices:

- Assistive listening devices (ALDs) help amplify the sounds you want to hear, especially where there's a lot of background noise. ALDs can be used with a hearing aid or cochlear implant to help a wearer hear certain sounds better.

- Augmentative and alternative communication (AAC) devices help people with communication disorders to express themselves. These devices can range from a simple picture board to a computer program that synthesizes speech from text.

- Alerting devices connect to a doorbell, telephone, or alarm that emits a loud sound or blinking light to let someone with hearing loss know that an event is taking place.

What Types of Assistive Listening Devices Are Available?

Several types of ALDs are available to improve sound transmission for people with hearing loss. Some are designed for large facilities such as classrooms, theaters, places of worship, and airports. Other types are intended for personal use in small settings and for one-on-one conversations. All can be used with or without hearing aids or a cochlear implant. ALD systems for large facilities include hearing loop systems, frequency-modulated (FM) systems, and infrared systems.

Hearing loop (or induction loop) systems use electromagnetic energy to transmit sound. A hearing loop system involves four parts:

1. A sound source, such as a public address system, microphone, or home television (TV) or telephone

2. An amplifier

3. A thin loop of wire that encircles a room or branches out beneath carpeting

4. A receiver worn in the ears or as a headset

Amplified sound travels through the loop and creates an electro-magnetic field that is picked up directly by a hearing loop receiver or a telecoil, a miniature wireless receiver that is built into many hearing aids and cochlear implants. To pick up the signal, a listener must be wearing the receiver and be within or near the loop. Because the sound is picked up directly by the receiver, the sound is much clearer, without as much of the competing background noise associated with many listening environments. Some loop systems are portable, making it possible for people with hearing loss to improve their listening environments, as needed, as they proceed with their daily activities. A hearing loop can be connected to a public address system, a television, or any other audio source. For those who don't have hearing aids with embedded telecoils, portable loop receivers are also available.

FM systems use radio signals to transmit amplified sounds. They are often used in classrooms, where the instructor wears a small microphone connected to a transmitter and the student wears the receiver, which is tuned to a specific frequency, or channel. People who have a telecoil inside their hearing aid or cochlear implant may also wear a wire around the neck (called a neckloop) or behind their aid or implant (called a silhouette inductor) to convert the signal into magnetic signals that can be picked up directly by the telecoil. FM systems can transmit signals up to 300 feet and are able to be used in many public places. However, because radio signals are able to penetrate walls, listeners in one room may need to listen to a different channel than those in another room to avoid receiving mixed signals. Personal FM systems operate in the same way as larger-scale systems and can be used to help people with hearing loss to follow one-on-one conversations.

Infrared systems use infrared light to transmit sound. A transmitter converts sound into a light signal and beams it to a receiver that is worn by a listener. The receiver decodes the infrared signal back to sound. As with FM systems, people whose hearing aids or cochlear implants have a telecoil may also wear a neckloop or silhouette inductor to convert the infrared signal into a magnetic signal, which can be picked up through their telecoil. Unlike induction loop or FM systems, the infrared signal cannot pass through walls, making it particularly useful in courtrooms, where confidential information is often discussed, and in buildings where competing signals can be a problem, such as classrooms or movie theaters. However, infrared systems cannot be used in environments with too many competing light sources, such as outdoors or in strongly lit rooms.

Personal amplifiers are useful in places in which the above systems are unavailable or when watching TV, being outdoors, or traveling in a car. About the size of a cell phone, these devices increase sound levels and reduce background noise for a listener. Some have directional microphones that can be angled toward a speaker or other source of sound. As with other ALDs, the amplified sound can be picked up by a receiver that the listener is wearing, either as a head-set or as earbuds.

What Types of Augmentative and Alternative Communication Devices Are Available for Communicating Face-to-Face?

The simplest AAC device is a picture board or touch screen that uses pictures or symbols of typical items and activities that make up a person's daily life. For example, a person might touch the image of a glass to ask for a drink. Many picture boards can be customized and expanded based on a person's age, education, occupation, and interests.

Keyboards, touch screens, and sometimes a person's limited speech may be used to communicate desired words. Some devices employ a text display. The display panel typically faces outward so that two people can exchange information while facing each other. Spelling and word prediction software can make it faster and easier to enter information.

Speech-generating devices go one step further by translating words or pictures into speech. Some models allow users to choose from several different voices, such as male or female, child or adult, and even some regional accents. Some devices employ a vocabulary of prerecorded words while others have an unlimited vocabulary, synthesizing speech as words are typed in. Software programs that convert personal computers into speaking devices are also available.

What Augmentative and Alternative Communication Devices Are Available for Communicating by Telephone?

For many years, people with hearing loss have used text telephone or telecommunications devices, called TTY or TDD machines, to communicate by phone. This same technology also benefits people with speech difficulties. A TTY machine consists of a typewriter keyboard that displays typed conversations onto a readout panel or printed on paper. Callers will either type messages to each other over the system or, if a call recipient does not have a TTY machine, use the national toll-free telecommunications relay service at 711 to communicate. Through the relay service, a communications assistant serves as a bridge between two callers, reading typed messages aloud to the person with hearing while transcribing what's spoken into type for the person with hearing loss.

With today's new electronic communication devices, however, TTY machines have almost become a thing of the past. People can place phone calls through the telecommunications relay service using almost any device with a keypad, including a laptop, personal digital assistant, and cell phone. Text messaging has also become a popular method of communication, skipping the relay service altogether.

Another system uses voice recognition software and an extensive library of video clips depicting American Sign Language (ASL) to translate a signer's words into text or computer-generated speech in real time. It is also able to translate spoken words back into sign language or text.

Finally, for people with mild to moderate hearing loss, captioned telephones allow you to carry on a spoken conversation, while providing a transcript of the other person's words on a readout panel or computer screen as backup.

What Types of Alerting Devices Are Available?

Alerting or alarm devices use sound, light, vibrations, or a combination of these techniques to let someone know when a particular event is occurring. Clocks and wake-up alarm systems allow a person to choose to wake up to flashing lights, horns, or a gentle shaking.

Visual alert signalers monitor a variety of household devices and other sounds, such as doorbells and telephones. When the phone rings, the visual alert signaler will be activated and will vibrate or flash a light to let people know. In addition, remote receivers placed around the house can alert a person from any room. Portable vibrating pagers can let parents and caretakers know when a baby is crying. Some baby-monitoring devices analyze a baby's cry and light up a picture to indicate if the baby sounds hungry, bored, or sleepy.

What Research Is Being Conducted on Assistive Technology?

The National Institute on Deafness and Other Communication Disorders (NIDCD) funds research into several areas of assistive technology, such as those described below.

- Improved devices for people with hearing loss

NIDCD-funded researchers are developing devices that help people with varying degrees of hearing loss communicate with others. One team has developed a portable device in which two or more users type messages to each other that can be displayed simultaneously in real time. Another team is designing an ALD that amplifies and enhances speech for a group of individuals who are conversing in a noisy environment.

- Improved devices for nonspeaking people

- More natural synthesized speech
  NIDCD-sponsored scientists are also developing a personalized text-to-speech synthesis system that synthesizes speech that is more intelligible and natural sounding to be incorporated in speech-generating devices. Individuals who are at risk of losing their speaking ability can prerecord their own speech, which is then converted into their personal synthetic voice.

- Brain–computer interface research
  A relatively new and exciting area of study is called brain–computer interface research. NIDCD-funded scientists are studying how neural signals in a person's brain can be translated by a computer to help someone communicate. For example, people with amyotrophic lateral sclerosis (ALS, or Lou Gehrig disease) or brainstem stroke lose their ability to move their arms, legs, or body. They can also become locked-in, where they are not able to express words, even though they are able to think and reason normally. By implanting electrodes on the brain's motor cortex, some researchers are studying how a person who is locked-in can control communication software and type out words simply by imagining the movement of his or her hand. Other researchers are attempting to develop a prosthetic device that will be able to translate a person's thoughts into synthesized words and sentences. Another group is developing a wireless device that monitors brain activity that is triggered by visual stimulation. In this way, people who are locked-in can call for help during an emergency by staring at a designated spot on the device.

Chapter 35

Therapists for Autism Spectrum Disorder

Chapter Contents

Section 35.1

Speech-Language Pathologists

This section includes text excerpted from "Speech-Language Pathologists," U.S. Bureau of Labor Statistics (BLS), U.S. Department of Labor (DOL), July 2, 2018.

Speech-language pathologists (SLPs) (sometimes called speech therapists) assess, diagnose, treat, and help to prevent communication and swallowing disorders in children and adults. Speech, language, and swallowing disorders result from a variety of causes, such as a stroke, brain injury, hearing loss, developmental delay, Parkinson disease (PD), a cleft palate, or autism.

Duties

SLPs typically do the following:

- Evaluate levels of speech, language, or swallowing difficulty
- Identify treatment options
- Create and carry out an individualized treatment plan that addresses specific functional needs
- Teach children and adults how to make sounds and improve their voices and maintain fluency
- Help individuals improve vocabulary and sentence structure used in oral and written language
- Work with children and adults to develop and strengthen the muscles used to swallow
- Counsel individuals and families on how to cope with communication and swallowing disorders

SLPs work with children and adults who have problems with speech and language, including related cognitive or social communication problems. They may be unable to speak at all, or they may speak with difficulty or have rhythm and fluency problems, such as stuttering. SLPs may work with people who are unable to understand language or with those who have voice disorders, such as inappropriate pitch or a harsh voice.

SLPs also must complete administrative tasks, including keeping accurate records and documenting billing information. They record their initial evaluations and diagnoses, track treatment progress, and note any changes in an individual's condition or treatment plan.

Some SLPs specialize in working with specific age groups, such as children or the elderly. Others focus on treatment programs for specific communication or swallowing problems, such as those resulting from strokes, trauma, or a cleft palate.

In medical facilities, speech-language pathologists work with physicians and surgeons, social workers, psychologists, occupational therapists, physical therapists, and other healthcare workers. In schools, they evaluate students for speech and language disorders and work with teachers, other school personnel, and parents to develop and carry out individual or group programs, provide counseling, and support classroom activities.

Section 35.2

Occupational Therapists

This section contains text excerpted from the following sources: Text in the section begins with excerpts from "Occupational Therapists," U.S. Bureau of Labor Statistics (BLS), U.S. Department of Labor (DOL), April 13, 2018; Text under the heading "Occupational Therapy Assistant Duties" is excerpted from "Occupational Therapy Assistants and Aides," U.S. Bureau of Labor Statistics (BLS), U.S. Department of Labor (DOL), April 13, 2018.

Occupational therapists treat injured, ill, or disabled patients through the therapeutic use of everyday activities. They help these patients develop, recover, improve, and maintain the skills needed for daily living and working.

Occupational Therapists Duties

Occupational therapists typically do the following:

- Review patients' medical history, ask the patients questions, and observe them doing tasks
- Evaluate a patient's condition and needs

- Develop a treatment plan for patients, identifying specific goals and the types of activities that will be used to help the patient work toward those goals

- Help people with various disabilities perform different tasks, such as teaching a stroke victim how to get dressed

- Demonstrate exercises—for example, stretching the joints for arthritis relief—that can help relieve pain in people with chronic conditions

- Evaluate a patient's home or workplace and, on the basis of the patient's health needs, identify potential improvements, such as labeling kitchen cabinets for an older person with poor memory

- Educate a patient's family and employer about how to accommodate and care for the patient

- Recommend special equipment, such as wheelchairs and eating aids, and instruct patients on how to use that equipment

- Assess and record patients' activities and progress for patient evaluations, billing, and reporting to physicians and other healthcare providers

Patients with permanent disabilities, such as cerebral palsy (CP), often need help performing daily tasks. Therapists show patients how to use appropriate adaptive equipment, such as leg braces, wheelchairs, and eating aids. These devices help patients perform a number of daily tasks, allowing them to function more independently.

Some occupational therapists work with children in educational settings. They evaluate disabled children's abilities, modify classroom equipment to accommodate children with disabilities, and help children participate in school activities. Therapists also may provide early intervention therapy to infants and toddlers who have, or are at risk of having, developmental delays.

Therapists who work with the elderly help their patients lead more independent and active lives. They assess patients' abilities and environment and make recommendations to improve the patients' everyday lives. For example, therapists may identify potential fall hazards in a patient's home and recommend their removal.

In some cases, occupational therapists help patients create functional work environments. They evaluate the workspace, recommend modifications, and meet with the patient's employer to collaborate on changes to the patient's work environment or schedule.

Occupational therapists also may work in mental-health settings, where they help patients who suffer from developmental disabilities, mental illness, or emotional problems. Therapists teach these patients skills such as managing time, budgeting, using public transportation, and doing household chores in order to help them cope with, and engage in, daily life activities. In addition, therapists may work with individuals who have problems with drug abuse, alcoholism, depression, or other disorders. They may also work with people who have been through a traumatic event, such as a car accident.

Some occupational therapists, such as those employed in hospitals, work as part of a healthcare team along with doctors, registered nurses, and other types of therapists. They may work with patients who have chronic conditions, such as diabetes, or help rehabilitate a patient recovering from hip replacement surgery. Occupational therapists also oversee the work of occupational therapy assistants and aides.

Occupational Therapy Assistant Duties

Occupational therapy assistants typically do the following:

- Help patients do therapeutic activities, such as stretches and other exercises

- Lead children who have developmental disabilities in play activities that promote coordination and socialization

- Encourage patients to complete activities and tasks

- Teach patients how to use special equipment—for example, showing a patient with Parkinson disease (PD) how to use devices that make eating easier

- Record patients' progress, report to occupational therapists, and do other administrative tasks

Occupational therapy aides typically do the following:

- Prepare treatment areas, such as setting up therapy equipment

- Transport patients

- Clean treatment areas and equipment

- Help patients with billing and insurance forms

- Perform clerical tasks, including scheduling appointments and answering telephones

Occupational therapy assistants collaborate with occupational therapists to develop and carry out a treatment plan for each patient. Plans include diverse activities such as teaching the proper way for patients to move from a bed into a wheelchair and advising patients on the best way to stretch their muscles. For example, an occupational therapy assistant might work with injured workers to help them get back into the workforce by teaching them how to work around lost motor skills. Occupational therapy assistants also may work with people who have learning disabilities (LD), teaching them skills that allow them to be more independent.

Assistants monitor activities to make sure that patients are doing them correctly. They record the patient's progress and provide feedback to the occupational therapist so that the therapist can change the treatment plan if the patient is not getting the desired results.

Occupational therapy aides typically prepare materials and assemble equipment used during treatment. They may assist patients with moving to and from treatment areas. After a therapy session, aides clean the treatment area, put away equipment, and gather laundry.

Occupational therapy aides fill out insurance forms and other paperwork and are responsible for a range of clerical tasks, such as scheduling appointments, answering the telephone, and monitoring inventory levels.

Chapter 36

Autism Spectrum Disorders Medications

Chapter Contents

Section 36.1

Parent Training Complements Medication for Treating Behavioral Problems in Children with Pervasive Developmental Disorders

This section includes text excerpted from "Parent Training Complements Medication for Treating Behavioral Problems in Children with Pervasive Developmental Disorders," National Institutes of Health (NIH), November 20, 2009. Reviewed October 2018.

Treatment that includes medication plus a structured training program for parents reduces serious behavioral problems in children with autism and related conditions, according to a study funded by the National Institute of Mental Health (NIMH). The study, which was part of the NIMH Research Units on Pediatric Psychopharmacology (RUPP) Autism Network, was published in the December 2009 issue of the *Journal of the American Academy of Child and Adolescent Psychiatry.*

Results from a previous RUPP study reported in 2002 showed that the antipsychotic medication risperidone (Risperdal) reduced such behavior problems as tantrums, aggression, and self-injury in children with autism. However, most children's symptoms returned when the medication was discontinued. Although effective, risperidone is associated with adverse effects such as weight gain, which can lead to metabolic changes, obesity and related health problems.

"Medication alone has been shown to help with some symptoms of autism, but its potential is limited," said NIMH Director Thomas R. Insel. "This study shows promise of a more effective treatment protocol that could improve life for children with autism and their families."

In the study, the RUPP group tested the benefits of medication alone compared to medication plus a parent training program that actively involves parents in managing their children's severely disruptive and noncompliant behavior. Parents were taught to modify their children's behavior and learned to enhance their children's daily living skills.

The 24-week, three-site trial included 124 children ages 4 to 13 with pervasive developmental disorders (PDD) such as autism, Asperger or related disorders accompanied by tantrums, aggression, and self-injury. The children were randomized to a combination of risperidone and parent training, or to risperidone only. Parents in combination therapy received an average of 11 sessions of training over the course of the study.

Although both groups improved over the six-month trial, the group receiving combination therapy showed greater reduction in behavioral problems like irritability, tantrums, and impulsiveness compared to the group receiving medication only. The combination therapy group also ended the trial taking an average dose of 1.98 milligrams (mg) per day of risperidone, compared to 2.26 mg/day in the medication-only group—a 14-percent lower dose. However, children in both groups gained weight, indicating "a need to learn more about the metabolic consequences of medications like risperidone," said the authors.

"The combination group was able to achieve its gains with a lower dose of medication. Plus, it appeared that the benefits of added behavioral treatment increased over time, a strong signal that actively including parents in the treatment of children with PDD could only benefit families, " said lead author Michael Aman, Ph.D., of the Ohio State University.

"Future studies will evaluate whether the benefits of parent training endure over a long period of time, " concluded the authors. The investigators also plan to apply the parent training to younger children with PDD to prevent the evolution of serious behavioral problems. Future studies may also look for ways in which the parent training program can be used in schools and community clinics.

Section 36.2

Citalopram No Better than Placebo Treatment for Children with Autism Spectrum Disorders

This section includes text excerpted from "Citalopram No Better than Placebo Treatment for Children with Autism Spectrum Disorders," National Institutes of Health (NIH), June 1, 2009. Reviewed October 2018.

Citalopram, a medication commonly prescribed to children with autism spectrum disorders (ASDs), was no more effective than a placebo at reducing repetitive behaviors, according to researchers funded by the National Institute of Mental Health (NIMH) and other National Institutes of Health (NIH) institutes. The study was published in the June 2009 issue of *Archives of General Psychiatry*.

"Parents of children with autism spectrum disorders face an enormous number of treatment options, not all of which are research-based," said NIMH Director Thomas R. Insel, M.D. "Studies like this help us to better understand which treatments are likely to be beneficial and safe."

The researchers say their findings do not support using citalopram to treat repetitive behaviors in children with ASD. Also, the greater frequency of side effects from this particular medication compared to placebo illustrates the importance of placebo-controlled trials in evaluating medications prescribed to this population.

Citalopram is in a class of antidepressant medications called selective serotonin reuptake inhibitors (SSRIs) that is sometimes prescribed for children with ASD to reduce repetitive behaviors. These behaviors, a hallmark of ASD, include stereotypical hand flapping, repetitive complex whole body movements (such as spinning, swaying, or rocking over and over, with no clear purpose), repetitive play, and inflexible daily routines.

Past research suggested that some children with ASD have abnormalities in the brain system that makes serotonin, a brain chemical that, among many other functions, plays an important role in early brain development. Children with obsessive-compulsive disorder (OCD) may also have serotonin abnormalities and have repetitive or inflexible behaviors. OCD is effectively treated with SSRIs, leading some researchers to wonder whether similar treatment may reduce repetitive behaviors in children with ASD. So far, studies have produced mixed results, but SSRIs remain among the most frequently prescribed medications for children with ASD.

Researchers in the Studies to Advance Autism Research and Treatment (STAART) network, funded by five NIH institutes, conducted a six-site, randomized controlled trial (RCT) comparing the effectiveness and safety of using the SSRI citalopram (Celexa) versus placebo to treat repetitive behaviors in children with ASD. The study included 149 participants, ages 5 to 17, who had autism, Asperger disorder, or pervasive developmental disorder-not otherwise specified (PDD-NOS).

After 12 weeks of treatment, roughly 1 out of 3 children in both groups—32.9 percent of those treated with citalopram and 34.2 percent those treated with placebo—showed fewer or less severe repetitive symptoms.

"Adverse symptoms were common in both groups, probably reflecting common childhood ailments as well as the changing nature of symptoms associated with ASD," according to Bryan King, M.D., director of child and adolescent psychiatry at Seattle Children's Hospital and lead author on the study. However, reports of increased energy, impulsiveness, decreased concentration, hyperactivity, diarrhea, insomnia, and dry skin were more common in the citalopram group.

According to the researchers, the study results may challenge the underlying premise that repetitive behaviors in children with ASD are similar to repetitive and inflexible behaviors in OCD.

Chapter 37

Web Technology for Behavioral Deficit of Autism

Autism is one of a group of disorders known as autism spectrum disorders (ASDs). It is characterized by developmental disabilities that cause substantial impairments in social interaction and communication and the presence of unusual behaviors and interests. It begins before age three and lasts throughout a person's life. Autism occurs in all racial, ethnic, and socioeconomic groups. It is also on the rise. New research indicates a possible mitigation strategy for autism. Deletions of genes or regions potentially involved in regulation of gene expression, suggests that defects in activity-dependent gene expression may be a cause of cognitive deficits in patients with autism. Therefore, disruption of activity-related synaptic development may be one mechanism common to at least a subset of seemingly heterogeneous autism-associated mutations. If the above hypothesis is true, then controlled environmental experiences coupled with calculated experiential exposure might be able to allow treatment through behavioral modification to facilitate learning in normal environments. But given the characteristics of autistic individuals, controlled environmental experiences are difficult to conduct. Reports from teachers, therapists, researchers, and parents indicate that many children with ASD show an affinity for computers. Research indicates that computer-based

This chapter includes text excerpted from "The Application of Modeling and Simulation to the Behavioral Deficit of Autism," National Aeronautics and Space Administration (NASA), 2010. Reviewed October 2018.

tasks can motivate people with autism and encourage learning. Efforts to incorporate the ability to interact with and control virtual characters (avatars) within a computer-generated environment are increasing. While there is good evidence that virtual environments are well accepted by individuals with ASD and of potential benefit to them, the use of the technology remains relatively unexplored. There is great potential to repurpose technology and simulation content developed for the U.S. military that combines 3-dimensional (3D) video game technology with the constructivist principles of coaching, scaffolding, and deliberate practice to help teach cultural awareness and nonverbal communications skills. This chapter describes a research effort designed to leverage this military technology, repurpose game assets and adapt learning strategies to support virtual social skills training within a computer game environment in an effort to diminish the impact of social impairments on the lives of people diagnosed with ASD. If successful, the potential return on investment is enormous, both in actual cost savings, and reduction of family suffering. Researching this area is an ethical imperative.

Autism

Autism is one of a group of disorders known as autism spectrum disorders (ASDs). They include autistic disorder, pervasive developmental disorder not otherwise specified (PDD-NOS, including atypical autism), and Asperger syndrome (AS). These conditions all have some of the same symptoms, but they differ in terms of when the symptoms start, the severity of the symptoms, and the exact nature of the symptoms. The three conditions, along with Rett syndrome (RTT) and childhood disintegrative disorder (CDD), make up the broad diagnosis category of pervasive developmental disorders (PDDs). ASD begins before the age of three and lasts throughout a person's life. It occurs in all racial, ethnic, and socioeconomic groups and is four times more likely to occur in boys than girls.

The Cost

Dr. Michael Ganz, MS, PhD, Assistant Professor of Society, Human development and Health at the Harvard School of Public Health, and respected expert on the societal costs associated with autism and its related disorders claims that autism is a very expensive disorder costing upwards of $35billion indirect (both medical and nonmedical) and indirect costs to care for all individuals diagnosed each year over their lifetimes. In a paper published in the *Archives of Pediatric Adolescent Medicine*, Dr. Ganz details the substantial costs resulting from lifetime care and lost productivity of individuals with autism, their caretakers and society in general. Direct costs measure the value of goods and services used and indirect costs measure the value of lost productivity due to autism. Physician and other professional services, hospital and emergency department services, drugs, equipment, and other supplies, and medically related travel and time costs are typical components of direct medical costs. Special education, transportation, child care and babysitting, respite care, out-of-home placement, home and vehicle modifications, and supported employment services are typical components of direct nonmedical costs. Indirect costs are the value of lost or impaired work time (income), benefits, and household services of individuals with autism and their caregivers because of missed time at work, reduced work hours, switching to a lower-paying but more flexible job, or leaving the workforce. Behavioral therapies, which are the largest component of direct medical costs, make up 6.5 percent of total discounted lifetime costs. Those costs, combined with very limited to nonexistent income for their adult children with autism combined with potentially lower levels of savings because of decreased income and benefits while employed, may create a large financial burden affecting not only those families but potentially society in general.

Autism Is Increasing

The Center for Disease Control and Prevention (CDC) states that it is clear that more children than ever before are being classified as having ASDs, however, it is unclear how much of this increase is due to changes in how ASDs are identified and classified in people, and how much is due to a true increase in prevalence. By current standards, ASDs are the second most common serious developmental disability after mental retardation/intellectual impairment. The impact of having a developmental disability is great for families affected and for the community services that provide intervention and support for these families. It is important that we treat common developmental disabilities, and especially ASDs, as conditions of urgent public health concern, do all we can to identify children's learning needs, and start intervention as early as possible to give all children the chance to reach their full potential. The CDC also states that ASDs can often be detected as early as 18 months and children in high-risk groups—children with a parent or sibling with an ASD—should be watched particularly closely. Studies have shown that among identical twins, if one child has autism, then the other will be affected about 75 percent of the time. In nonidentical twins, if one child has autism, than the other has it about 3 percent of the time. Also, parents who have a child with an ASD have a 2 to 8 percent chance of having a second child who is also affected.

Research Directions

New research conducted by Eric M. Morrow et al., of the Division of Genetics at Children's Hospital Boston and Harvard Medical School, states that the regulation of expression of some autism candidate genes by neuronal membrane depolarization, suggests the hypotheses that neural activity-dependent regulation of synapse development may be a mechanism common to several autism mutations. Early brain development is driven largely by intrinsic patterns of gene expression that do not depend on experience-driven synaptic activity. Postnatal brain development requires input from the environment that triggers the release of neurotransmitters and promotes critical aspects of synaptic maturation. During this process, neural activity alters the expression of hundreds of genes, each with a defined temporal course that may be particularly vulnerable to gene dosage changes. The connection between experience-dependent neural activity and gene expression in the postnatal period forms the basis of learning and memory, and autism symptoms typically emerge during these later stages of development. This finding that deletions of genes regulated by neuronal activity or regions potentially involved in regulation of gene expression in autism suggests that defects in activity-dependent gene expression may be a cause of cognitive deficits in patients with autism. Therefore, disruption of activity-related synaptic development maybe mechanism common to at least a subset of seemingly heterogeneous autism-associated mutations. If the above hypothesis is true, then controlled environmental experiences coupled with calculated experiential exposure might be able to allow treatment, behavioral modification, and learning to occur in normal environments.

The Use of Computers and Virtual Reality

Reality reports from teachers, therapists, researchers, and parents indicate that many children with ASD show an affinity for computers. Previous research has shown that computer-based tasks can motivate people with autism and encourage learning. The social and communication deficits of ASD make it difficult to engage in social interaction, and therefore, access to learning opportunities in these social settings is limited. Computer-based experiences in constructed social environments mitigate this deficiency. New research efforts incorporate the ability to interact with and/or control virtual characters (avatars) within a virtual environment. The Authorable Virtual Peers (AVP) program at Northwestern University uses language-based avatars to enable children diagnosed with ASD to learn about language and social interactions through collaborative storytelling. The use of avatars has also been found to increase facial recognition, emotion recognition, and social interaction skills for children with ASD through repeated practice of multiple different interactions. This affirms the commonly used approach of repeated practice in a natural setting to successfully teach skills to those with ASD.

- Virtual reality (VR) uses sight and sound more than touch: auditory and visual stimuli have been found to be most effective in teaching abstract concepts to people with autism.

- In the virtual environment, input stimuli can be modified to a tolerable level.

- The environment can be altered gradually to teach generalization and cross-recognition.

- Virtual reality offers a safe learning environment in which the individual may make mistakes that might be physically or socially hazardous in the real world.

A research study on autistic children conducted at the University of Haifa focused on the transfer of skills mastered within a virtual environment to the real world and found that the intelligence level of severity of the autism does not affect the ability to understand the system, and therefore, is an important way to improve their cognitive and social abilities. Six children with autism, ages 7 to 12, spent one month learning how to cross virtual streets, to wait for the virtual light at the crosswalk to change, and to look left and right for virtual cars using a simulation programmed by Yuval Naveh. The children in the study showed substantial improvement throughout the learning process. At the beginning of the study, the average child was able to use the second level of the software; by the end, they mastered the ninth level, which is characterized by more vehicles traveling at a higher speed. A local practice area with street and crosswalk, complete with traffic signals, was used for validation. The children's ability to cross the street safely was tested in this area, evaluating, for example, whether they stopped to wait on the sidewalk or waited for a green light before crossing. The children were brought to the practice area before and after their virtual learning. Here too, the children exhibited an improvement in their skills, following the training on the virtual street, with three of the children showing considerable improvement. One of the study participants, a 16-year old, had participated in the past in a road safety program in the school, but he was not able to learn how to cross the street safely. After learning the skill in a virtual environment, he knew how to stop on the sidewalk before stepping into the street, look at the color of the traffic light, cross only when the light was green, and cross without waiting too long.

Leveraging Current Modeling and Simulation Technology

While there is good evidence that virtual environments are well accepted by individuals with ASD and of potential benefit to them, the use of this technology remains relatively unexplored. New computer-based game technologies increasingly integrate a social as well as a cognitive component. There is potential to leverage this technology in an innovative new direction to provide a context that can scaffold social interactions and communications skills for children with ASD.

The ability to simulate, test, and assess cognitive and social skills within a virtual environment provides professionals with rigorous practice and guidance to increase their chances of success in situations that may not be safe or cost effective to performing a live training environment.

Simulations and games can supplement traditional training methods by providing challenges and experiences that closely approximate a complex situation in the real world, where students must think in real-time and the course of events will be determined by their decisions. Students with ASD may be able to develop a deeper understanding of the knowledge presented and retain that information better when it is learned through the process of repeatedly solving problems in realistic situations. This approach places the learner in a "real-world" environment, which allows the student to learn in context and apply what they have learned. It is this contextual experience of knowledge acquisition in an authentic environment that facilitates the learner to create their own constructs that can be applied to new and unfamiliar situations. There is also an opportunity to provide practical, hands-on experience in situations that cannot easily be practiced using real scenarios. There is also great potential to repurpose technology and simulation content developed for the U.S. military that combines 3D video game technology with the constructivist principles of coaching, scaffolding, and deliberate practice to help teach cultural awareness and nonverbal communications skills. The emerging importance of cultural identity and its inherent frictions make it imperative for soldiers and leaders to understand the societal and cultural norms of the populaces in which they operate and function. Much of this communication occurs through nonverbal channels, especially when language skills are minimal or absent. It is possible to leverage this military technology, repurpose game assets, and adapt learning strategies to support virtual social skills training within a 3D video game in an effort to diminish the impact of social impairments on the lives of people diagnosed with ASD.

Specific Application Strategies

The symptoms and characteristics of autism can present themselves in a wide variety of combinations. The uniqueness of each individual with autism and the context of their lives provide interesting design challenges for the successful creation and adoption of technologies for this domain. The first goal is to enable children with ASD to not only interact with virtual environment, but also to build social skills. Socially relevant scenarios can be designed to encourage human interaction with artificially intelligent avatars. Inside the virtual world, which includes settings commonly encountered in everyday life—such as restaurants, shops, offices, parks, and other social places—autistic individuals will be able to interact with other real people's avatars as practice. The user interface and scripts will be extremely clear and simple, and since previous ASD research has shown benefits of storytelling, each game scenario may consist of a short vignette design to elicit response from the student. Vignettes used for the project may include:

- Teaching the student how to interact through social stories, modeling, role-playing, and other activity-based learning

- Conflict resolution and managing disagreement with compromise and recognizing the opinions of others. Learning not to respond with aggression or immature mechanisms.

- Turn taking, and other socially acceptable mannerisms, such as verbal interactions, changing conversational topics, introductions to new people and others

Individuals with autism will encounter prototypical social contexts via a computer interface and will have to interact with 3D avatars within the game that have predefined roles, tasks, and visible body language. Within the context of the game scenario, the student will trigger events, which equate to learning objectives that they must successfully interact with to advance further into the game. Incremental learning objectives will eventually combine to form a fully collaborative social environment. The initial sequence of tasks will most likely follow a linear model, progressing from simple tasks to more complex ones. The effects of the student's actions will impact the behaviors of the other avatars within the scenario in a realistic fashion. Further, as the scenario reacts to the student's input, it will track performance and provide feedback concerning the consequences of particular actions and/or omissions. In terms of people with ASD learning social behaviors, errors do need to be made to support learning. Therefore, a balance must be made between allowing the user to make errors and clearly showing what options are available at any given time within the game.

A secondary goal is to begin the research and development of VR exercises aimed at triggering the release of neurotransmitters to promote critical aspects of synaptic maturation at an early age, to change the course of the disease. Rigorous scientific evaluation is necessary to estimate the likely benefits of this approach and its application to the individual. Research should also attempt to evaluate the contribution of this technology to any observed gains through comparison with traditional teaching approaches.

Web-based instruction and testing via "intelligent" computer simulations of typical social environments will prove an efficacious means for people with ASD to acquire social skills. Computer-based media allows people with autism continuous access to the curriculum, while concurrently allowing researchers to track the frequency of exposure and/or duration of exposure to a given skill (e.g., time logged onto vignettes and testing). It is expected that participants may engage in virtual skills training for longer durations when compared to traditional lecture-based curriculum.

For the parents, teachers, and families of autistic children, understanding and active participation can be critical to their development and eventual independence. Adolescents often play games. These games, whether played in isolation or in a group setting, may be an effective reinforcement for skills that can be practiced in the home with family members and peers. Combining skill instruction with the gaming experience offers the gamer a chance to repeatedly practice skills. Although the skills learned may be constrained to the capabilities of each individual, such strategies may prove to be the gateway to increased socialization and acceptance by peers.

The vision is to use online, PC-based games and immersive 3D environments that leverage existing U.S. Department of Defense (DoD) research and development in modeling, simulation, serious gaming, performance assessment, and after-action review technologies. The goal is to establish a seamless management and delivery capability to provide a distributed virtual environment where skills can be practiced and honed as a student interacts within each prescribed scenario. Virtual reality and gaming applications for social skills may prove to be less resource intensive than traditional in-vivo and "Video Self Modeling" training models. Further, this technology may provide a more engaging and socially controlled environment in which autistic individuals can practice social skills without excessive distractions. Attention must be paid to new collaborative technologies such as massive multiplayer environments that allow interactive experiences for groups as well as individuals. Automated support tools should be investigated to help teachers perform in-depth assessments of student performance and to identify and mitigate critical behavior by providing essential feedback. In this way, distributed and collaborative virtual environments can be incorporated into the continuum of ASD treatment to work in tandem with the full spectrum of other case-management interventions.

Based on positive outcomes from this effort, additional studies could also begin to look at which social skills acquired and practiced via virtual models will generalize to school, home, and community environments. Scenario authoring capabilities should also be investigated to provide the ability to modify and insert new resources into the virtual environment as required by the various ASD treatment interventions. The ability to tailor virtual scenarios to specific student needs is intended to help the student contextualize social situations and events. The application of this augmented virtual reality technology contained within the science of modeling and simulation could produce tremendous synergy in mitigating the treatment and educational interventions to reduce the rising cost in resources, as well as in pain and suffering. Researching this area is an ethical imperative.

Chapter 38

Research Studies and Autism Spectrum Disorder

Chapter Contents

Section 38.1

Participating in Autism Spectrum Disorder Research Studies

This section includes text excerpted from "Find a Study on Autism,"
Eunice Kennedy Shriver National Institute of Child Health and
Human Development (NICHD), January 31, 2017.

The *Eunice Kennedy Shriver* National Institute of Child Health
and Human Development (NICHD) conducts and supports a variety of
clinical research projects related to autism spectrum disorder (ASD).

Featured NICHD Clinical Trials

- Adaptive Interventions for Minimally Verbal Children with
  ASD in the Community (AIM-ASD) (clinicaltrials.gov/ct2/show/
  NCT01751698)

  This study will test the effects of behavioral therapies on communication and speaking among children ages five to eight who have ASD.

- Biomarkers of Developmental Trajectories and Treatment in
  Autism Spectrum Disorder (ASD) (J) (clinicaltrials.gov/ct2/show/
  NCT01874327)

  This study is evaluating the efficacy of a new classroom-based
  intervention to improve joint attention and joint engagement skills
  in infants who are at risk of developing ASD.

- Study of Oxytocin in Autism to Improve Reciprocal Social
  Behaviors (SOARS-B) (clinicaltrials.gov/ct2/show/NCT01944046)

  The purpose of this study is to learn about the effects of a treatment
  using the hormone oxytocin on social difficulties in children and adolescents with autism. This study will also provide additional information
  about the safety and tolerability of this treatment.

Autism Centers of Excellence Program

Autism Centers of Excellence (ACE) consists of research centers and
research networks around the country. Research centers perform multiple, interrelated, multidisciplinary studies at one location. Research

networks each conduct one study across several sites throughout the country.

Centers

- Center for Autism Research and Treatment (CART) (University of California, Los Angeles)
- Marcus Autism Center (MAC) (Emory University)
- Center for Autism Research Excellence (CARE) (Boston University)

Networks

- Adaptive Interventions for Minimally Verbal Children with ASD in the Community
- Autism Genetics: Increasing Representation of Human Diversity
- Early Biomarkers of Autism in Infants with Tuberous Sclerosis
- Intervention Effects of Intensity and Delivery Style for Toddlers with ASD
- A Longitudinal MRI Study of Infants at Risk for Autism
- Multigenerational Families and Environmental Risk for Autism Network
- Multimodal Developmental Neurogenetics of Females with ASD
- Study of Oxytocin in Autism to Improve Reciprocal Social Behaviors

Section 38.2

Baby Teeth Link Autism and Heavy Metals

This section includes text excerpted from "Baby Teeth Link Autism
and Heavy Metals, NIH Study Suggests," National Institutes of
Health (NIH), June 1, 2017.

Baby teeth from children with autism contain more toxic lead and
less of the essential nutrients zinc and manganese, compared to teeth
from children without autism, according to an innovative study funded
by the National Institute of Environmental Health Sciences (NIEHS),
part of the National Institutes of Health (NIH). The researchers studied twins to control genetic influences and focus on possible environmental contributors to the disease. The findings, published June 1,
2017, in the journal *Nature Communications*, suggest that differences
in early-life exposure to metals, or more importantly how a child's body
processes them, may affect the risk of autism.

The differences in metal uptake between children with and without autism were especially notable during the months just before and
after the children were born. The scientists determined this by using
lasers to map the growth rings in baby teeth generated during different
developmental periods.

The researchers observed higher levels of lead in children with
autism throughout development, with the greatest disparity observed
during the period following birth. They also observed a lower uptake of
manganese in children with autism, both before and after birth. The
pattern was more complex for zinc. Children with autism had lower
zinc levels earlier in the womb, but these levels then increased after
birth, compared to children without autism.

The researchers note that replication in larger studies is needed to
confirm the connection between metal uptake and autism.

"We think autism begins very early, most likely in the womb, and
research suggests that our environment can increase a child's risk. But
by the time children are diagnosed at age three or four, it's hard to go
back and know what the moms were exposed to," said Cindy Lawler,
Ph.D., head of the NIEHS Genes, Environment, and Health Branch
(GEH). "With baby teeth, we can actually do that."

Patterns of metal uptake were compared using teeth from 32 pairs
of twins and 12 individual twins. The researchers compared patterns in
twins where only one had autism, as well as in twins where both or neither had autism. Smaller differences in the patterns of metal uptake

occurred when both twins had autism. Larger differences occurred in twins where only one sibling had autism.

The findings build on prior research showing that exposure to toxic metals, such as lead, and deficiencies of essential nutrients, such as manganese, may harm brain development while in the womb or during early childhood. Although manganese is an essential nutrient, it can also be toxic at high doses. Exposure to both lead and high levels of manganese has been associated with autism traits and severity.

The study was led by Manish Arora, Ph.D., an environmental scientist and dentist at the Icahn School of Medicine at Mount Sinai (ISMMS) in New York. With support from NIEHS, Arora and colleagues had previously developed a method that used naturally shed baby teeth to measure children's exposure to lead and other metals while in the womb and during early childhood. The researchers use lasers to extract precise layers of dentine, the hard substance beneath tooth enamel, for metal analysis. The team previously showed that the amount of lead in different layers of dentine corresponds to lead exposure during different developmental periods.

Arora said that autism is a condition where both genes and environment play a role, but figuring out which environmental exposures may increase risk has been difficult.

"What is needed is a window into our fetal life," he said. "Unlike genes, our environment is constantly changing, and our body's response to environmental stressors not only depends on just how much we were exposed to, but at what age we experienced that exposure."

Prior studies relating toxic metals and essential nutrients to autism have faced key limitations, such as estimating exposure based on blood levels after autism diagnosis rather than before, or not being able to control for differences that could be due to genetic factors.

"A lot of studies have compared current lead levels in kids that are already diagnosed," said Lawler. "Being able to measure something the children were exposed to long before diagnosis is a major advantage."

The method of using baby teeth to measure past exposure to metals also holds promise for other disorders, such as attention deficit hyperactivity disorder. "There is growing excitement about the potential of baby teeth as a rich record of a child's early life exposure to both helpful and harmful factors in the environment," said David Balshaw, Ph.D., head of the NIEHS Exposure, Response, and Technology Branch (ERTB), which supported the development of the tooth method.

Section 38.3

Children's Visual Engagement Is Heritable and Altered in Autism

This section includes text excerpted from "Children's Visual
Engagement Is Heritable and Altered in Autism," National Institutes
of Health (NIH), July 12, 2017.

How children visually engage with others in social situations is a heritable behavior that is altered in children with autism, according to a study funded by the National Institutes of Health. The study appears in one of the issues of *Nature*. Autism spectrum disorder affects how a person acts, communicates and learns. In the United States, approximately 1 out of 68 children has the disorder.

Reduced attention to other people's eyes and faces is a behavior associated with autism, and it is often used to screen for and help diagnose the disorder. In a study, National Institutes of Health (NIH)-funded researchers from Washington University in St. Louis and Emory University in Atlanta explored the potential genetic foundation of this behavior, which can appear by the first six months of age and persist as children grow older.

"Research shows that autism likely has a genetic basis. Siblings of children diagnosed with autism and people with certain genetic mutations have a higher risk of developing the disorder, compared to the general population," said Diana Bianchi, M.D., director of the *Eunice Kennedy Shriver* National Institute of Child Health and Human Development (NICHD), which provided funding for the study along with the National Institute of Mental Health (NIMH). "Understanding how genes influence social behaviors will help researchers identify new or better ways to treat autism."

The study team conducted eye-tracking experiments in a group of 250 typically developing toddlers ages 18 to 24 months, including 82 identical twins (41 pairs), 84 nonidentical twins (42 pairs) and 84 nonsibling children (42 randomized pairs). They also evaluated 88 nontwin children diagnosed with autism.

Each child watched videos that showed either an actress speaking directly to the viewer or scenes of children interacting in daycare. In all video frames, children could look at the onscreen characters' eyes, mouth, body or surrounding objects. Special software captured how often the children looked at different regions, as well as the timing and direction of eye movements.

The team found that identical twins had synchronized visual patterns, compared to nonidentical twins and nonsibling pairs. Identical twins tended to shift their eyes at the same times and in the same direction. They also were more likely to look at the subject's eyes or mouth at the same moments.

Using a statistical measurement called the intraclass correlation coefficient (ICC), which measures how well individuals within a group resemble each other (with a value of 1 marking perfect agreement), the researchers found that identical twins had an ICC of 0.91 for eye-looking and 0.86 for mouth-looking. On the other hand, nonidentical twins had scores of 0.35 and 0.44, respectively, while nonsibling pairs had scores of 0.16 and 0.13.

"By comparing identical twins who share the same genes to nonidentical twins and randomly paired children who do not share the same genes, the study is one of the first to show that social visual behaviors are under genetic control," said Lisa Gilotty, Ph.D., chief of NIMH's Research Program on Autism Spectrum Disorders.

To explore this concept further, the researchers evaluated children with autism and discovered that they looked at eye and mouth regions—the most heritable visual traits—much less, compared to the other groups of children.

With these findings, researchers can explore which genes are involved in social visual engagement, how these genes interact with a child's environment to shape his/her social engagement, and how these genetic pathways are disrupted in neurodevelopmental disorders such as autism.

Section 38.4

Delayed Walking May Signal Spontaneous Gene Anomalies in Autism

This section includes text excerpted from "Delayed Walking May
Signal Spontaneous Gene Anomalies in Autism," National
Institute of Mental Health (NIMH), March 24, 2017.

A team of National Institute of Mental Health (NIMH) intramural
and grant-supported researchers has discovered a pattern of behavioral and genetic features seen in some cases of autism spectrum disorder (ASD) that could ultimately lead to identification of subgroups
and improved treatment.

Children diagnosed with ASD who had spontaneous, noninherited
changes in autism-linked genes showed "muted" core autism symptoms
relating to social behavior and language when compared to sex, age,
and intelligence quotient (IQ)-matched children with ASD without
known genetic abnormalities. A key clue was that children with the
spontaneous glitches—abnormal numbers of copies of genes or other
mutations linked to functional impairments—tended to start walking
later than usual, which is not typical of children with ASD. In fact, the
odds of a child in this sample having a spontaneous abnormal gene
finding increased by 17 percent for each month of delay in walking.

"Identifying individuals whose ASD is associated with a specific
type of genetic abnormality may lead us to distinct processes ultimately traceable to specific causes, which could be targeted by more
personalized interventions," explained Audrey Thurm, Ph.D., of the
NIMH Intramural Research Program (IRP). "In the meantime, our
results can increase awareness that among children with an ASD
diagnosis, certain characteristics like late walking are associated with
genetic abnormalities."

Thurm, NIMH grant-supported researcher Somer Bishop, Ph.D., of
the University of California San Francisco, and colleagues, report on
their identification of an emerging cluster of developmental, behavioral, and genetic markers in ASD, March 3, 2017 in the *American
Journal of Psychiatry.*

Prior to the study, the estimated 10–15 percent of children with
ASD who have noninherited, or *"de novo,"* gene copy number variations or suspected disrupting, severe mutations had not been found to
show specific patterns of ASD-related symptoms or delays in developmental milestones. The new discovery was made possible through a

combination of advances in genomics technology, allowing for a large number of "high confidence" suspect genes to be identified, as well as more rigorous matching of children with and without genetic abnormalities than in previous studies. For example, the new study controlled for potentially confounding effects of IQ, which has been previously found to be lower in children with ASD with *de novo* mutations.

Results showed that children with *de novo* mutations tended to be less impaired on core ASD symptoms than their peers with more typical ASD and no known genetic abnormalities. Children with *de novo* mutations also tended to have stronger verbal, language, and social-communication abilities—and clinicians involved in assessing the children were less confident in their ASD diagnoses for the subgroup with *de novo* mutations. Yet children with *de novo* mutations began walking, on average, at 19 months, compared to 13.6 months for children with typical ASD, when controlling for differences in nonverbal IQ.

"While all children in this study met diagnostic criteria for ASD, those with genetic abnormalities showed subtle, yet potentially important, differences in their behavioral profiles when compared to appropriately matched children with no such abnormalities," said Bishop. "These findings are in line with previous assertions that, as a group, *de novo* mutations may be best understood as conferring risk for neurodevelopmental problems more generally, rather than ASD core symptoms specifically."

Chapter 39

False or Misleading Claims for Treating Autism

One thing that is important to know about autism up front: There is no cure for autism. So, products or treatments claiming to "cure" autism do not work as claimed. The same is true of many products claiming to "treat" autism or autism-related symptoms. Some may carry significant health risks.

The U.S. Food and Drug Administration (FDA) plays an important role in warning these companies against making improper claims about their products' intended use as a treatment or cure for autism or autism-related symptoms.

About Autism

According to the Centers for Disease Control and Prevention (CDC), about 1 in 68 children has been identified with an autism spectrum disorder (ASD). ASDs are reported to occur in all racial, ethnic and socioeconomic groups, and are about 4.5 times more common among boys (1 in 42) than among girls (1 in 189).

This chapter contains text excerpted from the following sources: Text in this chapter begins with excerpts from "Autism: Beware of Potentially Dangerous Therapies and Products," U.S. Food and Drug Administration (FDA), November 9, 2017; Text beginning with the heading "Six Tip-Offs to Rip-Offs" is excerpted from "6 Tip-Offs to Rip-Offs: Don't Fall for Health Fraud Scams," U.S. Food and Drug Administration (FDA), December 13, 2017.

The National Institutes of Health (NIH) describe children with autism as having difficulties with social interaction, displaying problems with verbal and nonverbal communication, exhibiting repetitive behaviors and having narrow, obsessive interests. These behaviors can range in impact from mild to disabling.

"Autism varies widely in severity and symptoms," says Amy Taylor, M.D., M.H.S., a pediatrician at the FDA. "Existing autism therapies and interventions are designed to address specific symptoms and can bring about improvement," she adds.

In addition, the FDA has approved drugs that can help some people manage related symptoms of ASD. For example, the FDA has approved the use of antipsychotics such as risperidone (for patients ages 5–16) and aripiprazole (for patients ages 6–17) to treat irritability associated with autistic disorder. Before using any behavioral intervention or drug therapy that claims to be a treatment or cure for ASD, you should check with your healthcare professional.

The Association for Science in Autism Treatment (ASAT), a not-for-profit organization of parents and professionals committed to improving the education, treatment, and care of people with autism, says that since autism was first identified, there has been a long history of failed treatments and fads.

The FDA Cracks Down on False Claims

According to Commander Jason Humbert, M.H.S., R.N., a regulatory operations officer in the FDA's Office of Regulatory Affairs (ORA), the agency has warned and/or taken action against a number of companies that have made improper claims about their products' intended use as a treatment or cure for autism or autism-related symptoms. Some of these so-called therapies carry significant health risks and include:

- **"Chelation therapies."** These products claim to cleanse the body of toxic chemicals and heavy metals by binding to them and "removing" them from circulation. They come in a number of forms, including sprays, suppositories, capsules, liquid drops, and clay baths. FDA-approved chelating agents are approved for specific uses that do not include the treatment or cure of autism, such as the treatment of lead poisoning and iron overload, and are available by prescription only. FDA-approved prescription chelation therapy products should only be used under professional supervision. Chelating important minerals needed by the body can lead to serious and life-threatening outcomes.

- **Hyperbaric oxygen therapy (HBOT).** This involves breathing oxygen in a pressurized chamber and has been cleared by the FDA only for certain medical uses, such as treating decompression sickness suffered by divers.

- **Detoxifying clay baths.** Added to bath water, these products claim to draw out chemical toxins, pollutants, and heavy metals from the body. They are improperly advertised as offering "dramatic improvement" for autism symptoms.

- **Various products**, including raw camel milk and essential oils. These products have been marketed as a treatment for autism or autism-related symptoms, but have not been proven safe and effective for these advertised uses.

Humbert offers some quick tips to help you identify false or misleading claims.

- Be suspicious of products that claim to treat a wide range of diseases.

- Personal testimonials are no substitute for scientific evidence.

- Few diseases or conditions can be treated quickly, so be suspicious of any therapy claimed as a "quick fix."

- So-called miracle cures, which claim scientific breakthroughs or contain secret ingredients, may be a hoax.

The bottom line is this—if it's an unproven or little-known treatment, talk to your healthcare professional before buying or using these products.

Six Tip-Offs to Rip-Offs

Bogus product! Danger! Health fraud alert!

You'll never see these warnings on health products, but that's what you ought to be thinking when you see claims like "miracle cure," "revolutionary scientific breakthrough," or "alternative to drugs or surgery."

Health fraud scams have been around for hundreds of years. The snake oil salesmen of old have morphed into the deceptive, high-tech marketers of today. They prey on people's desires for easy solutions to difficult health problems—from losing weight to curing serious diseases such as cancer.

According to the FDA, a health product is fraudulent if it is deceptively promoted as being effective against a disease or health condition but has not been scientifically proven safe and effective for that purpose.

Scammers promote their products through newspapers, magazines, TV infomercials, and cyberspace. You can find health fraud scams in retail stores and on countless websites, in pop-up ads and spam, and on social media sites such as Facebook and Twitter.

Not Worth the Risk

Health fraud scams can do more than waste your money. They can cause serious injury or even death, says Gary Coody, R.Ph., the FDA's national health fraud coordinator. "Using unproven treatments can delay getting a potentially life-saving diagnosis and medication that actually works. Also, fraudulent products sometimes contain hidden drug ingredients that can be harmful when unknowingly taken by consumers."

Coody says fraudulent products often make claims related to:

- Weight loss
- Sexual performance
- Memory loss
- Serious diseases such as cancer, diabetes, heart disease, arthritis, and Alzheimer disease

A Pervasive Problem

Fraudulent products not only won't work—they could cause serious injury. In the past few years, FDA laboratories have found more than 100 weight-loss products, illegally marketed as dietary supplements, that contained sibutramine, the active ingredient in the prescription weight-loss drug Meridia. In 2010, Meridia was withdrawn from the U.S. market after studies showed that it was associated with an increased risk of heart attack and stroke.

Fraudulent products marketed as drugs or dietary supplements are not the only health scams on the market. The FDA found a fraudulent and expensive light therapy device with cure-all claims to treat fungal meningitis, Alzheimer disease, skin cancer, concussions, and many other unrelated diseases. Generally, making health claims about a medical device without FDA clearance or approval of the device is illegal.

"Health fraud is a pervasive problem," says Coody, "especially when scammers sell online. It's difficult to track down the responsible parties. When the FDA finds them and tells them their products are illegal, some will shut down their website. Unfortunately, however, these same products may reappear later on a different website, and sometimes may reappear with a different name."

Tip-Offs

The FDA offers some tip-offs to help you identify rip-offs.

- **One product does it all.** Be suspicious of products that claim to cure a wide range of diseases. A New York firm claimed its products marketed as dietary supplements could treat or cure senile dementia, brain atrophy, atherosclerosis, kidney dysfunction, gangrene, depression, osteoarthritis, dysuria, and lung, cervical, and prostate cancer. In October 2012, at the FDA's request, U.S. marshals seized these products.

- **Personal testimonials.** Success stories, such as, "It cured my diabetes" or "My tumors are gone," are easy to make up and are not a substitute for scientific evidence.

- **Quick fixes.** Few diseases or conditions can be treated quickly, even with legitimate products. Beware of language such as, "Lose 30 pounds in 30 days" or "eliminates skin cancer in days."

- **"All natural."** Some plants found in nature (such as poisonous mushrooms) can kill when consumed. Moreover, the FDA has found numerous products promoted as "all natural" that contain hidden and dangerously high doses of prescription drug ingredients or even untested active artificial ingredients.

- **"Miracle cure."** Alarms should go off when you see this claim or others like it such as, "new discovery," "scientific breakthrough" or "secret ingredient." If a real cure for a serious disease were discovered, it would be widely reported through the media and prescribed by health professionals—not buried in print ads, TV infomercials, or on Internet sites.

- **Conspiracy theories.** Claims such as "The pharmaceutical industry and the government are working together to hide information about a miracle cure" are always untrue and unfounded. These statements are used to distract consumers from the obvious, common-sense questions about the so-called miracle cure.

Even with these tips, fraudulent health products are not always easy to spot. If you're tempted to buy an unproven product or one with questionable claims, check with your doctor or other healthcare professional first.

Part Six

Education and Autism Spectrum Disorder

Chapter 40

Understanding the Special Education Process

Chapter Contents

Section 40.1

Autism Awareness and Acceptance in Early Childhood Education

This section includes text excerpted from "Autism Awareness and Acceptance in Early Childhood Education," Administration for Children and Families (ACF), U.S. Department of Health and Human Services (HHS), November 14, 2017.

Autism spectrum disorder (ASD) affects about 1 in 68 children in the United States, with more children being identified than ever before. The early childhood community has a unique opportunity to touch the lives of these children and their families in ways that can make a real difference.

What Is Autism Spectrum Disorder?

Autism spectrum disorder (ASD) is a developmental disability that can affect social communication and behavioral development. ASD is a spectrum disorder which means that each child is affected differently and has unique strengths, challenges, and needs. ASD begins before the age of three and lasts throughout a person's life, although symptoms may improve over time. Early identification of ASD is important so children and families can attain the services and support they need as soon as possible. With awareness, acceptance, and appropriate supports, children with ASD can reach their incredible potential.

ASD affects about 1 in 68 children in the United States, with more children being identified than ever before. The early childhood community has a unique opportunity to touch the lives of these children and their families in ways that can make a real difference.

What Is the Role of Early Care and Education Providers?

While diagnosing and providing specific interventions for young children with ASD is the role of specialists, early childhood providers can play an active role in supporting children with autism and other developmental disabilities. By using developmentally appropriate practices, tracking developmental milestones, communicating with parents, and being aware of community-based resources, early care, and education providers can make important contributions to the lives of young children with ASD and their families.

Administration for Children and Families (ACF) is dedicated to providing early education providers with the information they need to better understand ASD and support the children in their care.

What Services are Available to Young Children with Autism Spectrum Disorder under IDEA?

The Individuals with Disabilities Education Act (IDEA) is a federal law that requires that all children suspected of having a disability be evaluated without cost to families to determine if they have a disability and are eligible for services under IDEA. For children under three years of age, these services are provided through a State's IDEA Part C early intervention system. For children older than three, IDEA Part B services are available through the public school system.

The National Dissemination Center for Children with Disabilities (NICHCY) provides information and resources about IDEA (www. parentcenterhub.org/idea). For information on early intervention services in your state, visit the Early Childhood Technical Assistance (ECTA) Center (ectacenter.org/contact/ptccoord.asp).

Section 40.2

504 Education Plans

This section includes text excerpted from "Parent and Educator Resource Guide to Section 504 in Public Elementary and Secondary Schools," U.S. Department of Education (ED), December 2016.

Section 504 is a federal law that prohibits disability discrimination by recipients of federal financial assistance. All public schools and school districts, as well as all public charter schools and magnet schools, that receive federal financial assistance from the department must comply with Section 504.

Section 504 provides a broad spectrum of protections against discrimination on the basis of disability. For example, all qualified elementary and secondary public school students who meet the definition of an individual with a disability under Section 504 are entitled to receive regular or special education and related aids and services that are designed to meet their individual educational needs as adequately as the needs of students without disabilities are met. Section 504 also requires, among other things, that a student with a disability receive an equal opportunity to participate in athletics and extracurricular activities, and to be free from bullying and harassment based on disability.

The Meaning of Disability under Section 504

Below is a discussion of what it means to be a student or individual with a disability, and of related terms that help to comprehensively define disability as it is used in Section 504 and its implementing regulations.

Disability. Under Section 504, an individual with a disability (also referred to as a student with a disability in the elementary and secondary education context) is defined as a person who:

1. has a physical or mental impairment that substantially limits a major life activity;

2. has a record of such an impairment; or

3. is regarded as having such an impairment.

The determination of whether a student has a physical or mental impairment that substantially limits a major life activity (and therefore, has a disability) must be made on a case by case basis. In addition, when determining if someone meets the definition of a disability, the definition must be understood to provide broad coverage of individuals.

Physical or mental impairments. Section 504 defines a physical or mental impairment as any:

- physiological disorder or condition,

- cosmetic disfigurement, or

- anatomical loss affecting one or more of the following body systems: neurological; musculoskeletal; special sense organs; respiratory, including speech organs; cardiovascular; reproductive; digestive; genitourinary; hemic and lymphatic; skin; and endocrine.

The Section 504 definition of physical and mental impairment also includes any mental or psychological disorder. The definition does not include all specific diseases and conditions that may be physical or mental impairments because of the difficulty of ensuring the completeness of such a list.

Major Life Activities

The major life activities include certain acts a person does (such as hearing, speaking, lifting) and a person's bodily functions (such as lung disease that affects a person's respiratory system, or a traumatic brain injury (TBI) that affects the function of the brain).

The list of major life activities under Section 504 includes, but is not limited to, the activities listed below.

- Caring for oneself
- Performing manual tasks
- Seeing
- Hearing
- Eating
- Sleeping
- Walking
- Standing
- Lifting
- Bending
- Speaking
- Breathing
- Learning
- Reading
- Concentrating
- Thinking
- Communicating
- Working

Major bodily functions are also major life activities under the law, and these major bodily functions include functions of the bowel, bladder, and brain; normal cell growth; and the immune, endocrine (for example, thyroid, pituitary, and pancreas), respiratory, reproductive, circulatory, digestive, and neurological systems.

These lists, however, do not provide every possible major life activity or bodily function; therefore, if an activity or bodily function is not listed in the Amendments Act, it might still be considered a major life activity under Section 504.

For example, if a school provides a form with a list of major life activities to consider during an evaluation process, a student may still have a physical or mental impairment that substantially limits a major life activity even if the activity is not listed on the school's form.

School staff should note, in particular, that a student may have a disability and be eligible for Section 504 services even if his or her disability does not limit the major life activity of learning.

Therefore, rather than considering only how an impairment affects a student's ability to learn, school staff must also consider how the impairment affects any major life activity of the student and, if necessary, assess what is needed to ensure that students have an equal opportunity to participate in the school's programs.

An Overview of a Free Appropriate Public Education

Section 504 and the Individuals with Disabilities Education Act (IDEA) contain requirements for free appropriate public education (FAPE) for students with disabilities, but there are some differences. Under the IDEA, FAPE is a statutory term. It requires a school district to develop an individualized education program (IEP) for each eligible student with a disability that sets out, among other information, the student's program of special education and related services.

All elementary and secondary school students who are qualified individuals with disabilities, as defined by Section 504, and who need special education and/or related aids and services are entitled to FAPE. Under Section 504, FAPE is the provision of regular or special education and related aids and services that are designed to meet the individual educational needs of students with disabilities as adequately as the needs of nondisabled students are met and are based on adherence to procedures governing educational setting, evaluation and placement, and procedural safeguards. Implementation of an IEP developed in accordance with the IDEA is one means of meeting the Section 504 FAPE standard.

Though not explicitly required by the department's Section 504 regulations, school districts often document the elements of an individual student's FAPE under Section 504 in a document, typically referred to as a Section 504 Plan.

A written Section 504 Plan is often a useful way to document that the school district engaged in a process to identify and address the needs of a student with a disability and to communicate, to school personnel, the information needed for successful implementation. Office for Civil Rights (OCR) encourages schools to document a student's Section 504 services in a written plan to help avoid misunderstandings or confusion about what Section 504 services the school offered the student. Note, however, that IDEA-eligible students with disabilities who have an IEP are not required to also have a Section 504 plan even though they are protected under Section 504. For these students, the IEP developed and implemented in accordance with the IDEA is sufficient.

Under Section 504, FAPE must be provided free of charge to students with disabilities. Schools may impose fees on a student with a disability only if the fees are equally imposed on students without disabilities. For example, fees to cover the cost of a field trip that apply to all students are fees a school can charge to a student with a disability

Key features of FAPE under Section 504 include:

- Evaluation and placement procedures that guard against misclassification or inappropriate placement of students;

- Periodic reevaluation of students who have been provided special education or related services and prior to a significant change in placement;

- Provision of regular or special education and related aids and services that are designed so that the individual educational needs of students with disabilities are met as adequately as the needs of nondisabled students are met;

- Education of students with disabilities with nondisabled students—to the maximum extent that this arrangement is appropriate for the needs of students with disabilities;

- A system of procedural safeguards (that is designed to inform parents of a school district's actions or decisions and to provide parents with a process for challenging those actions or decisions) that include notice; an opportunity for parents to review their child's records; an impartial due process hearing (with an opportunity for participation by the student's parents or guardians and representation by counsel); and a review procedure.

Section 40.3

Individualized Education Plan

This section includes text excerpted from "A Guide to the
Individualized Education Program," U.S. Department of
Education (ED), March 23, 2007. Reviewed October 2018.

Each public school child who receives special education and related
services must have an Individualized Education Program (IEP). Each
IEP must be designed for one student and must be a truly individualized document. The IEP creates an opportunity for teachers, parents,
school administrators, related services personnel, and students (when
appropriate) to work together to improve educational results for children with disabilities. The IEP is the cornerstone of a quality education
for each child with a disability.

To create an effective IEP, parents, teachers, other school
staff—and often the student—must come together to look closely
at the student's unique needs. These individuals pool knowledge,
experience and commitment to design an educational program
that will help the student be involved in, and progress in, the general curriculum. The IEP guides the delivery of special education
supports and services for the student with a disability. Without
a doubt, writing—and implementing—an effective IEP requires
teamwork.

This section explains the IEP process, which can be considered to
be one of the most critical elements to ensure effective teaching, learning, and better results for all children with disabilities. It is designed
to help teachers, parents, and anyone involved in the education of a
child with a disability-develop and carry out an IEP. The information in this section is based on what is required by the United States
special education law—the Individuals with Disabilities Education
Act, or IDEA.

The IDEA requires certain information to be included in each child's
IEP. It is useful to know, however, that states and local school systems
often include additional information in IEPs in order to document that
they have met certain aspects of federal or state law. The flexibility
that states and school systems have to design their own IEP forms is
one reason why IEP forms may look different from school system to
school system or state to state. Yet each IEP is critical in the education
of a child with a disability.

The Basic Special Education Process under IDEA

The writing of each student's IEP takes place within the larger picture of the special education process under IDEA. Before taking a detailed look at the IEP, it may be helpful to look briefly at how a student is identified as having a disability and needing special education and related services and, thus, an IEP.

Step 1. Child is identified as possibly needing special education and related services.

"Child Find." The state must identify, locate, and evaluate all children with disabilities in the state who need special education and related services. To do so, states conduct "Child Find" activities. A child may be identified by "Child Find," and parents may be asked if the "Child Find" system can evaluate their child. Parents can also call the "Child Find" system and ask that their child be evaluated.

or

Referral or request for evaluation. A school professional may ask that a child be evaluated to see if she or he has a disability. Parents may also contact the child's teacher or other school professional to ask that their child be evaluated. This request may be verbal or in writing. Parental consent is needed before the child may be evaluated. Evaluation needs to be completed within a reasonable time after the parent gives consent.

Step 2. Child is evaluated.

The evaluation must assess the child in all areas related to the child's suspected disability. The evaluation results will be used to decide the child's eligibility for special education and related services and to make decisions about an appropriate educational program for the child. If the parents disagree with the evaluation, they have the right to take their child for an Independent Educational Evaluation (IEE). They can ask that the school system pay for this IEE.

Step 3. Eligibility is decided.

A group of qualified professionals and the parents look at the child's evaluation results. Together, they decide if the child is a "child with a disability," as defined by IDEA. Parents may ask for a hearing to challenge the eligibility decision.

Step 4. Child is found eligible for services.

If the child is found to be a "child with a disability," as defined by IDEA, she or he is eligible for special education and related services.

Within 30 calendar days after a child is determined eligible, the IEP team must meet to write an IEP for the child.

Step 5. IEP meeting is scheduled.

The school system schedules and conducts the IEP meeting. School staff must:

- contact the participants, including the parents;

- notify parents early enough to make sure they have an opportunity to attend;

- schedule the meeting at a time and place agreeable to parents and the school;

- tell the parents the purpose, time, and location of the meeting;

- tell the parents who will be attending; and

- tell the parents that they may invite people to the meeting who have the knowledge or special expertise about the child.

Step 6. IEP meeting is held and the IEP is written.

The IEP team gathers to talk about the child's needs and write the student's IEP. Parents and the student (when appropriate) are part of the team. If the child's placement is decided by a different group, the parents must be part of that group as well.

Before the school system may provide special education and related services to the child for the first time, the parents must give consent. The child begins to receive services as soon as possible after the meeting.

If the parents do not agree with the IEP and placement, they may discuss their concerns with other members of the IEP team and try to work out an agreement. If they still disagree, parents can ask for mediation, or the school may offer mediation. Parents may file a complaint with the state education agency and may request a due process hearing, at which time mediation must be available.

Step 7. Services are provided.

The school makes sure that the child's IEP is being carried out as it was written. Parents are given a copy of the IEP. Each of the child's teachers and service providers has access to the IEP and knows his or her specific responsibilities for carrying out the IEP. This includes the accommodations, modifications, and supports that must be provided to the child, in keeping with the IEP.

Step 8. Progress is measured and reported to parents.

The child's progress toward the annual goals is measured, as stated in the IEP. His or her parents are regularly informed of their child's progress and whether that progress is enough for the child to achieve the goals by the end of the year. These progress reports must be given to parents at least as often as parents are informed of their nondisabled children's progress.

Step 9. IEP is reviewed.

The child's IEP is reviewed by the IEP team at least once a year, or more often if the parents or school ask for a review. If necessary, the IEP is revised. Parents, as team members, must be invited to attend these meetings. Parents can make suggestions for changes, can agree or disagree with the IEP goals, and agree or disagree with the placement.

If parents do not agree with the IEP and placement, they may discuss their concerns with other members of the IEP team and try to work out an agreement. There are several options, including additional testing, an independent evaluation, or asking for mediation (if available) or a due process hearing. They may also file a complaint with the state education agency.

Step 10. Child is reevaluated.

At least every three years the child must be reevaluated. This evaluation is often called a "triennial." Its purpose is to find out if the child continues to be a "child with a disability," as defined by IDEA, and what the child's educational needs are. However, the child must be reevaluated more often if conditions warrant or if the child's parent or teacher asks for a new evaluation.

Contents of the Individualized Education Plan

By law, the IEP must include certain information about the child and the educational program designed to meet his or her unique needs. In a nutshell, this information is:

- **Current performance.** The IEP must state how the child is currently doing in school (known as present levels of educational performance). This information usually comes from the evaluation results such as classroom tests and assignments, individual tests given to decide eligibility for services or during reevaluation, and observations made by parents, teachers, related service providers, and other school staff. The statement about

335

"current performance" includes how the child's disability affects his or her involvement and progress in the general curriculum.

- **Annual goals.** These are goals that the child can reasonably accomplish in a year. The goals are broken down into short-term objectives or benchmarks. Goals may be academic, address social or behavioral needs, relate to physical needs, or address other educational needs. The goals must be measurable-meaning that it must be possible to measure whether the student has achieved the goals.

- **Special education and related services.** The IEP must list the special education and related services to be provided to the child or on behalf of the child. This includes supplementary aids and services that the child needs. It also includes modifications (changes) to the program or supports for school personnel-such as training or professional development that will be provided to assist the child.

- **Participation with nondisabled children.** The IEP must explain the extent (if any) to which the child will not participate with nondisabled children in the regular class and other school activities.

- **Participation in state and district-wide tests.** Most states and districts give achievement tests to children in certain grades or age groups. The IEP must state what modifications in the administration of these tests the child will need. If a test is not appropriate for the child, the IEP must state why the test is not appropriate and how the child will be tested instead.

- **Dates and places.** The IEP must state when services will begin, how often they will be provided, where they will be provided, and how long they will last.

- **Transition service needs.** Beginning when the child is age 14 (or younger, if appropriate), the IEP must address (within the applicable parts of the IEP) the courses she or he needs to take to reach his or her postschool goals. A statement of transition services needs must also be included in each of the child's subsequent IEPs.

- **Needed transition services.** Beginning when the child is age 16 (or younger, if appropriate), the IEP must state what transition services are needed to help the child prepare for leaving school.

- **Age of majority.** Beginning at least one year before the child reaches the age of majority, the IEP must include a statement that the student has been told of any rights that will transfer to him or her at the age of majority. (This statement would be needed only in states that transfer rights at the age of majority.)

- **Measuring progress.** The IEP must state how the child's progress will be measured and how parents will be informed of that progress.

A sample IEP form will be presented, along with the federal regulations describing the "Content of the IEP," to help you gain a fuller understanding of what type of information is important to capture about a child in an IEP. It is useful to understand that each child's IEP is different. The document is prepared for that child only. It describes the individualized education program designed to meet that child's needs.

The Individualized Education Plan Team Members

- By law, certain individuals must be involved in writing a child's Individualized Education Program. These are identified in the figure at the left. Note that an IEP team member may fill more than one of the team positions if properly qualified and designated. For example, the school system representative may also be the person who can interpret the child's evaluation results.

- These people must work together as a team to write the child's IEP. A meeting to write the IEP must be held within 30 calendar days of deciding that the child is eligible for special education and related services.

- Each team member brings important information to the IEP meeting. Members share their information and work together to write the child's Individualized Education Program. Each person's information adds to the team's understanding of the child and what services the child needs.

- Parents are key members of the IEP team. They know their child very well and can talk about their child's strengths and needs as well as their ideas for enhancing their child's education. They can offer insight into how their child learns, what his or her interests are, and other aspects of the child that

337

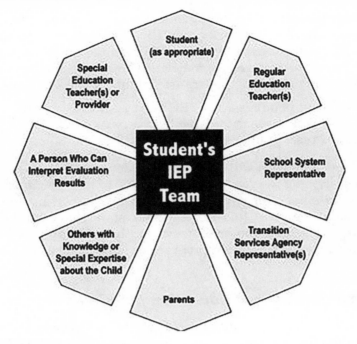

Figure 40.1. *IEP Team Members*

only a parent can know. They can listen to what the other team members think their child needs to work on at school and share their suggestions. They can also report on whether the skills the child is learning at school are being used at home.

- Teachers are vital participants in the IEP meeting as well. At least one of the child's regular education teachers must be on the IEP team if the child is (or may be) participating in the regular education environment. The regular education teacher has a great deal to share with the team. For example, she or he might talk about:

  - the general curriculum in the regular classroom;

  - the aids, services or changes to the educational program that would help the child learn and achieve; and

  - strategies to help the child with behavior, if behavior is an issue.

The regular education teacher may also discuss with the IEP team the supports for school staff that are needed so that the child can:

- advance toward his or her annual goals;

- be involved and progress in the general curriculum;

- participate in extracurricular and other activities; and

- be educated with other children, both with and without disabilities.

Supports for school staff may include professional development or more training. Professional development and training are important for teachers, administrators, bus drivers, cafeteria workers, and others who provide services for children with disabilities.

The child's special education teacher contributes important information and experience about how to educate children with disabilities. Because of his or her training in special education, this teacher can talk about such issues as:

- how to modify the general curriculum to help the child learn;

- the supplementary aids and services that the child may need to be successful in the regular classroom and elsewhere;

- how to modify testing so that the student can show what she or he has learned; and

- other aspects of individualizing instruction to meet the student's unique needs.

Beyond helping to write the IEP, the special educator has responsibility for working with the student to carry out the IEP. She or he may:

- work with the student in a resource room or special class devoted to students receiving special education services;

- team teach with the regular education teacher; and

- work with other school staff, particularly the regular education teacher, to provide expertise about addressing the child's unique needs.

Another important member of the IEP team is the individual who can interpret what the child's evaluation results mean in terms of designing appropriate instruction. The evaluation results are very useful in determining how the child is currently doing in school and what areas of need the child has. This IEP team member must be able to talk about the instructional implications of the child's evaluation results, which will help the team plan appropriate instruction to address the child's needs.

The individual representing the school system is also a valuable team member. This person knows a great deal about special education services and educating children with disabilities. She or he can talk about the necessary school resources. It is important that this individual have the authority to commit resources and be able to ensure that whatever services are set out in the IEP will actually be provided.

The IEP team may also include additional individuals with knowledge or special expertise about the child. The parent or the school system can invite these individuals to participate on the team. Parents, for example, may invite an advocate who knows the child, a professional with special expertise about the child and his or her disability, or others (such as a vocational educator who has been working with the child) who can talk about the child's strengths and/or needs. The school system may invite one or more individuals who can offer special expertise or knowledge about the child, such as a paraprofessional or related services professional. Because an important part of developing an IEP is considering a child's need for related services, related service professionals are often involved as IEP team members or participants. They share their special expertise about the child's needs and how their own professional services can address those needs. Depending on the child's individual needs, some related service professionals attending the IEP meeting or otherwise helping to develop the IEP might include occupational or physical therapists, adaptive physical education providers, psychologists, or speech-language pathologists (SLPs).

When an IEP is being developed for a student of transition age, representatives from transition service agencies can be important participants. Whenever a purpose of meeting is to consider needed transition services, the school must invite a representative of any other agency that is likely to be responsible for providing or paying for transition services. This individual can help the team plan any transition services the student needs. She or he can also commit the resources of the agency to pay for or provide needed transition services. If she or he does not attend the meeting, then the school must take alternative steps to obtain the agency's participation in the planning of the student's transition services.

And, last but not least, the student may also be a member of the IEP team. If transition service needs or transition services are going to be discussed at the meeting, the student must be invited to attend. More and more students are participating in and even leading their own IEP meetings. This allows them to have a strong voice in their own education and can teach them a great deal about self-advocacy and self-determination.

Section 40.4

Individuals with Disabilities Education Act Summary

This section includes text excerpted from "About IDEA," U.S. Department of Education (ED), December 15, 2015. Reviewed October 2018.

The Individuals with Disabilities Education Act (IDEA) is a law that makes available a free appropriate public education to eligible children with disabilities throughout the nation and ensures special education and related services to those children.

The IDEA governs how states and public agencies provide early intervention, special education, and related services to more than 6.5 million eligible infants, toddlers, children, and youth with disabilities.

Infants and toddlers, birth through age 2, with disabilities and their families receive early intervention services under IDEA Part C. Children and youth ages 3 through 21 receive special education and related services under IDEA Part B.

Additionally, the IDEA authorizes:

- Formula grants to states to support special education and related services and early intervention services.

- Discretionary grants to state educational agencies, institutions of higher education, and other nonprofit organizations to support research, demonstrations, technical assistance and dissemination, technology development, personnel preparation and development, and parent-training and parent-information centers.

The Congress reauthorized the IDEA in 2004 and amended the IDEA through Public Law 114-95, the Every Student Succeeds Act, in December 2015.

In the law, Congress states:

"Disability is a natural part of the human experience and in no way diminishes the right of individuals to participate in or contribute to society. Improving educational results for children with disabilities is an essential element of our national policy of ensuring equality of opportunity, full participation, independent living, and economic self-sufficiency for individuals with disabilities."

Individuals with Disabilities Education Act Purpose

The stated purpose of the IDEA is:

- to ensure that all children with disabilities have available to them a free appropriate public education that emphasizes special education and related services designed to meet their unique needs and prepare them for further education, employment, and independent living;

- to ensure that the rights of children with disabilities and parents of such children are protected;

- to assist states, localities, educational service agencies, and federal agencies to provide for the education of all children with disabilities;

- to assist states in the implementation of a statewide, comprehensive, coordinated, multidisciplinary, interagency system of early intervention services for infants and toddlers with disabilities and their families;

- to ensure that educators and parents have the necessary tools to improve educational results for children with disabilities by supporting system improvement activities; coordinated research and personnel preparation; coordinated technical assistance, dissemination, and support; and technology development and media services;

- to assess, and ensure the effectiveness of, efforts to educate children with disabilities.

History of the Individuals with Disabilities Education Act

On November 29, 1975, President Gerald Ford signed into law the Education for All Handicapped Children Act (EAHCA) (Public Law

94-142), now known as the Individuals with Disabilities Education Act. In adopting this landmark civil rights measure, Congress opened public school doors for millions of children with disabilities and laid the foundation of the country's commitment to ensuring that children with disabilities have opportunities to develop their talents, share their gifts, and contribute to their communities.

The law guaranteed access to a free appropriate public education in the least restrictive environment to every child with a disability. Subsequent amendments, as reflected in the IDEA, have led to an increased emphasis on access to the general education curriculum, the provision of services for young children from birth through five, transition planning, and accountability for the achievement of students with disabilities. The IDEA upholds and protects the rights of infants, toddlers, children, and youth with disabilities and their families.

In the last 40+ years, we have advanced our expectations for all children, including children with disabilities. Classrooms have become more inclusive and the future of children with disabilities is brighter. Significant progress has been made toward protecting the rights of, meeting the individual needs of, and improving educational results and outcomes for infants, toddlers, children, and youths with disabilities.

Since 1975, we have progressed from excluding nearly 1.8 million children with disabilities from public schools to providing more than 6.9 million children with disabilities special education and related services designed to meet their individual needs.

More than 62 percent of children with disabilities are in general education classrooms 80 percent or more of their school day, and early intervention services are being provided to more than 340,000 infants and toddlers with disabilities and their families.

Section 40.5

Free Appropriate Public Education under Section 504

This section includes text excerpted from "Free Appropriate Public Education under Section 504," U.S. Department of Education (ED), August 2010. Reviewed October 2018.

Section 504 of the Rehabilitation Act of 1973 protects the rights of individuals with disabilities in programs and activities that receive federal financial assistance, including federal funds. Section 504 provides that: "No otherwise qualified individual with a disability in the United States . . . shall, solely by reason of her or his disability, be excluded from the participation in, be denied the benefits of, or be subjected to discrimination under any program or activity receiving Federal financial assistance . . ."

The U.S. Department of Education (ED) enforces Section 504 in programs and activities that receive funds from ED. Recipients of these funds include public school districts, institutions of higher education, and other state and local education agencies. ED has published a regulation implementing Section 504 (34 C.F.R. Part 104) and maintains an Office for Civil Rights (OCR), with 12 enforcement offices and a headquarters office in Washington, D.C., to enforce Section 504 and other civil rights laws that pertain to recipients of funds.

The Section 504 regulation requires a school district to provide a "free appropriate public education" (FAPE) to each qualified person with a disability who is in the school district's jurisdiction, regardless of the nature or severity of the person's disability.

This section answers the following questions about FAPE according to Section 504:

- Who is entitled to a free appropriate public education?

- How is an appropriate education defined?

- How is a free education defined?

Who Is Entitled to Free Appropriate Public Education?

All qualified persons with disabilities within the jurisdiction of a school district are entitled to a free appropriate public education. The ED Section 504 regulation defines a person with a disability as "any person who: (i) has a physical or mental impairment which substantially limits one or more major life activities, (ii) has a record of such an impairment, or (iii) is regarded as having such an impairment."

For elementary and secondary education programs, a qualified person with a disability is a person with a disability who is:

- of an age during which it is mandatory under state law to provide such services to persons with disabilities;

- of an age during which persons without disabilities are provided such services; or

- entitled to receive a free appropriate public education under the Individuals with Disabilities Education Act (IDEA).

In general, all school-age children who are individuals with disabilities as defined by Section 504 and IDEA are entitled to FAPE.

How Is an Appropriate Education Defined?

An appropriate education may comprise education in regular classes, education in regular classes with the use of related aids and services, or special education and related services in separate classrooms for all or portions of the school day. Special education may include specially designed instruction in classrooms, at home, or in private or public institutions, and may be accompanied by related services such as speech therapy, occupational and physical therapy, psychological counseling, and medical diagnostic services necessary to the child's education.

An appropriate education will include:

- Education services designed to meet the individual education needs of students with disabilities as adequately as the needs of nondisabled students are met;

- Education of each student with a disability with nondisabled students, to the maximum extent appropriate to the needs of the student with a disability;

- Evaluation and placement procedures established to guard against misclassification or inappropriate placement of students, and a periodic reevaluation of students who have been provided special education or related services; and

- Establishment of due process procedures that enable parents and guardians to:

345

- receive required notices;

- review their child's records; and

- challenge identification, evaluation and placement decisions.

Due process procedures must also provide for an impartial hearing with the opportunity for participation by parents and representation by counsel, and a review procedure.

How Is a Free Education Defined?

Recipients operating federally funded programs must provide education and related services free of charge to students with disabilities and their parents or guardians. Provision of a free education is the provision of education and related services without cost to the person with a disability or his or her parents or guardians, except for fees equally imposed on nondisabled persons or their parents or guardians.

If a recipient is unable to provide a free appropriate public education itself, the recipient may place a person with a disability in, or refer such person to, a program other than the one it operates.

However, the recipient remains responsible for ensuring that the education offered is an appropriate education, as defined in the law, and for coverage of financial obligations associated with the placement.

The cost of the program may include tuition and other related services, such as room and board, psychological and medical services necessary for diagnostic and evaluative purposes, and adequate transportation. Funds available from any public or private source, including insurers, may be used by the recipient to meet the requirements of FAPE.

If a student is placed in a private school because a school district cannot provide an appropriate program, the financial obligations for this placement are the responsibility of the school district. However, if a school district makes available a free appropriate public education and the student's parents or guardian choose to place the child in a private school, the school district is not required to pay for the student's education in the private school. If a recipient school district places a student with a disability in a program that requires the student to be away from home, the recipient is responsible for the cost of room and board and nonmedical care.

To meet the requirements of FAPE, a recipient may place a student with a disability in, or refer such student to, a program not operated by the recipient. When this occurs, the recipient must ensure that adequate transportation is provided to and from the program at no greater personal or family cost than would be incurred if the student with a disability were placed in the recipient's program.

Free Appropriate Public Education Provisions in the Individuals with Disabilities Education Act

Part B of IDEA requires participating states to ensure that a free appropriate public education (FAPE) is made available to eligible children with disabilities in mandatory age ranges residing in the state. To be eligible, a child must be evaluated as having one or more of the disabilities listed in IDEA and determined to be in need of special education and related services. Evaluations must be conducted according to prescribed procedures. The disabilities specified in IDEA include: mental retardation, hearing impairments including deafness, speech or language impairments, visual impairments including blindness, emotional disturbance, orthopedic impairments, autism, traumatic brain injury (TBI), other health impairments, specific learning disabilities, deaf-blindness, and multiple disabilities. Additionally, states and local education agencies (LEAs) may adopt the term "developmental delay" for children aged three through nine (or a subset of that age range) who are experiencing a developmental delay as defined by the state and need special education and related services.

The requirements for FAPE under IDEA are more detailed than those under Section 504. In specific instances detailed in the Section 504 regulation (for example, with respect to reevaluation procedures and the provision of an appropriate education), meeting the requirements of IDEA is one means of meeting the requirements of the Section 504 regulation.

IDEA requirements apply to states receiving financial assistance under IDEA. States must ensure that their political subdivisions that are responsible for providing or paying for the education of children with disabilities meet IDEA requirements. All states receive IDEA funds. Section 504 applies to any program or activity receiving ED financial assistance.

Section 40.6

Protection of Student Education under Section 504

This section includes text excerpted from "Protecting Students with Disabilities," U.S. Department of Education (ED), September 25, 2018.

Students Protected under Section 504

Section 504 covers qualified students with disabilities who attend schools receiving federal financial assistance. To be protected under Section 504, a student must be determined to:

1. Have a physical or mental impairment that substantially limits one or more major life activities; or

2. Have a record of such an impairment; or

3. Be regarded as having such an impairment.

Section 504 requires that school districts provide a free appropriate public education (FAPE) to qualified students in their jurisdictions who have a physical or mental impairment that substantially limits one or more major life activities.

What Is a Physical or Mental Impairment That Substantially Limits a Major Life Activity?

The determination of whether a student has a physical or mental impairment that substantially limits a major life activity must be made on the basis of an individual inquiry. The Section 504 regulatory provision at 34 C.F.R. 104.3(j)(2)(i) defines a physical or mental impairment as any physiological disorder or condition, cosmetic disfigurement, or anatomical loss affecting one or more of the following body systems: neurological; musculoskeletal; special sense organs; respiratory, including speech organs; cardiovascular; reproductive; digestive; genitourinary; hemic and lymphatic; skin; and endocrine; or any mental or psychological disorder, such as mental retardation, organic brain syndrome, emotional or mental illness, and specific learning disabilities. The regulatory provision does not set forth an exhaustive list of specific diseases and conditions that may constitute physical or mental impairments because of the difficulty of ensuring the comprehensiveness of such a list.

Major life activities, as defined in the Section 504 regulations at 34 C.F.R. 104.3(j)(2)(ii), include functions such as caring for one's self, performing manual tasks, walking, seeing, hearing, speaking, breathing, learning, and working. This list is not exhaustive. Other functions can be major life activities for purposes of Section 504. In the Amendments Act, Congress provided additional examples of general activities that are major life activities, including eating, sleeping, standing, lifting, bending, reading, concentrating, thinking, and communicating. Congress also provided a nonexhaustive list of examples of "major bodily functions" that are major life activities, such as the functions of the immune system, normal cell growth, digestive, bowel, bladder, neurological, brain, respiratory, circulatory, endocrine, and reproductive functions. The Section 504 regulatory provision, though not as comprehensive as the Amendments Act, is still valid—the Section 504 regulatory provision's list of examples of major life activities is not exclusive, and an activity or function not specifically listed in the Section 504 regulatory provision can nonetheless be a major life activity.

Does the Meaning of the Phrase "Qualified Student with a Disability" Differ on the Basis of a Student's Educational Level, i.e., Elementary and Secondary versus Postsecondary?

Yes. At the elementary and secondary educational level, a "qualified student with a disability" is a student with a disability who is: of an age at which students without disabilities are provided elementary and secondary educational services; of an age at which it is mandatory under state law to provide elementary and secondary educational services to students with disabilities; or a student to whom a state is required to provide a free appropriate public education under the Individuals with Disabilities Education Act (IDEA).

At the postsecondary educational level, a qualified student with a disability is a student with a disability who meets the academic and technical standards requisite for admission or participation in the institution's educational program or activity.

Does the Nature of Services to Which a Student Is Entitled under Section 504 Differ by Educational Level?

Yes. Public elementary and secondary recipients are required to provide a free appropriate public education to qualified students with

349

disabilities. Such an education consists of regular or special education and related aids and services designed to meet the individual educational needs of students with disabilities as adequately as the needs of students without disabilities are met.

At the postsecondary level, the recipient is required to provide students with appropriate academic adjustments and auxiliary aids and services that are necessary to afford an individual with a disability an equal opportunity to participate in a school's program. Recipients are not required to make adjustments or provide aids or services that would result in a fundamental alteration of a recipient's program or impose an undue burden.

Once a Student Is Identified as Eligible for Services under Section 504, Is That Student Always Entitled to Such Services?

Yes, as long as the student remains eligible. The protections of Section 504 extend only to individuals who meet the regulatory definition of a person with a disability. If a recipient school district reevaluates a student in accordance with the Section 504 regulatory provision at 34 C.F.R. 104.35 and determines that the student's mental or physical impairment no longer substantially limits his/her ability to learn or any other major life activity, the student is no longer eligible for services under Section 504.

Are Current Illegal Users of Drugs Excluded from Protection under Section 504?

Generally, yes. Section 504 excludes from the definition of a student with a disability, and from Section 504 protection, any student who is currently engaging in the illegal use of drugs when a covered entity acts on the basis of such use. (There are exceptions for persons in rehabilitation programs who are no longer engaging in the illegal use of drugs).

Are Current Users of Alcohol Excluded from Protection under Section 504?

No. Section 504's definition of a student with a disability does not exclude users of alcohol. However, Section 504 allows schools to take disciplinary action against students with disabilities using drugs or alcohol to the same extent as students without disabilities.

Evaluation

At the elementary and secondary school level, determining whether a child is a qualified disabled student under Section 504 begins with the evaluation process. Section 504 requires the use of evaluation procedures that ensure that children are not misclassified, unnecessarily labeled as having a disability, or incorrectly placed, based on inappropriate selection, administration, or interpretation of evaluation materials.

What Is an Appropriate Evaluation under Section 504?

Recipient school districts must establish standards and procedures for initial evaluations and periodic reevaluations of students who need or are believed to need special education and/or related services because of disability. The Section 504 regulatory provision at 34 C.F.R. 104.35(b) requires school districts to individually evaluate a student before classifying the student as having a disability or providing the student with special education. Tests used for this purpose must be selected and administered so as best to ensure that the test results accurately reflect the student's aptitude or achievement or other factor being measured rather than reflect the student's disability, except where those are the factors being measured. Section 504 also requires that tests and other evaluation materials include those tailored to evaluate the specific areas of educational need and not merely those designed to provide a single intelligence quotient. The tests and other evaluation materials must be validated for the specific purpose for which they are used and appropriately administered by trained personnel.

How Much Is Enough Information to Document That a Student Has a Disability?

At the elementary and secondary education level, the amount of information required is determined by the multidisciplinary committee (MDC) gathered to evaluate the student. The committee should include persons knowledgeable about the student, the meaning of the evaluation data, and the placement options. The committee members must determine if they have enough information to make a knowledgeable decision as to whether or not the student has a disability. The Section 504 regulatory provision at 34 C.F.R. 104.35(c) requires that school districts draw from a variety of sources in the evaluation process so that the possibility of error is minimized. The information

351

obtained from all such sources must be documented and all significant factors related to the student's learning process must be considered. These sources and factors may include aptitude and achievement tests, teacher recommendations, physical condition, social and cultural background, and adaptive behavior. In evaluating a student suspected of having a disability, it is unacceptable to rely on presumptions and stereotypes regarding persons with disabilities or classes of such persons. Compliance with the IDEA regarding the group of persons present when an evaluation or placement decision is made is satisfactory under Section 504.

What Process Should a School District Use to Identify Students Eligible for Services under Section 504? Is It the Same Process as That Employed in Identifying Students Eligible for Services under the IDEA?

School districts may use the same process to evaluate the needs of students under Section 504 as they use to evaluate the needs of students under the IDEA. If school districts choose to adopt a separate process for evaluating the needs of students under Section 504, they must follow the requirements for evaluation specified in the Section 504 regulatory provision at 34 C.F.R. 104.35.

May School Districts Consider "Mitigating Measures" Used by a Student in Determining Whether the Student Has a Disability under Section 504?

No. As of January 1, 2009, school districts, in determining whether a student has a physical or mental impairment that substantially limits that student in a major life activity, must not consider the ameliorating effects of any mitigating measures that student is using. This is a change from prior law. Before January 1, 2009, school districts had to consider a student's use of mitigating measures in determining whether that student had a physical or mental impairment that substantially limited that student in a major life activity. In the Amendments Act, however, Congress specified that the ameliorative effects of mitigating measures must not be considered in determining if a person is an individual with a disability.

Congress did not define the term "mitigating measures" but rather provided a nonexhaustive list of "mitigating measures." The mitigating measures are as follows: medication; medical supplies, equipment or appliances; low-vision devices (which do not include ordinary eyeglasses or contact lenses); prosthetics (including limbs and devices); hearing aids and cochlear implants or other implantable hearing devices; mobility devices; oxygen therapy equipment and supplies; use of assistive technology; reasonable accommodations or auxiliary aids or services; and learned behavioral or adaptive neurological modifications.

Congress created one exception to the mitigating measures analysis. The ameliorative effects of the mitigating measures of ordinary eyeglasses or contact lenses shall be considered in determining if an impairment substantially limits a major life activity. "Ordinary eyeglasses or contact lenses" are lenses that are intended to fully correct visual acuity or eliminate refractive error, whereas "low-vision devices" (listed above) are devices that magnify, enhance, or otherwise augment a visual image.

Does Office for Civil Rights (OCR) Endorse a Single Formula or Scale That Measures Substantial Limitation?

No. The determination of substantial limitation must be made on a case-by-case basis with respect to each individual student. The Section 504 regulatory provision at 34 C.F.R. 104.35 (c) requires that a group of knowledgeable persons draw upon information from a variety of sources in making this determination.

Are There Any Impairments Which Automatically Mean That a Student Has a Disability under Section 504?

No. An impairment in and of itself is not a disability. The impairment must substantially limit one or more major life activities in order to be considered a disability under Section 504.

Can a Medical Diagnosis Suffice as an Evaluation for the Purpose of Providing FAPE?

No. A physician's medical diagnosis may be considered among other sources in evaluating a student with an impairment or believed to have an impairment which substantially limits a major life activity. Other sources to be considered, along with the medical diagnosis, include aptitude and achievement tests, teacher recommendations, physical condition, social and cultural background, and adaptive behavior. The Section 504 regulations require school districts to draw upon a variety of sources in interpreting evaluation data and making placement decisions.

Does a Medical Diagnosis of an Illness Automatically Mean a Student Can Receive Services under Section 504?

No. A medical diagnosis of an illness does not automatically mean a student can receive services under Section 504. The illness must cause a substantial limitation on the student's ability to learn or another major life activity. For example, a student who has a physical or mental impairment would not be considered a student in need of services under Section 504 if the impairment does not in any way limit the student's ability to learn or other major life activity, or only results in some minor limitation in that regard.

How Should a Recipient School District Handle an outside Independent Evaluation? Do All Data Brought to a Multidisciplinary Committee Need to Be Considered and Given Equal Weight?

The results of an outside independent evaluation may be one of many sources to consider. Multidisciplinary committees must draw from a variety of sources in the evaluation process so that the possibility of error is minimized. All significant factors related to the subject student's learning process must be considered. These sources and factors include aptitude and achievement tests, teacher recommendations, physical condition, social and cultural background, and adaptive behavior, among others. Information from all sources must be documented and considered by knowledgeable committee members. The weight of the information is determined by the committee given the student's individual circumstances.

What Should a Recipient School District Do If a Parent Refuses to Consent to an Initial Evaluation under the Individuals with Disabilities Education Act, but Demands a Section 504 Plan for a Student without Further Evaluation?

A school district must evaluate a student prior to providing services under Section 504. Section 504 requires informed parental permission for initial evaluations. If a parent refuses consent for an initial evaluation and a recipient school district suspects a student has a disability, the IDEA and Section 504 provide that school districts may use due process hearing procedures to seek to override the parents' denial of consent.

Who in the Evaluation Process Makes the Ultimate Decision Regarding a Student's Eligibility for Services under Section 504?

The Section 504 regulatory provision at 34 C.F.R.104.35 (c) (3) requires that school districts ensure that the determination that a student is eligible for special education and/or related aids and services be made by a group of persons, including persons knowledgeable about the meaning of the evaluation data and knowledgeable about the placement options. If a parent disagrees with the determination, she or he may request a due process hearing.

Once a Student Is Identified as Eligible for Services under Section 504, Is There an Annual or Triennial Review Requirement? If So, What Is the Appropriate Process to Be Used? or Is It Appropriate to Keep the Same Section 504 Plan in Place Indefinitely after a Student Has Been Identified?

Periodic reevaluation is required. This may be conducted in accordance with the IDEA regulations, which require reevaluation at three-year intervals (unless the parent and public agency agree that reevaluation is unnecessary) or more frequently if conditions warrant, or if the child's parent or teacher requests a reevaluation, but not more than once a year (unless the parent and public agency agree otherwise).

Is a Section 504 Reevaluation Similar to an IDEA Reevaluation? How Often Should It Be Done?

Yes. Section 504 specifies that reevaluations in accordance with the IDEA is one means of compliance with Section 504. The Section 504 regulations require that reevaluations be conducted periodically. Section 504 also requires a school district to conduct a reevaluation prior to a significant change of placement. OCR considers an exclusion from the educational program of more than 10 school days a significant change of placement. OCR would also consider transferring a student from one type of program to another or terminating or significantly reducing a related service a significant change in placement.

What Is Reasonable Justification for Referring a Student for Evaluation for Services under Section 504?

School districts may always use regular education intervention strategies to assist students with difficulties in school. Section 504 requires recipient school districts to refer a student for an evaluation for possible special education or related aids and services or modification to regular education if the student, because of disability, needs or is believed to need such services.

A Student Is Receiving Services That the School District Maintains Are Necessary under Section 504 in Order to Provide the Student with an Appropriate Education. the Student's Parent No Longer Wants the Student to Receive Those Services. If the Parent Wishes to Withdraw the Student from a Section 504 Plan, What Can the School District Do to Ensure Continuation of Services?

The school district may initiate a Section 504 due process hearing to resolve the dispute if the district believes the student needs the services in order to receive an appropriate education.

A Student Has a Disability Referenced in the IDEA, but Does Not Require Special Education Services. Is Such a Student Eligible for Services under Section 504?

The student may be eligible for services under Section 504. The school district must determine whether the student has an impairment which substantially limits his or her ability to learn or another major life activity and, if so, make an individualized determination of the child's educational needs for regular or special education or related aids or services. For example, such a student may receive adjustments in the regular classroom.

How Should a Recipient School District View a Temporary Impairment?

A temporary impairment does not constitute a disability for purposes of Section 504 unless its severity is such that it results in a substantial limitation of one or more major life activities for an extended period of time. The issue of whether a temporary impairment is substantial enough to be a disability must be resolved on a case-by-case basis, taking into consideration both the duration (or expected duration) of the impairment and the extent to which it actually limits a major life activity of the affected individual.

In the Amendments Act, Congress clarified that an individual is not "regarded as" an individual with a disability if the impairment is transitory and minor. A transitory impairment is an impairment with an actual or expected duration of 6 months or less.

Is an Impairment That Is Episodic or in Remission a Disability under Section 504?

Yes, under certain circumstances. In the Amendments Act, Congress clarified that an impairment that is episodic or in remission is a disability if it would substantially limit a major life activity when active. A student with such an impairment is entitled to a free appropriate public education under Section 504.

Section 40.7

Including Children with ASD in Regular Classrooms

This section includes text excerpted from "IDEA Series: The Segregation of Students with Disabilities," National Council on Disability (NCD), February 7, 2018.

The legal and scientific basis for special education services points to the positive outcomes for students with disabilities when they receive an inclusive versus segregated education. Yet nationally, students with disabilities, in particular students of color and students in urban settings, as well as students with specific disability labels (such as autism or intellectual disability), continue to be removed from general education, instructional, and social opportunities and to be segregated disproportionately when compared to White students who live in suburban and rural areas and those who have less intensive academic support needs.

Key Findings

For this report, national student placement patterns, as well as federal and state policies, were reviewed to understand the state of special education service delivery and administrative guidance. This was supplemented by a review of research and input from families and educators about their experiences in educating students with disabilities. It's found that, although states are required to first consider that a student with a disability should attend the school that they would attend if they did not have a disability and only if the student's needs cannot be met, this consideration was not always present. States are expected to only remove the student to the extent needed to implement the student's individual plan and meet individually designed goals. Further, research demonstrates that inclusive education results in the best learning outcomes; there is no research that supports the value of a segregated special education class and school. The emerging picture, however, is one in which the opportunity for students to participate in their neighborhood school alongside their peers without disabilities is influenced more by the zip code in which they live, their race, and disability label, than by meeting the federal law defining how student placements should be made. While there are states and examples of schools that are indeed meeting the learning needs of students—even those with extensive support needs—that is more the exception than the rule. While the federal government monitors and reviews state performance on a number of indicators, including placement practices, there do not appear to be sanctions or strong guidance that directs states to attend to this concern.

Key Recommendations

It is recommended that Congress support full funding for special education, and that any funding authorized by Congress emphasize the delivery of special education services in general education settings. Further, discretionary grants for research and development should establish expectations for inclusive school practices, particularly those that address personnel development and organizational changes to sustain effective education services that address the needs of all students in an equitable manner to achieve equitable outcomes. This report also recommends that the U.S. Department of Education (ED) stand boldly in its support of inclusive education, and maintain data collection on the amount of time students spend in general education and the location of student placements. Funding opportunities for national centers and significant projects should ensure that recipients plan to:

- prepare teachers, administrators, and related service providers to implement effective schoolwide, equity-based educational services; and

- build state and local capacity for sustainable inclusive education practices. States should be expected to carefully analyze their placement data, and consider it with respect to disproportionate placement practices for students by disability label and race, across their local jurisdictions.

Benefits to Students with Disabilities

Data shows us that when students are included, they have more access to the general curriculum and effective instruction, achieve at higher rates of academic performance, and acquire better social and behavioral outcomes. In addition, when educated in inclusive classrooms, peers without disabilities experience either a positive academic and social impact or at least no negative impact on academic achievement. Since 1990, research studies have demonstrated a variety of benefits for students with intellectual and developmental disabilities who are educated in general education classes. Membership and participation benefits include increased student engagement, improved communication, improved expressive language and literacy skills, more satisfying and diverse friendships, higher levels of social engagement with peers without disabilities, less disruptive behavior, and more social competence. The National Longitudinal Transition Study (NLTS) examined the outcomes of 11,000 students with a range of disabilities, and found that more time spent in a general education classroom was positively correlated with (a) fewer absences from school, (b) fewer referrals for disruptive behavior, and (c) better outcomes after high school in the areas of employment and independent living. Although students with extensive support needs (i.e., students with intellectual disabilities, multiple disabilities, autism) have higher rates of segregated schooling, research shows that these students actually acquire more academic benefits when included in general education instruction, particularly increases in literacy skills. Hehir et al. describe several studies that demonstrate significant improvement for students with disabilities who require extensive supports in the areas of language and math who spent a larger portion of their day in general education classes with peers without disabilities—compared to those who spent a smaller proportion of their school day with peers without disabilities in general education classes.

Benefits to Students without Disabilities

A large-scale study by Waldron, Cole, and Majd demonstrated that students without disabilities made comparable or greater gains in math and reading when taught in general education classes with students who had learning disabilities and were engaged in the same instruction; a few other studies also found a positive impact on the academic achievement of peers without disabilities when students with and without disabilities are taught together. A review of international research discovered that the vast majority of studies conducted in the United States, Australia, Canada, and Ireland demonstrated either a positive effect or no negative effect on the academic, social, and personal development of students without disabilities when they were educated with peers who had intellectual, learning, or other disabilities.

Other benefits to students without disabilities who learn in general education classes with students who need extensive supports include reduced fear of human differences, increased comfort and awareness of differences, growth in social cognition, improvements in self-concept, growth of ethical principles, and caring friendships. Teachers, parents, and para-educators also believe that students without disabilities benefit when educated with peers who have extensive support needs by developing greater empathy, greater awareness and tolerance of differences, learning to help others, and acquiring specific skills (e.g., sign language).

Opportunity to Learn: Special versus Regular Classes

Early studies, such as those described by Helmstetter et al., found that teachers in general education classes offer more instruction, a comparable amount of 1:1 instructional time, more academic content, and are more likely to use peers without disabilities to support instruction than teachers in special education classes. When comparing special versus regular education classes, they found significant differences in the amount of time spent in noninstructional activity: in special education classes, 58 percent of the time was not devoted to instruction, in contrast with only 35 percent of noninstructional time in general education classes. Along these lines, Soukup, Wehmeyer, Bashinski, and Boyaird found that students who spent a greater amount of time in the general education classroom worked more of the time on grade-level standards and were more likely to have higher access to the general curriculum than students with low general education participation rates.

In an analysis of self-contained classes, Kurth, Born, and Love examined special education classes that were spacious, well staffed by educators and paraprofessionals, and supplied with adequate resources. Despite these supports and resources, they found a remarkable lack of time that students spent in instruction, and the instruction that did occur was provided primarily by paraprofessionals. There were few opportunities for students to respond to instructional cues, a high level of distractions in the classroom, a lack of communication supports for students, and a lack of individualization of instruction.

In contrast, McDonnell, Thorson, and McQuivey compared the instructional contexts for students with and without disabilities in general education setting. They found that in general education settings, students with disabilities were 13 times more likely than their peers without disabilities to receive instruction directed exclusively toward them during whole-class activities, and 23 times more likely to receive 1:1 instruction when educated in general education classes. Research consistently paints a picture that depicts students with disabilities who are educated in segregated special education placements as receiving less instruction, having fewer opportunities to learn, and fewer opportunities to use knowledge and skills during instruction and other meaningful activities.

Chapter 41

Classroom Management for Students with Autism Spectrum Disorders

Managing a classroom for students with autism spectrum disorders (ASDs) creates some challenges for teachers. Traditional classroom-management techniques such as structure, routines, rules, and lesson plans may need to be adjusted to meet the students' needs and accommodate the additional staff members who will provide collaborative instruction and programming for the students. In addition, teachers may need to implement nontraditional techniques such as visual aids, behavior plans, and data-collection systems in a classroom with students on the autism spectrum. Every child with ASD is unique, however, so classroom management should be handled on a case-by-case basis depending on the student's level of functioning and behavioral characteristics.

The following general strategies may be helpful in creating classroom-management systems that maximize instruction and learning and minimize chaos and confusion:

"Classroom Management for Students with ASD," © 2016 Omnigraphics. Reviewed October 2018.

Staff Collaboration

In the school setting, most students with ASD receive instruction and support from a team of staff members, including general education teachers, special education teachers, and paraprofessionals. Effective classroom management strategies can help coordinate the efforts of this team of educators and enable students with ASD to function better at school. Suggestions for improving staff collaboration include:

- Preparing a written plan for classroom roles and responsibilities, such as taking attendance, preparing for snack time, or leading the art lesson

- Displaying a job chart that outlines individual and shared tasks

- Assigning each staff member to specific students, activities, or areas of the classroom to eliminate confusion

- Matching staff strengths and interests with classroom activities

- Establishing a schedule for breaks and lunch hours to ensure that enough staff members are available during key periods

- Holding a weekly debriefing session to discuss the needs and issues of students, review teaching and communication strategies, and adjust classroom schedules and responsibilities

Structure and Schedules

Many children with ASD feel more comfortable and function more effectively in a structured, consistent classroom environment. Experts suggest establishing a daily routine that encourages independence. In the morning, for instance, the students' routine might include lining up, entering the classroom, greeting the teacher, hanging up their coats, unpacking their book bags, and taking their seats.

Students with ASD may also benefit from a customized daily schedule in visual form. This schedule would include such tasks and activities as independent work time, one-on-one instruction, fine motor skills development, sensory play, social skills instruction, and structured recreation activities. A personalized schedule can help reduce anxiety by letting students with ASD know what to expect.

Visual Strategies

There are many steps teachers can take in setting up the classroom environment to meet the needs of students with ASD. One recommended approach is to incorporate visual aids, which have been shown to help children with autism process information and learn more easily than oral or written instructions. Visual aids can be used to label areas of the classroom, post rules for appropriate behavior, or provide directions for activities. Pictures, symbols, and visual cues also play an important role in augmentative and alternative communication (AAC) techniques that can enhance learning for students with ASD.

Behavior Intervention Plans

Written behavior plans are another important element of classroom management for students with ASD. These plans should be developed in consultation with parents and shared with all members of the classroom staff so that everyone responds to targeted behavior in a consistent manner. Behavior plans should identify any inappropriate or challenging behaviors, designate preferred alternative behaviors, and list strategies for modifying the behaviors.

Accommodations for Sensory Issues

Many students with ASD experience problems with sensory processing. Each child's specific sensory issues should be identified and addressed as part of the classroom management system. Some possible accommodations to help children with sensory issues include:

- Providing inflatable seat cushions or pillows to enable them to move around while remaining seated

- Offering opportunities for movement, such as jumping on a mini-trampoline or chewing gum

- Eliminating flickering fluorescent lights and distracting sources of noise

- Allowing them to skip loud and crowded school assemblies or take a break if they feel overwhelmed

- Allowing them to eat lunch in a quiet room with a friend or a teacher rather than in a busy cafeteria

- Providing a quiet area for them to relax, listen to music, look out the window, or play with a toy for a few minutes to calm down and refocus

Data-Collection Systems

Finally, classroom management for students with ASD includes putting a system in place to measure and record the students' progress toward meeting the objectives in their Individualized Education Plans (IEP). All members of the classroom staff should be familiar with this data-collection system.

Reference

"Guidelines for Educating Students with Autism Spectrum Disorders," Virginia Department of Education (VDOE), October 2010.

Chapter 42

Social Interaction Education for Students with Autism Spectrum Disorders

Social interaction can be challenging for people with autism spectrum disorders (ASDs). Programs designed to help children with autism develop social skills and learn to interact with other children are an increasingly common component of special education services. Studies have shown that students with ASD who participate in social interaction education programs with typically developing classmates experience significant improvements in language, appropriate conversation, social skills, and classroom behavior. These programs also offer benefits to typically developing children in terms of promoting acceptance and positive attitudes toward people with disabilities.

Designing an Effective Program

To increase the likelihood of successful outcomes, programs for facilitating social interaction between typically developing children and children with autism should be tailored to the individual students, settings, and circumstances involved. Since not all children are well suited for involvement in these programs, the participants must be

---

selected carefully. The students with autism should have enough communication skills to follow simple directions and use two- to three-word phrases. The socially competent children should be open to involvement in the program, possess good role-model qualities, and demonstrate an ability to interact positively with students with autism.

Prior to launching the social interaction program, the typically developing students should be educated about the characteristics and behaviors of children with autism. For instance, they might watch a child-friendly video that explains ways to help and support classmates with autism. Promoting an understanding of autism helps general education students approach interactions with greater confidence and a positive attitude. For the children with ASD, any aggressive or challenging behaviors should be brought under control prior to participation in the social interaction program. Typically developing children are unlikely to be willing to interact with children who hit them, scream at them, or exhibit other disruptive behaviors.

Although the general education students should be encouraged to be accepting, responsive, and patient toward their peers with autism, none of the children should be pressured to form intimate friendships. The foundations of such relationships—including mutual interests and compatibility—may not be present in associations between children with and without autism, and it is important for the expectations of the social interaction program to be realistic.

Some additional suggestions to help develop an effective social interaction education program include the following:

- Encourage social interactions in settings where they are most likely to occur naturally, such as an integrated classroom, playground, or lunchroom.

- Allow the students to interact during regular daily activities when classmates would ordinarily be talking with one another.

- Incorporate items and materials that have natural interactive qualities, such as building toys or collaborative art projects.

- Include visual aids to serve as prompts. In a sharing activity, for instance, students could use a small sign with a picture and the phrase "May I have it?"

- Break down social interaction skills into component parts, and help the student with autism master each task before working on the entire skill.

- Prioritize skills that have the greatest potential impact and can be used with a variety of people and situations.

- Review and practice skills even after the child with ASD has mastered them in order to avoid their forgetting and needing additional instruction.

- Generalize skills learned in a specific setting or under certain conditions so that they can be practiced and used with other people and in other environments.

- Emphasize the quality of social interactions over the frequency or duration. A long, rehearsed response is less meaningful than a short, spontaneous request or comment.

- Provide ongoing instruction, feedback, and supervision of the social interactions.

- Collect and analyze data on social interactions between students with and without autism in both structured and unstructured settings to decide whether the program is effective or may need modification.

References

1. "Considerations for Social Interaction with Autistic Students," TeacherVision, 2016.

2. "Social Training with Peers Helps Kids with Autism," Autism Speaks, April 8, 2015.

Chapter 43

Secondary School Experiences of Students with Autism Spectrum Disorders

This chapter provides a description of students' secondary school experiences and does not address questions regarding the appropriateness of particular experiences or school practices for students with autism nor is there an intention to imply causality from the data presented in this chapter.

Secondary school students with autism take a range of courses in a given semester, with many taking academic, vocational, and other types of courses, such as life skills. Most take classes in both general and special education settings, although they are more likely to take courses in a special than a general education setting.

The curriculum used to instruct the majority of students with autism who are in general education academic classes often is modified to some degree. Reports of most other teacher-directed aspects of the class, such as instructional groupings, materials used, and

This chapter includes text excerpted from "Secondary School Experiences of Students with Autism," Institute of Education Sciences (IES), U.S. Department of Education (ED), April 2007. Reviewed October 2018.

instructional experiences outside the classroom, are largely the same for students with autism as for their classmates.

This similarity of teacher-directed experiences of students with autism and their peers in general education academic classes contrasts sharply with the differences between the groups in their participation in those classes. Students with autism are consistently reported to be less likely to participate in their general education academic classes than are their classmates.

In addition to academic subjects in general education settings, students with autism take general education vocational classes. Similar to experiences in general education academic courses, many students with autism in general education vocational classes experience the same instructional practices as the class as a whole.

Almost 9 in 10 secondary students with autism take at least one nonvocational special education course in a semester. The use of a general education curriculum without modification is rare in such classes; the large majority of students with autism receive a curriculum with some degree of modification or specialization, or they have no curriculum at all. Students are more likely to receive individual or small group instruction in special education than in general education classes. A variety of instructional materials and equipment are used in nonvocational special education classes, augmented by instructional activities that occur outside the classroom. More than half of those with autism participate in class discussions, respond orally to questions, and work with a peer or group at least sometimes in their nonvocational special education courses.

Almost all secondary students with autism are reported to receive some type of accommodation, modification, support, technology aid, or related service. Additional time to complete assignments and tests and modified tests and assignments are among the more frequent types of accommodations. Instructional support often is provided through monitoring of students' progress by special education teachers and individual help from teacher aides, instructional assistants, or personal aides. Technology aids are less frequently provided than other types of supports and services. In addition to the accommodations and supports they receive in their classes, students with autism receive a variety of related services, addressing a wide range of needs and functional issues. Speech-language pathology services are the most frequently received type of service. Almost half of the secondary students with autism have a case manager provided from or through their school to help coordinate and oversee services.

Chapter 44

Preparing for Postsecondary Education

More and more high-school students with disabilities are planning to continue their education in postsecondary schools, including vocational and career schools, two- and four- year colleges, and universities. As a student with a disability, you need to be well informed about your rights and responsibilities as well as the responsibilities postsecondary schools have toward you. Being well informed will help ensure you have a full opportunity to enjoy the benefits of the postsecondary education experience without confusion or delay.

The information in this chapter, provided by the Office for Civil Rights (OCR) in the U.S. Department of Education (ED), explains the rights and responsibilities of students with disabilities who are preparing to attend postsecondary schools. This chapter also explains the obligations of a postsecondary school to provide academic adjustments, including auxiliary aids and services, to ensure the school does not discriminate on the basis of disability.

OCR enforces Section 504 of the Rehabilitation Act of 1973 (Section 504) and Title II of the Americans with Disabilities Act of 1990 (ADA) (Title II), which prohibit discrimination on the basis of disability. Practically every school district and postsecondary school in the

This chapter includes text excerpted from "Students with Disabilities Preparing for Postsecondary Education," U.S. Department of Education (ED), September 2011. Reviewed October 2018.

United States is subject to one or both of these laws, which have similar requirements.*

Although Section 504 and Title II apply to both school districts and postsecondary schools, the responsibilities of postsecondary schools differ significantly from those of school districts.

Moreover, you will have responsibilities as a postsecondary student that you do not have as a high school student. OCR strongly encourages you to know your responsibilities and those of postsecondary schools under Section 504 and Title II. Doing so will improve your opportunity to succeed as you enter postsecondary education.

The following questions and answers provide more specific information to help you succeed.

As a Student with a Disability Leaving High School and Entering Postsecondary Education, Will I See Differences in My Rights and How They Are Addressed?

Yes. Section 504 and Title II protect elementary, secondary, and postsecondary students from discrimination. Nevertheless, several of the requirements that apply through high school are different from the requirements that apply beyond high school. For instance, Section 504 requires a school district to provide a free appropriate public education (FAPE) to each child with a disability in the district's jurisdiction. Whatever the disability, a school district must identify an individual's educational needs and provide any regular or special education and related aids and services necessary to meet those needs as well as it is meeting the needs of students without disabilities.

Unlike your high school, however, your postsecondary school is not required to provide FAPE. Rather, your postsecondary school is required to provide appropriate academic adjustments as necessary to ensure that it does not discriminate on the basis of disability. In addition, if your postsecondary school provides housing to nondisabled students, it must provide comparable, convenient, and accessible housing to students with disabilities at the same cost.

* *You may be familiar with another federal law that applies to the education of students with disabilities—the Individuals with Disabilities Education Act (IDEA). That law is administered by the Office of Special Education Programs (OSEP) in the Office of Special Education and Rehabilitative Services (OSERS) in the U.S. Department of Education (ED). The IDEA and its individualized education program (IEP) provisions do not apply to postsecondary schools.*

Other important differences that you need to know, even before you arrive at your postsecondary school, are addressed in the remaining questions.

May a Postsecondary School Deny My Admission Because I Have a Disability?

No. If you meet the essential requirements for admission, a postsecondary school may not deny your admission simply because you have a disability.

Do I Have to Inform a Postsecondary School That I Have a Disability?

No. But if you want the school to provide an academic adjustment, you must identify yourself as having a disability. Likewise, you should let the school know about your disability if you want to ensure that you are assigned to accessible facilities. In any event, your disclosure of a disability is always voluntary.

What Academic Adjustments Must a Postsecondary School Provide?

The appropriate academic adjustment must be determined based on your disability and individual needs. Academic adjustments may include auxiliary aids and services, as well as modifications to academic requirements as necessary to ensure equal educational opportunity. Examples of adjustments are: arranging for priority registration; reducing a course load; substituting one course for another; providing note takers, recording devices, sign language interpreters, extended time for testing, and, if telephones are provided in dorm rooms, a teletypewriter (TTY) in your dorm room; and equipping school computers with screen-reading, voice recognition, or other adaptive software or hardware.

In providing an academic adjustment, your postsecondary school is not required to lower or substantially modify essential requirements. For example, although your school may be required to provide extended testing time, it is not required to change the substantive content of the test. In addition, your postsecondary school does not have to make adjustments that would fundamentally alter the nature of a service, program, or activity, or that would result in an undue financial or administrative burden. Finally, your postsecondary school does not have to provide personal attendants, individually prescribed devices, readers for personal use or study, or other devices or services of a personal nature, such as tutoring and typing.

If I Want an Academic Adjustment, What Must I Do?

You must inform the school that you have a disability and need an academic adjustment. Unlike your school district, your postsecondary school is not required to identify you as having a disability or to assess your needs.

Your postsecondary school may require you to follow reasonable procedures to request an academic adjustment. You are responsible for knowing and following those procedures. In their publications providing general information, postsecondary schools usually include information on the procedures and contacts for requesting an academic adjustment. Such publications include recruitment materials, catalogs, and student handbooks, and are often available on school websites. Many schools also have staff whose purpose is to assist students with disabilities. If you are unable to locate the procedures, ask a school official, such as an admissions officer or counselor.

When Should I Request an Academic Adjustment?

Although you may request an academic adjustment from your postsecondary school at any time, you should request it as early as possible. Some academic adjustments may take more time to provide than others. You should follow your school's procedures to ensure that the school has enough time to review your request and provide an appropriate academic adjustment.

Do I Have to Prove That I Have a Disability to Obtain an Academic Adjustment?

Generally, yes. Your school will probably require you to provide documentation showing that you have a current disability and need an academic adjustment.

What Documentation Should I Provide?

Schools may set reasonable standards for documentation. Some schools require more documentation than others. They may require you to provide documentation prepared by an appropriate professional, such as a medical doctor, psychologist, or other qualified diagnostician. The required documentation may include one or more of the following: a diagnosis of your current disability, as well as supporting information, such as the date of the diagnosis, how that diagnosis was reached, and the credentials of the diagnosing professional; information on how your disability affects a major life activity; and information on how the disability affects your academic performance. The documentation should provide enough information for you and your school to decide what is an appropriate academic adjustment.

An individualized education program (IEP) or Section 504 plan, if you have one, may help identify services that have been effective for you. This is generally not sufficient documentation, however, because of the differences between postsecondary education and high school education. What you need to meet the new demands of postsecondary education may be different from what worked for you in high school. Also, in some cases, the nature of a disability may change.

If the documentation that you have does not meet the postsecondary school's requirements, a school official should tell you in a timely manner what additional documentation you need to provide. You may need a new evaluation in order to provide the required documentation.

Who Has to Pay for a New Evaluation?

Neither your high school nor your postsecondary school is required to conduct or pay for a new evaluation to document your disability and need for an academic adjustment. You may, therefore, have to pay or find funding to pay an appropriate professional for an evaluation. If you are eligible for services through your state vocational rehabilitation agency, you may qualify for an evaluation at no cost to you. You may locate your state vocational rehabilitation agency at rsa.ed.gov by clicking on "Info about RSA," then "People and Offices," and then "State Agencies/Contacts."

Once the School Has Received the Necessary Documentation from Me, What Should I Expect?

To determine an appropriate academic adjustment, the school will review your request in light of the essential requirements for the relevant program. It is important to remember that the school is not required to lower or waive essential requirements. If you have requested a specific academic adjustment, the school may offer that academic adjustment, or it may offer an effective alternative. The school may also conduct its own evaluation of your disability and needs at its own expense.

You should expect your school to work with you in an interactive process to identify an appropriate academic adjustment. Unlike the experience you may have had in high school, however, do not expect your postsecondary school to invite your parents to participate in the process or to develop an Individualized Education Program (IEP) for you.

What If the Academic Adjustment We Identified Is Not Working?

Let the school know as soon as you become aware that the results are not what you expected. It may be too late to correct the problem if you wait until the course or activity is completed. You and your school should work together to resolve the problem.

May a Postsecondary School Charge Me for Providing an Academic Adjustment?

No. Nor may it charge students with disabilities more for participating in its programs or activities than it charges students who do not have disabilities.

What Can I Do If I Believe the School Is Discriminating against Me?

Practically every postsecondary school must have a person—frequently called the Section 504 Coordinator, ADA Coordinator, or Disability Services Coordinator—who coordinates the school's compliance with Section 504, Title II, or both laws. You may contact that person for information about how to address your concerns.

The school must also have grievance procedures. These procedures are not the same as the due process procedures with which you may be familiar from high school. But the postsecondary school's grievance procedures must include steps to ensure that you may raise your concerns fully and fairly, and must provide for the prompt and equitable resolution of complaints.

School publications, such as student handbooks and catalogs, usually describe the steps that you must take to start the grievance process. Often, schools have both formal and informal processes. If you decide to use a grievance process, you should be prepared to present all the reasons that support your request.

If you are dissatisfied with the outcome of the school's grievance procedures or wish to pursue an alternative to using those procedures, you may file a complaint against the school with OCR or in a court.

Students with disabilities who know their rights and responsibilities are much better equipped to succeed in postsecondary school. ED encourages you to work with the staff at your school because they, too, want you to succeed. Seek the support of family, friends, and fellow students, including those with disabilities. Know your talents and capitalize on them, and believe in yourself as you embrace new challenges in your education.

Part Seven

Living with Autism Spectrum Disorder and Transitioning to Adulthood

Chapter 45

Managing Challenging Autism Spectrum Disorders Behaviors

Most people with autism spectrum disorders (ASDs) will display challenging behaviors at times. Common types of challenging behaviors that may occur with autism include physical or verbal aggression, disruption, noncompliance, tantrums, self-injury, destruction of property, obsessions or compulsions, repetitive rituals, sexual inappropriateness, and eloping (running away from home, school, or another safe place). Although autism does not cause challenging behaviors directly, the core symptoms of ASD—including difficulties with social interaction, verbal and nonverbal communication, sensory processing, and motor skills—can create feelings of confusion, frustration, anxiety, and lack of control that may result in challenging behaviors.

Researchers believe that some challenging behaviors with autism are biologically driven and may involve impulses or reflexes that are beyond the person's control. But some people with ASD may use challenging behavior as a form of communication to express their needs or concerns. The key to understanding challenging behavior is to determine its purpose or function. Some of the common functions of challenging behavior in people with ASD include escaping from a situation, avoiding a task, getting attention, obtaining an object, gaining control over an environment, responding to pain or discomfort, or attempting to calm down or self-regulate.

Although some behaviors may be biologically driven, much behavior is learned over time and shaped by experiences. As a result, parents, teachers, and medical professionals who work with people with ASD can often employ positive interventions to change challenging behavior into appropriate behavior. The response to challenging behavior can have a significant impact on how the person with ASD behaves upon encountering a similar situation in the future. Specialized approaches aimed at improving challenging behavior are often aimed at helping a person with ASD recognize their own environmental triggers, communicate their needs in a more acceptable manner, and develop self-regulation abilities.

Addressing Challenging Behaviors

It is vital to address challenging behaviors as soon as possible to prevent them from getting worse and to ensure a good quality of life for the individual with ASD and his or her family. Effective function-based behavior interventions should be positive, consistent, and continued even after the challenging behavior begins to abate. Reshaping challenging behaviors into appropriate adaptive behaviors requires commitment, because any subtle adjustments that caregivers make to accommodate the problem behaviors can accumulate over time and make the behaviors harder to change. Even if certain behaviors mostly seem annoying rather than truly problematic, they can still create tension at home, at school, and in the community if they are allowed to become more pronounced or frequent over time.

Challenging behaviors can make life more difficult for the person with ASD and his or her family. They can prevent the person from taking advantage of opportunities for growth and development, such as play dates, recreational activities, and job options. They can also affect the person's health and well-being by causing physical pain or injury and creating psychological stress, anxiety, or depression. They can impair social relationships with family members, friends, and classmates, and they can disrupt academic learning as well as long-term employability.

For parents, teachers, and caregivers of people with ASD, challenging behaviors can increase stress, worry, anxiety, and depression. They can also create fear of harm or physical danger, as well as lead to embarrassment, withdrawal, and social isolation. Challenging behaviors can also create financial hardships by forcing a parent to stop working, causing damage to property, or generating medical bills. For all of these reasons, it is vital to address challenging behaviors with positive interventions.

Building a Support Team

To determine the function of a challenging behavior and design an effective intervention, a team approach is needed. Ideally, the support team should include the person with autism, their parents or caregivers, a case manager from a school or state service agency, and a pediatrician or primary-care physician who has a relationship with the family. The doctor may wish to include additional specialists or therapists—such as an audiologist, gastroenterologist, allergist, nutritionist, or immunologist—on the team to focus on specific areas of concern. The support team should also include:

- A Board Certified Behavior Analyst (BCBA) with expertise in understanding, evaluating, and developing support strategies to address challenging behaviors. These providers use applied behavior analysis techniques to determine the environmental factors that precipitate the behavior and develop positive reinforcement strategies to reshape the behavior.

- A psychologist or psychiatrist to evaluate emotional and mental-health concerns and provide training and supports for the person with ASD and their family.

- A speech-language pathologist (SLP) to evaluate the communication abilities and deficits of the person with ASD and help them develop functional communication skills.

- A physical therapist or occupational therapist to evaluate motor skills, sensory processing differences, and other physical concerns and develop interventions and coping strategies to help an individual with ASD feel more comfortable in their surroundings.

Combining the different perspectives of these professionals can enable parents or caregivers to create a positive behavior intervention plan that addresses physical, mental, and learning concerns in order to help the person with ASD adapt more successfully.

Strategies for Positive Behavior Intervention

The essential elements of an effective behavior intervention plan include clarity, consistency, simplicity, and continuation even as the behavior improves. Research has shown that positive behavior supports, rather than punishment (which can actually increase aggression and strain the relationship with the caregiver), are most helpful in teaching appropriate behaviors and self-regulation skills. Since many skills take time to develop, changes in behavior may take time as well. In fact, challenging behavior may get worse or more frequent before it gets better. Experts recommend setting priorities and starting with the most dangerous behaviors first. They also suggest setting realistic goals and starting with small steps that grow larger over time.

Positive behavior supports are intended to increase desirable behaviors, instill a sense of what is expected, and build a sense of pride and personal responsibility in the person with ASD. Some tips include providing positive feedback, celebrating successes, and validating concerns. Experts also suggest providing clear expectations, ignoring the challenging behavior when it occurs, and rewarding desired behavior and instances of self-control. Finally, it may be helpful to allow the person with ASD to take breaks, offer them a safe place to calm down and refocus, and provide accommodations as needed.

Making changes to the environment can also help eliminate challenging behavior and promote desired behavior. If places, situations, or relationships seem to promote good behavior, it may be helpful to expand access to them. On the other hand, it is a good idea to avoid situations and places that seem to increase frustration and anxiety and trigger challenging behavior. Creating a more successful environment for people with ASD also involves providing structure and routines, using visual supports, eliminating distractions or upsetting stimuli, and providing an escape from crowded or noisy activities.

Managing a Crisis Situation

In a crisis situation, when a person with ASD is behaving aggressively or destructively, it is usually not possible to reason with them or teach them appropriate alternative behaviors. Instead, the focus of parents and other caregivers needs to be on ensuring the safety of the person with ASD, as well as protecting other people and personal property. It may be helpful to develop a crisis-management plan to help anticipate troubling situations, prevent them from escalating, and keep everyone involved safe.

Strategies for managing a behavioral crisis and staying safe include identifying triggers, developing tools for ensuring safety in various settings, establishing procedures for de-escalation, and collecting data to evaluate and revamp the plan. If the situation becomes dangerous for the individual with ASD or others, it may be helpful to know the location of the nearest emergency room or facility for hospitalization and treatment. If it becomes necessary to involve law enforcement, experts suggest preparing a card to hand out to police officers that provides information about autism and the person's specific behavior issues. Finally, for people with ASD who are over the age of eighteen, parents or caregivers should make sure that their crisis-management plan includes a document that secures guardianship in case they need to make medical decisions for them.

Long-Term Solutions

Although positive interventions can help individuals with autism learn the skills they need to succeed and thrive, sometimes challenging behaviors such as aggression or self-injury exceed the resources and support families are able to provide. Parents who are exhausted, discouraged, or afraid may not be well equipped to follow a positive behavioral intervention plan. In that case, parents and other caregivers may need to consider alternative solutions, such as placing the person with ASD in a residential setting where they can receive the support they need.

Reference

"Challenging Behaviors Tool Kit," Autism Speaks, 2016.

Chapter 46

Safety and Children with Disabilities

We all want to keep our children safe and secure and help them to be happy and healthy. Preventing injuries and harm is not very different for children with disabilities compared to children without disabilities. However, finding the right information and learning about the kinds of risks children might face at different ages is often not easy for parents of children with disabilities. Each child is different—and the general recommendations that are available to keep children safe should be tailored to fit your child's skills and abilities.

There are steps that parents and caregivers can take to keep children with disabilities safe.

To keep all children safe, parents and caregivers need to:

- know and learn about what things are unique concerns or a danger for their child

- plan ways to protect their child and share the plan with others

- remember that their child's needs for protection will change over time

What Parents and Caregivers Can Do

Parents or caregivers can talk to their child's doctor or healthcare professional about how to keep him or her safe. Your child's teacher

This chapter includes text excerpted from "Keeping Children with Disabilities Safe," Centers for Disease Control and Prevention (CDC), June 22, 2018.

or child care provider might also have some good ideas. Once you have ideas about keeping your child safe, make a safety plan and share it with your child and other adults who might be able to help if needed.

Here are some things to think about when making a safety plan for your child:

Moving Around and Handling Things

Does your child have challenges with moving around and handling things around them? Sometimes children are faced with unsafe situations, especially in new places. Children who have limited ability to move, see, hear, or make decisions, and children who do not feel or understand pain might not realize that something is unsafe, or might have trouble getting away.

Take a look around the place where your child will be to make sure every area your child can reach is safe for your child. Check your child's clothing and toys—are they suitable for his or her abilities, not just age and size? For example, clothing and toys that are meant for older children might have strings that are not safe for a child who cannot easily untangle themselves, or toys might have small parts that are not safe for children who are still mouthing toys.

Safety Equipment

Do you have the right kind of safety equipment? Safety equipment is often developed for age and size, and less for ability.

For example, a major cause of child death is motor vehicle crashes. Keeping your child safe in the car is important. When choosing the right car seat, you might need to consider whether your child has difficulties sitting up or sitting still in the seat, in addition to your child's age, height, and weight. If you have a child with disabilities, talk to your healthcare professional about the best type of car seat or booster seat and the proper seat position for your child. You can also ask a certified child passenger safety technician who is trained in special needs.

Other examples of special safety equipment:

- Life jackets may need to be specially fitted for your child.

- Smoke alarms that signal with a light and vibration may be better in a home where there is a child who cannot hear.

- Handrails and safety bars can be put into homes to help a child who has difficulty moving around or a child who is at risk for falling.

Speak to your healthcare professional about the right equipment for your child and have this equipment ready and available before you may need it.

Talking and Understanding

Does your child have problems with talking or understanding? Children who have problems communicating might have limited ability to learn about safety and danger.

For example, children who cannot hear might miss spoken instructions. Children who have trouble understanding or remembering might not learn about safety as easily as other children. Children who have a hard time communicating might not be able to ask questions about safety. Adults might think that children with disabilities are aware of dangers when they actually are not.

Parents and caregivers may need to find different ways to teach their children about safety, such as:

• Showing them what to do

• Using pretend play to rehearse

• Practicing on a regular basis

Parents and caregivers may need to find different ways to let their children communicate that they are in danger. For example, you might teach your child to use a whistle, bell, or alarm can alert others to danger. Tell adults who take care of your child about the ways to communicate with your child if there is any danger.

It's also useful to contact your local fire department and explain any special circumstances you have, so that they don't have to rely on the child or others to explain their special needs in case of an emergency.

Making Decisions

Does your child have problems with making decisions? Children might have limited ability to make decisions either because of developmental delays or limits in their thinking skills, or in their ability to stop themselves from doing things that they want, but should not do.

For example, children with attention deficit hyperactivity disorder (ADHD) or fetal alcohol spectrum disorders (FASDs) might be very impulsive and fail to think about the results of their actions. People often put more dangerous things higher up, so that little children cannot reach them. Your older child might be able to reach something that she or he is not ready to handle safely. Check your child's environment, particularly new places.

Some children might also have problems distinguishing when situations and people are safe or dangerous. They might not know what to do. Parents and caregivers can give children specific instructions on how to behave in certain situations that might become dangerous.

Moving and Exploring

Does your child have enough chances to move and explore? Children with disabilities often need some extra protection. But just like all children, they also need to move and explore so that they can develop healthy bodies and minds.

Some parents of children with special needs worry about their children needing extra protection. It is not possible to protect children from every bump and bruise. Exploring can help children learn what's safe and what might be difficult or dangerous. Being fit and healthy can help children stay safe, and an active lifestyle is important for long-term health.

Children with disabilities might find it hard to take part in sports and active play—for example, equipment may need to be adjusted, coaches may need extra information and support to help a child with a disability, or a communication problem may make it more difficult for some children to play as part of a team.

Talk to your child's teachers, potential coaches, care providers, or health professional about ways to find the right balance between being safe and being active.

Chapter 47

Home Modifications for People with Autism

If the home is to better support the life of an individual who experiences significant autism spectrum disorder (ASD), there are a few "must-haves." Each individual is unique, but environments where people experiencing autism can live, learn, work, and play successfully share many common characteristics. If you ask the right questions and get the fundamental patterns right, then the whole environment will work better for everyone. The home will be a safer place, the individual will have more opportunity and choice, other supports can be more effective, and the family can be more stable and resilient to other stresses.

Autism-Friendly Home: Reducing Risk and Anticipating Activities

Many people with ASD share common characteristics, including sensory and perception problems, organizational problems, communication issues, and impaired thinking abilities. Unfortunately, conventionally available home environments can be confusing, overstimulating, frightening, upsetting, or too restrictive for these individuals.

This chapter includes text excerpted from "Making Homes That Work—A Resource Guide for Families Living with Autism Spectrum Disorder + Co-Occurring Behaviors," U.S. Department of Health and Human Services (HHS), September 2, 2011. Reviewed October 2018.

An individual's preferred activities and their coping mechanisms can result in property damage, put people at risk, or irritate the neighbors. These become labeled "problem behaviors." The real problem is often the inadequacy of the house. Failures of the environment should not be presumed to be someone's fault.

Providing a home environment that anticipates common use patterns will result in a more ASD-friendly home that works and makes sense for the person with an ASD, reduces stress and workload, and improves health and safety. Every home is full of items that can hurt people. Ensuring the health and safety needs of a person with disability should, at a minimum, meet the life and health/safety requirements of modern building code. Look at individual circumstances and address any unique safety concerns.

Eliminate Obvious Hazards

- Secure toxins such as paints, solvents, fuels, chemicals, medications, or poisons such as insecticides, cleaning products, detergents, or bleach in closed and locked cabinets.

- Firearms and ammunition must be under lock and key.

- Install scald-prevention devices on tubs and in showers. Drowning is the most common form of accidental death among people with autism. Secure pools, hot tubs, fountains, ponds, or other potentially dangerous water hazards in or around your home with lockable covers or fences.

- Inspect your landscape and remove poisonous plants or other toxic materials from the yard.

- Remove or encapsulate any lead paint per local regulations. Install carbon dioxide and particle smoke detectors in bedrooms, hallways, and living spaces. Select units that give voice commands such as "Leave the Home" to help avoid confusion. Consider installing "rate of rise" detectors in kitchens and garages.

- Installing arc-fault and ground-fault electrical receptacles will reduce the risk of electrocution from misuse of outlets.

- Grab bars, furniture, exercise/adaptive equipment, swings, or other wall- or ceiling-mounted toys and/or devices need to be solidly attached to adequate backing or framing. When needed, fall protection should be installed.

Address Personal Risks and Dangers

Many individuals with ASD have co-occurring conditions that require specific environmental modifications. Do seizures happen? Does the person hurt themselves or others? Are there sensitivities to food or does the person have an eating disorder?

In general, it is a good idea to consider the following:

- As much as possible, protect the head from injury in the event of a seizure, fall, or predictably dangerous behavior.
- Drop seizures suggest the use of built-in or padded furnishings without sharp corners or hard edges.
- Round corners on walls and countertops.
- Pad headboards and bed frames if needed.
- Eliminate places where individuals can get their heads or bodies stuck (e.g., between the headboard and the mattress or the toilet and tub).
- Eliminate access to easily ingested nonnutritive or toxic substances.

Install Finishes That Are Easily Cleaned

Surfaces should be user-friendly and attractive, but nonabsorbent. When a person has open cuts, scrapes, blisters, or burns, there is a greater need to clean and disinfect surfaces and other materials on a daily basis.

Provide Control

Provide increased opportunity to regulate the quality of light and air. Individuals experiencing ASD are often very sensitive to drafts, temperature, and air quality. Zoned heating, ventilation, and air-conditioning (HVAC) systems, individual mini-units and high-quality air-filtration systems (HEPA filters) are options. Lighting can be fitted with dimmers and curtains are available to provide the full range of light control.

Anticipate Unconventional Use

The parts of the home that tend to be most frequently damaged and wear quickly are window coverings and drapes, floor coverings, wall and cabinet finishes, and hardware. Alternatives to conventional window furnishings include internal blinds, commercial breakaway curtains, or curtains Velcroed to the wall or looped over a reinforced rod. Flooring and other finish surfaces should be durable, smooth, and easy to clean.

Most homes have painted drywall surfaces with a lightly textured finish. These walls are easily damaged and difficult to clean repeatedly. If surface damage is occurring, use semi-gloss or graffiti-resistant paints. Epoxy paint is a good choice in wet areas or areas of extreme use, such as around beds, recreation areas, or transitions. Industrial-quality wall coverings may also work. These include vinyl, polyvinyl chloride (PVC), and wallpaper reinforced with Kevlar. Plastic electrical switch and outlet-cover plates are easily broken. Cover plates made from nylon or Lexan are more durable and not expensive.

Anticipate Water Play

Water is almost always a source of interest. Inside the home, select faucets that direct water into a basin and cannot be manipulated to redirect water onto the wall, floor, or countertop. If the individual enjoys playing with water, try to make that activity safe and nondamaging. The bathroom is an obvious location for water play, as is the kitchen. If outdoor water play with hoses or sprinklers is a preferred activity, the runoff and splashing will need to be managed to prevent damage and maintain safety.

For example, if a person is splashing in the sink or tub, make sure nearby areas are protected. A wet room with a floor drain and sealed surfaces will safely support most water play. The shower door and curtains should be solidly attached and the doors properly adjusted. Any joints should be caulked and maintained. Shower curtain rods need to be strong enough to bear weight and should be attached solidly to the wall. Velcro loops that hold the curtain in the rod can be easily reattached if pulled loose without damage.

Address Problem Doors

Swinging doors are frequently a problem. They can be slammed and if this happens repeatedly the hinges and door frame will break. They are a danger because a slamming door can hit people and pinch fingers. There are reasonable alternatives. Commercial-quality pocket doors and breakaway curtains are two of the best choices. Fiberglass bifold doors with appropriate high-quality hardware can also be considered.

If doors are subject to repeated slamming or attempts at forced entry, make sure the jamb, hinges, and stops are solidly attached to the wall's framing. Protect the wall from damage caused by the door knob. Bumpers attached to the door can reduce the noise of slamming, and smoke seals attached to the jamb can slow a closing door. A sweep attached to the bottom of the door that drags on the floor can work in many cases.

Select Appropriate Furnishings

Some individuals with autism like to spin, swing, rock, or bounce. Accommodate this interest outside by using swings and other moving equipment that they prefer. Whenever possible, provide cover from the weather to extend usable times. Equipment will need to be upgraded and changed as the individual grows and interests change. Providing opportunities indoors to enjoy this activity is more challenging. Ceiling-mounted swinging chairs, rope swings, rocking chairs, and gliders can accommodate this interest. When installing these items, place solid anchor points into framing when attaching to walls, floors, or ceilings. Use fasteners, safety chains, or straps that are rated for commercial use. Sports equipment such as high-jump mats can be made into couches with pillows and slipcovers.

Cloth-covered furniture and cushions are difficult to maintain and frequently become damaged or stained and absorb unpleasant odors. If furniture damage is an issue, use solid wood or plywood furniture glued, screwed, and/or bolted together. Construct furniture to be thoroughly cleanable and avoid having places where food can be trapped. Institutional-quality couches and chairs often address these concerns. Vinyl cushions or foam rubber covered in ballistic nylon, often used in boats and equipment seats, may prove appropriate in some cases.

Connected Home
Increasing Visibility and Connections

The overarching concern of families is the health and safety of their family member living with ASD. Fundamental to ensuring their safety is awareness of the person's whereabouts and the ability to monitor what they are doing. In many homes, this requires being with the person most of the time, or constantly checking in. The need for constant vigilance can be overwhelming and is a common cause of caregiver fatigue. Caregivers need to be able to see, hear, and monitor activities inside and outside the home. At the same time, healthy awareness means monitoring without controlling the individual's every move or watching every minute. Modifications should provide ways for you to be aware when they are venturing on. Families can relax when they know where their family member is and what they are up to. In most cases, this will mean providing a secure perimeter. In all cases there should be a definite boundary that everyone knows is the limit of safe activity.

Visibility and Openings between Rooms

It is common to find families struggling to overcome the visual barriers in the home. This is especially the case in older homes that were designed with many separate rooms. Interior windows or "re-lites," with tempered glass or even without glass, can help solve this. Where more direct connections are necessary, walls can be opened to create a series of visually and physically interconnected rooms. Pocket doors or curtains can provide separation when desired without losing floor space or having the safety hazards of swing doors.

Connections for Needed Caregiving

It is especially important to make good visual and acoustic connections if there are safety risks, seizures, or medical issues. In cases that require night-time monitoring or assistance, it can be helpful to locate the individual's bedroom adjacent to the parent's or caregiver's room, then make an opening directly between the two. Circulation patterns can be designed to allow the individual with ASD more independence during the day, while maintaining a direct visual, acoustic, and physical connection between rooms at night.

Using Technology to Monitor Safety

Alarms and sensors can improve a family's or caregiver's ability to monitor remotely. Door and window alarms are the most common strategy, and they are most useful for passively monitoring a person's whereabouts. Infrared or motion detectors can be used to track movement, which may be useful in supporting eating disorders, elopement, or problematic interactions with siblings. If it is necessary to monitor a physical condition such as seizures, you may want to install sensors in the bed or on the floor. Webcams, security cameras, and computer technology are often useful and even more appropriate outside. They can allow a person to be in the yard with less direct or even unnecessary supervision. In the house, cameras can be useful in situations in which there are significant or life-threatening health issues, but be careful not to rely too heavily on technology and cameras. Technology breaks and becomes obsolete. Ask yourself what information you need, and if there are simpler and less intrusive ways to gather it. A window cut in the wall that gives a view of the yard from the kitchen will always be reliable.

The Essential Bathroom
Solving the Most Common Challenge

Modifications to the bathroom are the most common need of families. It is safe to say that the more significant the autism experience, the more pressure and stress build up around bathroom mechanics. Balancing the activities that need to occur in the bathroom—such as toileting, bathing, and grooming—with recreational and therapeutic activities, such as water play or soaking, may be challenging. Bathrooms are subject to water damage, rot, and mold. Water also poses safety risks for slip and fall, drowning, and burns. Bathrooms can require certain protocols that don't always make sense for people with ASD. Over time, a list of autism-friendly bathroom modifications has been developed that comprise "The Essential Bathroom."

Enough Space

Cramped bathrooms can trigger defensiveness and discourage participation in toileting or bathing activities. In some cases, it is simply the constrained area of the toileting space that presents the barrier to use. Often there is a need to reorganize the bathroom or appropriate adjacent square footage so that the bathroom can be transformed to address tactile defensiveness, claustrophobia, or sensory overload.

Address Safety

Address safety issues such as slip and fall, scald prevention, electrical shock, and broken glass. Install nonskid flooring such as nonskid tile, covered commercial-grade vinyl with nonskid wax, or epoxy. Install weight-bearing bars with solid backing. Ground Fault Interrupter (GFI) outlets, tempered glass and mirrors and tempering/balancing valves are also mandatory.

Install a Floor Drain

Splashing water makes the floor slippery; mopping it up to prevent damage and improve safety is labor intensive. The most effective way

399

to control spilled water is to drain it away. By installing a floor drain, water splashed or poured onto the floor can drain away. Installing a floor drain is a very worthwhile and simple modification that can make a big difference.

Use Commercial- or Institutional-Grade Fixtures

This is especially important for the toilet. Installing a wall-mounted unit with the tank and flush mechanism in the wall is recommended. The tank is no longer a problem because it is hidden in the wall. Wall-hung toilets open floor space and provide toe space that allows a care-giver to assume good ergonomic posture when providing assistance. It also makes cleaning around the toilet easier. This type of toilet is readily available and is standard in many places in the world.

Anchor Fixtures and Grab Bars

Most bathroom accessories are too flimsy to hold up in a bathroom that is used intensely. Standard residential plumbing installations also don't anticipate the kinds of force that can be applied with nontraditional activities or to help a person stand or stay seated with every use. If you substitute weight-bearing grab bars for towel bars, one of the problems is solved. Institutional-grade fixtures have special features and extra strength, and they are a worthwhile alternative.

It is important to make strong connections to the wall structure when the wall is open. It costs very little to add extra wood backing before the finish is applied. A good option is installing a continuous sheet of plywood to allow for complete flexibility for solid attachment later. This is not a "standard" construction practice, so it's necessary to communicate very clearly with builders before the wall is closed in.

Operable Windows and Natural Light

Bathrooms are not always located on exterior walls, but if at all possible, find a way to include natural light and natural ventilation. This is essential to maintaining a healthy, welcoming bathroom when it is intensively used. Exhaust fans alone cannot meet all the needs, but if that is all you have, pick a quiet one with high cubic feet per minute (CFM) and vent it to the outside.

A Secondary Heat Source

Radiant heating in the floor, heat lamps, or forced-air electric heaters are some of the best preventives to mold and eliminating slipping hazards. It has the benefit of creating a more welcoming bathroom for people who are temperature sensitive.

Eliminate Registers and Other Floor Openings

Floor registers collect water and dirt, and are difficult to clean when the toilet overflows. Move registers to the walls whenever possible.

Walking Loop
A Route for Pacing and Stress Relief

Many people experiencing ASD benefit from large muscle movement by walking, pacing, rocking, running, or jumping. To accommodate these activities in the home, look for the opportunity to create a "walking loop." Ideally, this is a path that circles through and/or around several rooms of the home.

In addition to sensory integration and stress relief, a walking loop can give an individual more control over social interactions. The loop makes it easy for them to enter a room, stay, leave, or return later on their own terms. To support this kind of control and interaction, try to connect private spaces such as bedrooms and sitting rooms to more public spaces such as living, dining, entry, or kitchens. In some cases, the loop can give caregivers a path to move away from stressful situations or confrontations.

Getting a Walking Loop to Happen in a Home

If you are designing a new home, the loop should be integrated in the layout of rooms. In an existing home, creating a loop often takes more creativity. In traditional houses, the stair is often central to the plan layout, and a loop can easily be developed by connecting rooms around the stair. Other plan types may not prove to be so easy to adapt, but it is usually possible to find a set of rooms that can be interconnected to form a loop.

Most often this involves opening walls or creating passageways that can be arranged so that it allows the individual to circle the rooms or walk down a hall to a room with a turnaround space. Paths need to go where the action is, and lead to safe rooms away from activity. Avoid dead ends such as hallways to locked rooms. Avoid pinch points where two people can't pass each other without giving ground. Whenever possible, make loops that can also connect the person to outside areas.

401

Places of Control + Layers of Freedom
Providing Choice and Options for Engagement

People with autism usually struggle with social interactions. Many prefer being alone. If they feel safe and can interact on their own terms, they are more likely to engage with others and pursue the things they like to do.

Safe Places and Predictability

Create private places that make the person feel safe and in control. Having the opportunity to retreat, when needed, often results in the person regaining control and being better able to choose more, not less, social interaction. Provide places to display information or post a schedule. Having this information at hand supports routines and allows everyone to know when supports are scheduled; and if there are changes, this helps people to feel in control.

The bedroom is the most obvious place of control, although it should not be the only one. Provide the person with as much control as possible in his or her bedroom, including control of the door, choice of favorite colors, and control of light, air, and sounds. Provide furnishings, entertainments systems, and toys that are preferred. Support coping strategies whenever possible. Frequently, white noise can mitigate sensory overload. Try fans, low music, or a television in the background.

Find places within the home outside of the bedroom, such as the bathroom or a sitting room, where the individual has opportunities for meaningful control and choices structured for voluntary participation. Create the bathroom as a safe place they can use independently. One simple modification that allows independent use of the bathroom is the installation of a bidet toilet seat, which reduces the need for caregiver assistance.

Layers of Freedom

Other areas of the home can be layered to provide opportunities as interests emerge and capacity is built. For example, physical or sensory cues that establish routines for use and participation in the laundry room, garage, or kitchen activities can build confidence and encourage independence. This idea extends beyond the interior to include the whole property. Enclosing a porch or patio provides an opportunity for an individual to go there independently and feel safe and secure. Moving from the porch to the yard can include other interesting activities such as a swing, hammock, or table. Providing layers of freedom builds an individual's capacity and confidence to engage in activities they enjoy.

Be sure each place of control meets the standards of the Autism Friendly Home and satisfies the unique needs and interests of the individual. For example, if the person makes holes in the wall or breaks windows or doors, their opportunity to live freely in those places is compromised. If the person has seizures or engages in self-injury, the risk to their health and safety must be addressed first before a meaningful opportunity for control or freedom is possible.

Eliminate Fear Triggers

Recognize an individual's fears as legitimate and determine if there are physical solutions. For example, add lights if there are dark spaces or dark hallways that are frightening. These lights can be motion activated. Add soundproofing or sound-absorbent materials if noise is alarming or an irritant. Listen for and mitigate household noises from appliances and equipment that may be frightening. Provide screening and fencing to prevent animals from entering the yard. Don't allow fear to be in control.

Control Access and Define Boundaries

Access may need to be controlled or shared in areas where safety is an issue or where the individual is still acquiring the skills and capacity for independence. Defining boundaries might include fencing the yard or restricting access to things in the yard that can be dangerous, such as a pool, hot tub, air-conditioning unit, or garbage and recycling. The exterior doors are important boundaries and may need to be controlled and monitored. Delayed or restricted egress can raise safety concerns and rights issues. These strategies need to be carefully evaluated in terms of risk/benefit for everyone involved. Safe egress from a building must always be maintained.

Make Home the Preferred Place

Try to make the home the individual's preferred place by accommodating enjoyable and interesting activities inside and around the home. Provide the opportunity to choose from a variety of activities that meet the person's preferences. Think about the seasons as well. Indoor activities may need to expand during winter months and outdoor activities in the summer. When planning, be open to changing interests and capacities, have patience, and recognize that ritual and routine are comforting and reassuring.

Tools for Housekeeping
Keeping Things Clean, Tidy, and Smelling Good

Individuals with autism often have a way of disorganizing the world around them. Chaos can lead to exhaustion for the caregiver and frustration for the individual, sometimes manifesting itself as aggression or property damage. People acquire life skills at different rates. It is important to be patient and support an individual's development of new capacities at their own speed. Two common strengths of people with autism are the ability to follow routines and an excellent memory for detail. A well-organized and thoughtfully designed environment can harness these strengths. In some cases, the sheer quantity of soiled clothes and laundry can be overwhelming and create what seems to be a never-ending task. The extra expense of cleaners, large garbage containers, supplies, and additional electricity to keep up the house can compound financial and personal stress.

Adequate Storage

The need for appropriate storage and adequate display space cannot be overemphasized. In many cases, homes fall into disorder simply because these two needs are not being met. Only store items intended for engagement in the "reach" zone. An area approximately three to six feet above the floor is the place where most grabbing, handling, rubbing, and pawing occur. Put stops on the edges of shelves to keep things from falling off. Two old adages work surprisingly well: "Everything in its place and a place for everything." Creative labeling helps organization and visual patterns can support rituals in a positive way. "Out-of-sight is out-of-mind" can be extremely effective: add screens and doors to cover things until they are needed or wanted. A refrigerator concealed behind a cabinet door can also eliminate the need for a point of control.

Limit the Opportunity for Clutter to Migrate

Installing dressers in closets will free up floor space and support safety. You may need to add a lockable door to allow for shared control of some possessions. Although, at times, access to closets and contents may need to be shared. Locks should be a temporary solution. In other rooms of the house—such as the kitchen, laundry room, or garage—some things may need to be locked permanently for safety reasons. Limit access to places where garbage and trash cans are stored. Good storage for toys or water- and bathroom-related items also needs to be provided.

Building in Routine

Reduce anxiety by arranging rooms in ways that help put tasks in order and cue what activity comes next, and where. Where possible, create a visual, nonverbal physical path to communicate the sequence of an intended activity. For example, if a person is going to take a shower, have the clothes hamper on the way to the bathroom door. Placing towel storage just outside the shower encourages patterned use. For people struggling to know where they are in space, providing strong visual cues throughout the home will help them understand patterns of use and support positive routines. Changes in floor coverings helps to identify various rooms.

Bad Smells

Odors can convey how a home is maintained and sometimes people pass judgment based on what they smell. Odors are a common problem and emanate from many sources. Garbage, especially if it contains diapers, soiled laundry and linens, mops, sponges, rags, and other housekeeping tools all contribute to bad odors. Drooling, spilling, incontinence, and other body odors can cause furniture, carpet, drapes, and other absorbent surfaces to take on undesirable smells. Changing areas are soiled often and require continual cleaning. If an individual picks or smears, this too contributes to the clean-up problem.

Flooring

Flooring is almost always a major contributing factor when undesirable smells are a concern. Avoid carpeting. Sheet vinyl is an affordable and reliable solution, but can look institutional if overused. If you use vinyl, select a product that can be welded at the seams and covered up the wall. There are cushioned-back products that are waterproof and will help quiet and soften the floor, but they cannot be covered to protect the joint between the floor surface and wall. In all cases, sealing the joints where liquid will accumulate and protecting any absorbent materials is critical. Seal the transitions between wall and floor. Self-adhering vinyl plank flooring yields good results provided it is well-sealed at the perimeter, edges, and transitions. Regardless of the flooring you choose, it must be well-maintained.

Negative Air Pressure or Air Seals

Using low-sone (quiet) fans or other ventilating systems, can negatively pressurize a room by pulling air out and odors in from the rest of the house with its exhaust system. Keep smells down with frequent air changes by using portable fans and opening doors and windows. Good ventilation in bathrooms is essential, but it also is necessary in the kitchen and laundry. Some individuals are particularly sensitive to food smells and off-gassing from cleaning products. Remove soiled mops, sponges, and towels from living areas and store these and other cleaning products and equipment in a ventilated closet. Use airtight containers for wet or soiled materials.

Eliminate Floor Registers

Eliminate floor registers if at all possible; most can be relocated to the wall. These are dirty in the best of circumstances because everything goes down and they are virtually uncleanable. When the heat comes on everything is blown back into the room. For an individual with toileting issues, a dark hole in the floor is a bad idea.

Make a Changing Area

Does the individual require frequent clothing changes or diapering? How has changing been accommodated to date? Are you using the bed? When changing soiled clothing, especially for older family members, it is best to do this activity in or near the bathroom. However, caregivers need adequate space, and most bathrooms are not big enough to accommodate this activity. A bathroom changing table saves steps and makes sense. It puts the resources needed to do the job close at hand. Soiled clothing can be transferred directly to airtight hampers or bins. Access to water, fresh air, and appropriate surfaces will result in fewer bad smells, save time, and reduce stress for everyone.

Laundry and Clean-Up

Most families living with ASD end up doing a lot of laundry. High quality, high-efficiency washers and dryers rated for commercial use actually save money when compared with the repair and replacement costs associated with residential appliances. A large utility sink is also helpful. Constant mopping, wiping down, and sanitizing contribute to caregiver fatigue. Floor sinks make handling mops and buckets more ergonomic and they have large drains that are harder to clog when doing heavy cleaning or pericare. A mop/cleaning station may be a good solution.

Be aware that odors from cleaning products can be a major problem for many individuals with autism, particularly those who are extremely sensitive to strong smells and experience physical distress as a result. Use caution when selecting and using these products.

Chapter 48

Grandparents Play Key Role in Lives of Children with Autism Spectrum Disorder

All families can benefit from connecting with resources that offer information, guidance, and support to help them meet the challenges of parenthood and family life.

- Family support services are community-based services that assist and support parents in their role as caregivers. Family support services promote parental competency and healthy child development by helping parents enhance their strengths and resolve problems that can lead to child maltreatment, developmental delays, and family disruption.

- Family preservation services are short-term services designed to help families cope with significant stresses or problems that interfere with their ability to nurture their children. The goal of

This chapter contains text excerpted from the following sources: Text in this chapter begins with excerpts from "Introduction to Family Support and Preservation," Child Welfare Information Gateway, U.S. Department of Health and Human Services (HHS), August 20, 2013. Reviewed October 2018; Text beginning with the heading "What Are Family Support Services?" is excerpted from "Frequently Asked Questions: Supporting and Preserving Families" Child Welfare Information Gateway, U.S. Department of Health and Human Services (HHS), August 28, 2018.

family preservation services is to maintain children with their families, or to reunify them, whenever it can be done safely.

Family support and preservation services may be provided to different types of families involved with the child welfare system—birth or biological families, kinship families, foster families, and adoptive families—to enhance family functioning and ensure child safety. In family support and preservation services, the worker assists the family in identifying strengths, needs, and current resources in order to create a plan to address their concerns and help them achieve their goals. Assessment is incorporated throughout the process and may take a number of different forms, but always with the family as partners in the process.

What Are Family Support Services?

Family support services are community-based services that assist and support parents in their role as caregivers. Family support services promote parental competence and healthy child development by helping parents enhance their strengths and resolve problems that can lead to child maltreatment, developmental delays, and family disruption.

Who Can Benefit from Family Support Services?

Family support services provide support and assistance to parents across the service continuum. While they are most often intended for families prior to involvement with formal service systems such as child welfare, these services also may be used to support and assist families who have experienced child maltreatment or family disruption. In addition, family support services may be helpful for families receiving in-home services, for those seeking to reunify with a child who has been in out-of-home care, for kinship families caring for their relative children, and for families formed by adoption.

What Are Family Preservation Services?

Family preservation services are short-term, family-focused, and community-based services designed to help families cope with significant stresses or problems that interfere with their ability to nurture their children. The goal of family preservation services is to maintain children with their families or to reunify them, whenever it can be done safely.

410

Who Can Benefit from Family Preservation Services?

Family preservation services have been used successfully for families at risk of disruption, as well as those seeking to reunify, including families receiving child welfare, juvenile justice, or mental health services.

Chapter 49

Pets for Easing Social Anxiety in Kids with Autism

When animals are present, children with autism spectrum disorders (ASDs) have lower readings on a device that detects anxiety and other forms of social arousal when interacting with their peers.

According to a study funded in part by the National Institutes of Health (NIH), companion animals—like dogs, cats, or the guinea pigs in the study—may prove to be a helpful addition to treatment programs designed to help children with ASDs improve their social skills and interactions with other people.

The study, published online in *Developmental Psychobiology*, was conducted by Marguerite O'Haire, Ph.D., from the Center for the Human–Animal Bond in the College of Veterinary Medicine of Purdue University in West Lafayette, Indiana, and colleagues in the School of Psychology at the University of Queensland in Brisbane, Australia.

"Previous studies suggest that in the presence of companion animals, children with autism spectrum disorders function better socially," said James Griffin, Ph.D., of the Child Development and Behavior Branch at NIH's *Eunice Kennedy Shriver* National Institute of Child Health and Human Development (NICHD). "This study provides physiological evidence that the proximity of animals eases the stress that children with autism may experience in social situations."

This chapter includes text excerpted from "Animals' Presence May Ease Social Anxiety in Kids with Autism," National Institutes of Health (NIH), May 20, 2015. Reviewed October 2018.

This study is among several funded under a public–private partnership established in 2008 between the NICHD and WALTHAM Centre for Pet Nutrition, a division of Mars Inc., to establish a human-animal interaction research program to support studies relevant to child development, health, and the therapeutic use of animals.

"By providing support for these research studies, we hope to generate more definitive answers about how human-animal interaction affects health," he said.

ASDs affect the structure and function of the brain and nervous system. People with these conditions have difficulty communicating and interacting with other people. They also have restricted and repetitive interests and behaviors.

For the current study, Dr. O'Haire and her colleagues measured skin conductance, the ease at which an unnoticeable electric charge passes through a patch of skin, in children with ASDs and in typically developing children. Researchers divided the 114 children, ages 5 to 12 years old, into 38 groups of three. Each group included one child with ASD and two of their typically developing peers.

Each child wore a wristband fitted with a device that measures skin conductance. When people are feeling excited, fearful, or anxious, the electric charge travels faster through the skin, providing an objective way for researchers to gauge social anxiety and other forms of psychological arousal.

For the first few minutes, the children read a book silently, giving researchers a baseline measure of skin conductance while carrying out a nonstressful, familiar task. Next, each child was asked to read aloud from the book in the presence of the two peers in their group, a task designed to measure their level of apprehension during social situations.

The researchers then brought toys in the room and allowed the children 10 minutes of free play time. These situations may be stressful for children with ASDs, who may have difficulty relating socially to their typically developing peers.

Finally, the researchers brought two guinea pigs into the room and allowed the children to have 10 minutes of supervised play with the animals. The researchers chose guinea pigs because of their small size and docile nature—much easier to manage in a classroom than larger animals.

The researchers found that, compared to the typically developing children, the children with autism had higher skin conductance levels when reading silently, reading aloud, and in the group toy session. These higher levels are consistent with reports from parents and teachers, and from other studies, that children with ASDs are more likely to be anxious in social situations than typically developing children.

When the session with the guinea pigs began, however, skin conductance levels among the children with ASDs dropped significantly. The researchers speculate that because companion animals offer unqualified acceptance, their presence makes the children feel more secure.

Whereas human counterparts inherently pass social judgment, animals are often perceived as sources of unconditional, positive support, the researchers wrote.

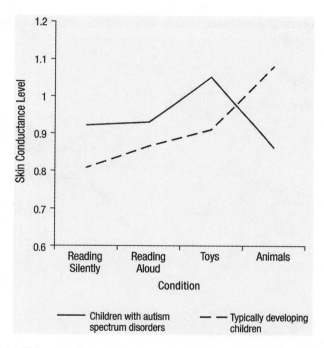

Figure 49.1. *Skin Conductance Level during Various Activities*

Skin conductance levels of children with ASD rose for the first three conditions, but fell during the play session with guinea pigs.

For reasons the researchers cannot explain, skin conductance levels in the typically developing children rose during the session with the guinea pigs. The researchers believe that these higher readings may indicate excitement at seeing the animals, rather than any nervousness or apprehension.

Dr. O'Haire added that earlier studies have shown that children with ASDs were less likely to withdraw from social situations when companion animals are present. These studies, along with some of the findings, indicate that animals might "play a part in interventions seeking to help children with autism develop their social skills," she said. She cautioned, however, that the findings do not mean that parents of children with ASDs should rush to buy an animal for their children. Further research is needed to determine how animals might be used in programs aimed at developing social skills.

"Our study was conducted in a supervised setting, by researchers experienced in working with kids with autism spectrum disorders who understand the needs and requirements of the animals," Dr. O'Haire said. She added that careful supervision was provided during the study, to ensure the welfare of the children as well as the animals.

Chapter 50

Feeding Problems and Toilet Training for Children with ASD

What Are Potential Feeding Problems for Typically Developing Children and Children with Autism Spectrum Disorder?

Feeding problems are common in typically developing children and can occur more frequently in children with autism spectrum disorder (ASD). When compared to children without ASD, children with ASD tend to:

- refuse more foods
- require more special utensils
- require food be presented in specific ways
- prefer food with less texture
- eat fewer foods

This chapter includes text excerpted from "Autism Case Training—Case Study II: A Closer Look," Centers for Disease Control and Prevention (CDC), June 20, 2018.

In addition, children with ASD may have pica, compulsive eating, mouth packing, or gagging and emesis. They may also associate discomfort with a certain food if the pain occurred just before or after consuming the food. Thus, they may repeatedly refuse that particular food item.

When Evaluating a Child with an Autism Spectrum Disorder Who Has Feeding Issues, What Medical Problems Should Be Considered before Assigning a Purely Behavioral Diagnosis?
Medical Problems

Consider the following medical problems

- Gastroesophageal reflux disease (GERD)
- Dental pain
- Oral motor dysfunction
- Food allergy
- Lactose intolerance

Other Problems to Consider

Other problems to consider for a child with ASD and feeding problems include:

- Developmental delay
- Obsessions/rituals related to food (color, texture) and environment (silverware, plates)
- Anxiety
- Sensory issues
- Learned behaviors (parental response to escalating behavior)

What Would Your Next Steps Be If You Suspect a Nutritional Deficiency?
Malnutrition

Because children with ASD have narrow food preferences, there is a concern about malnutrition. Adequate evidence to support these concerns is lacking. However, questions about a particular nutrient deficiency (i.e., iron) may require further evaluation.

Treatment Plan

Your history and physical exam will determine your diagnostic evaluation and treatment plan.

- If you suspect a nutritional deficiency, such as anemia, you may consider laboratory studies to evaluate for this.

- A nutrition consult may help to determine a child's nutritional needs and make recommendations to the family. Providing the family with strategies to promote healthy eating habits is essential for the picky eater.

- For severe feeding problems (i.e., resulting in failure to thrive), you may need to employ the help of trained professionals in this area. These can include psychologists, occupational therapists, and speech therapists who are often part of a multidisciplinary team that specializes in feeding problems.

What Would You Recommend to Help a Parent Encourage Positive Eating Habits?

Encourage parents to establish routine meal and snack times. At mealtime:

- Minimize distractions (shut off television, telephone)

- Keep meals calm and strive for an enjoyable experience

- Adults should sit down with children and eat the same foods

- Offer the child what everyone else is eating, but also provide one of their preferred foods

- Refrain from pleading and threatening to get the child to eat

- After the family is finished, allow the child to leave the table

- Food should not be provided until the next scheduled meal/snack

What Are Some Barriers Children with ASD May Encounter When Toilet Training?

There are several barriers to toilet training children with ASD.

1. Most obvious may be their communication delays, which inhibit their ability to verbalize when they have soiled or if they need to use the bathroom.

2. In addition to expressive language delays, they may have difficulties with language comprehension. Therefore, they may not understand what is expected of them for the toileting process.

3. A social reward system, used in typically developing children, may be ineffective for children with ASD because of their difficulties with social relationships. During the toileting process, typically developing children are praised for toileting in the potty and have a sense of accomplishment for a job well done. children with ASD may not possess the social motivation to please their parents by stooling in the toilet. They may not understand the difference between their diaper and the toilet.

4. A strict adherence to routines can also make toileting difficult. Children with ASD often have difficulty with changes in their routine, so adding toileting to their daily schedule can be disruptive.

5. Although not considered part of the diagnostic criteria for ASD, sensory issues often have a significant effect on children with ASD. Many sensory issues can arise during the toileting process:

   - Sitting on the toilet seat unclothed is a new experience that may require a gradual approach.

   - They may not recognize toileting cues (e.g., urge to defecate), making it difficult to rely on their own body's signals for using the toilet.

   - Flushing the toilet may be an issue if they are overly sensitive to sound.

6. Because of the many new experiences that go along with toileting, children with ASD and their parents can become very anxious about the entire process, adding another barrier to successful toilet training.

What Medical Issues May Impact the Toileting Process?

For any child with toileting problems, it is important to rule out constipation as a contributing problem. As constipation is a frequent issue, ask parents about it regularly.

Remember to review the child's medication list for potential side effects (e.g., constipation with atypical neuroleptics).

Other medical problems to consider include urinary tract infections, tethered cord, or possible sexual abuse or trauma (may result from self-stimulation behavior).

What Might You Recommend to Help with Bowel Training?
Bowel Training

Toilet training is an important milestone for any child to reach, but it can be especially challenging for a child with ASD. Providing careful guidance to the family of a child with ASD can make this process less difficult.

There are several techniques that can be employed, including timed sitting, visual supports such as picture icons, and awareness of sensory issues.

Timed Sits

If the child with ASD is not able to communicate the need to use the bathroom, timed sits can be introduced.

- For several days before having the child sit on the toilet, the parent or caregiver should record the child's bowel habits—times that the child stools and frequency of wet diapers. With this information, they can identify patterns to the child's stooling.

- Have the child sit on the toilet fully clothed, then gradually remove clothing with subsequent sits. Provide some type of positive reinforcement for cooperative sitting on the toilet, such as a favorite book or toy. A timer can be used to help the child know how long they are expected to sit there.

Visual Cues

Children with ASD usually respond better to visual cues than to verbal ones.

- Breaking down the steps of toileting into pictures can help the child understand what is expected of him or her.

- Parents can use standard pictures or they may take pictures of their child going through the different steps and use those.

- Parents can post a photograph of a toilet around the house and encourage the child to point to it when she or he needs to go.

Chapter 51

Practical Oral Care for People with ASD

Providing oral care to people with autism requires adaptation of the skills you use every day. In fact, most people with mild or moderate forms of autism can be treated successfully in the general practice setting. This chapter will help you make a difference in the lives of people who need professional oral care.

Autism is a complex developmental disability that impairs communication and social, behavioral, and intellectual functioning. Some people with the disorder appear distant, aloof or detached from other people or from their surroundings. Others do not react appropriately to common verbal and social cues, such as a parent's tone of voice or smile. Obsessive routines, repetitive behaviors, unpredictable body movements, and self-injurious behavior may all be symptoms that complicate dental care.

Autism varies widely in symptoms and severity, and some people have coexisting conditions such as intellectual disability or epilepsy. They can be among the most challenging of patients, but following the suggestions in this chapter can help make their dental treatment successful.

This chapter includes text excerpted from "Practical Oral Care for People with Autism," National Institute of Dental and Craniofacial Research (NIDCR), July 2009. Reviewed October 2018.

Oral Health Problems in Autism and Strategies for Care

People with autism experience a few unusual oral health conditions. Although commonly used medications and damaging oral habits can cause problems, the rates of caries and periodontal disease in people with autism are comparable to those in the general population. Communication and behavioral problems pose the most significant challenges in providing oral care.

Damaging oral habits are common and include bruxism; tongue thrusting; self-injurious behavior such as picking at the gingiva or biting the lips; and pica—eating objects and substances such as gravel, cigarette butts, or pens. If a mouth guard can be tolerated, prescribe one for patients who have problems with self-injurious behavior or bruxism.

Dental cavity risk increases in patients who have a preference for soft, sticky, or sweet foods; damaging oral habits; and difficulty brushing and flossing.

Tooth eruption may be delayed due to phenytoin (PHT)-induced gingival hyperplasia. Phenytoin is commonly prescribed for people with autism. Trauma and injury to the mouth from falls or accidents occur in people with seizure disorders. Suggest a tooth-saving kit for group homes. Emphasize to caregivers that traumas require immediate professional attention and explain the procedures to follow if a permanent tooth is knocked out. Also, instruct caregivers to locate any missing pieces of a fractured tooth, and explain that radiographs of the patient's chest may be necessary to determine whether any fragments have been aspirated.

Physical abuse often presents as oral trauma. Abuse is reported more frequently in people with developmental disabilities than in the general population. If you suspect that a child is being abused or neglected, state laws require that you call your Child Protective Services agency. Assistance is also available from the Childhelp® National Child Abuse Hotline at 800-422–4453 or the Child Welfare Information Gateway (www.childwelfare.gov).

Making a difference in the oral health of a person with autism may go slowly at first, but determination can bring positive results—and invaluable rewards. By adopting the strategies discussed in this chapter, you can have a significant impact not only on your patients' oral health, but on their quality of life as well.

Chapter 52

Transition to Adulthood for Individuals with Autism Spectrum Disorders

Chapter Contents

Section 52.1

Transition Plan

This section contains text excerpted from the following sources: Text in this section begins with excerpts from "Autism Spectrum Disorder (ASD)—Living with ASD," Centers for Disease Control and Prevention (CDC), April 26, 2018; Text under the heading "Adolescents with Autism Spectrum Disorders" is excerpted from "The Feasibility of Using Electronic Health Records (EHRs) and Other Electronic Health Data for Research on Small Populations," Office of the Assistant Secretary for Planning and Evaluation (ASPE), September 2013. Reviewed October 2018.

For many people with an autism spectrum disorder (ASD) and their families, daily life is not easy. However, finding resources and planning for the future can help families improve their quality of life.

Family Issues

Living with a person with an ASD affects the entire family—parents, siblings, and, in some families, grandparents, aunts, uncles, and cousins. Meeting the complex needs of a person with an ASD can put families under a great deal of stress—emotional, financial, and sometimes even physical. Respite care can give parents and other family caregivers a needed break and help maintain family well-being.

Healthy Living

To stay healthy, people with disabilities need the same basic healthcare as everyone else. They need to eat well, exercise, get enough rest, drink plenty of water, and have complete access to healthcare, including regular physical and dental check-ups. It is important to find healthcare providers who are comfortable with persons who have an ASD.

Sometimes when people with disabilities have a behavioral change or behavioral issue, it may be because they have a medical problem they cannot describe. For instance, head banging could be related to a disability, or it could be due to a headache or toothache. For this reason, it is important to find out if there is a physical problem before making changes in a person's treatment or therapy.

Safety

Safety is important for everyone. We all need to be safe in order to live full and productive lives. People with disabilities can be at higher risk for injuries and abuse. It is important for parents and other family members to teach their loved one how to stay safe and what to do if they feel threatened or have been hurt in any way. It can sometimes be helpful to give a person with a disability a bracelet or other item that has his or her name, address, phone number, and disability on it in case she or he gets lost.

Transitions

For some people with disabilities and their parents, change can be difficult. Planning ahead of time may make transitions easier for everyone.

The transition from high school to adulthood can be especially challenging. There are many important, life-changing decisions to make, such as whether to go to college or a vocational school or whether to enter the workforce, and if so, how and where. It is important to begin thinking about this transition in childhood, so that educational transition plans are put in place—preferably by age 14, but no later than age 16—to make sure the individual has the skills she or he needs to begin the next phase of life. The transition of healthcare from a pediatrician to a doctor who treats adults is another area that needs a plan.

Adolescents with Autism Spectrum Disorders

Autism spectrum disorders (ASDs) are a group of developmental disabilities that range from mild to severe and are characterized by social impairment, difficulty communicating, and repetitive motions or other unusual behaviors. These characteristics are usually noticeable before the age of three and remain as a lifelong chronic condition with both medical and psychological implications. ASDs include autistic disorder, Asperger disorder, pervasive developmental disorder—not otherwise specified (PDD-NOS), Rett syndrome (RTT), and childhood disintegrative disorder (CDD).

Based on data from the 14 sites in its Autism and Developmental Disabilities Monitoring (ADDM) Network, the Centers for Disease Control (CDC) estimates 1 in 88 8-year-old children have ASDs. Prevalence in these sites had increased 23 percent from two years earlier and 78 percent since 2002. Although there is disagreement about whether the true prevalence has increased (since guidelines for diagnosis have changed, more services are available, and awareness of ASD has increased), the CDC numbers are based on evaluation records, not parental reports. Measuring ASD prevalence continues to be a challenge due to the complexity of the disorder, the lack of consistent and reliable diagnostic standards, and changes in the definition of such conditions. ASD prevalence is about five times higher in boys than in girls (ratio of 4.5 boys to 1 girl). Prevalence is also significantly higher among non-Hispanic white children than among black and Hispanic children. Intellectual ability is highly variable, with 38 percent reported as intellectually disabled, 24 percent as borderline, and 38 percent with average or above average intellectual ability.

There are controversies about what should be included in the category of autism spectrum disorders. The National Institutes of Health (NIH) classifies Rett syndrome as an ASD, but some argue that it is more similar to nonautistic spectrum disorders such as fragile X syndrome or Down syndrome. Unlike other ASDs, Rett syndrome is also almost always in girls. There is also debate over whether Asperger disorder is a separate disorder or simply a less severe form of autism. The next revision of the *American Psychiatric Association's Diagnostic and Statistical Manual (DSM)* has dropped individual classifications for autistic disorder, Asperger disorder, childhood disintegrative disorder, and PDD-NOS, grouping all of them under "autism spectrum disorder"—a term that is already widely used. APA has said this change will help "more accurately and consistently diagnose children with autism." Rett syndrome will be dropped from the *DSM* altogether. There is concern among the Asperger and Rett communities that these changes will result in a loss of identity among individuals with these specific disorders and that it may affect health insurance coverage and school funding for special education.

The exact causes of ASDs remain unknown, but research suggests genetics and environment both play important roles. Researchers are studying factors such as family medical conditions, parental age and other demographic factors, exposure to toxins, and complications during birth or pregnancy. The CDC and IOM studies have found no link to childhood immunizations.

Health and Healthcare Issues

Among children with various developmental disabilities, autism has been found associated with the highest levels of health and functional impairment indicators. Over 95 percent of children with autism also have co-occurring conditions such as attention deficit disorder, attention deficit-hyperactivity disorder, learning disability, mental retardation, stuttering, and other developmental delays. Children With autism are also at elevated risk for depression, anxiety, and behavioral problems, often as a result of difficulty being understood or bullying.

Children with ASDs are also more likely than other children to be obese and to have a variety of conditions—respiratory disorders, food and skin allergies, epilepsy, schizophrenia, bowel disorders, cranial anomalies, type 1 diabetes, muscular dystrophy, and sleep disorders. As a result, children with ASDs use more healthcare services, therapy, counseling, and medication than children without ASDs. Prevalence of prescription medications for children with ASD is high: surveys indicate one-half to two-thirds are prescribed at least one medication of any type, and about 45 percent prescribed at least one psychotropic medication. The most commonly prescribed psychotropic medications are antidepressants, stimulants, and antipsychotics.

The significant amount of care needed for many children with ASDs means many of their parents have needed to reduce or stop work to provide care, spending an average of 10 hours per week providing or coordinating care. As a result, families of children with ASDs are more likely to report financial problems and to need additional income to support their child's medical care compared to families with children with other special healthcare needs that do not involve emotional, developmental, or behavioral problems. Among children with special healthcare needs, children with ASD were much more likely to have unmet healthcare needs for specific healthcare services and family support services. Having a medical home has been found to help reduce the financial burden on families of children with ASDs. However, children with ASDs are less likely than children without ASDs to receive care within a medical home.

Transition to Adulthood

Most research on ASDs focuses on the identification, assessment, and treatment of children. Few studies examine their transition into the adult world. The healthcare transition between adolescence and adulthood requires planning in order to maximize lifelong functioning and well-being. This process would ideally include ensuring uninterrupted, developmentally appropriate healthcare services as the person moves from adolescence to adulthood. For those with ASDs, there are a number of special considerations for this transitional period. The transition period from pediatric to adult care and from child to adult special services will have lifelong implications for their education, employment, social activities, and health. Because their conditions range in severity, a wide range of individualized adult services and supports is needed for this population.

Two key aspects of transition planning for teens with ASDs are helping them take increased responsibility for their healthcare, and plan for the transfer of care from a pediatric to an adult provider. Unfortunately, providers who care for adults often lack training and experience in dealing with this transitioning population. For those whose disability is impaired enough to interfere with the ability to make financial or medical decisions, parents can file for a petition to maintain guardianship. Most Individuals diagnosed with autism during childhood remain dependent into adulthood on their parents or caregivers for support in education, accommodation, and occupational situations.

Teens with ASDs who are transitioning to adulthood need help in understanding their disability, opportunities to talk about topics such as safety, substance abuse and sexuality, education about how to take medications and make routine healthcare appointments, and continual insurance coverage. An adult provider also needs to be identified, and the adolescent's medical records transferred. None of this is simple.

Unfortunately, healthcare transition planning is not common for youth with ASDs. One national survey found only 14 percent had a discussion with their pediatrician about transitioning to an adult provider, and fewer than 25 percent had discussed retaining health insurance. Being from a racial or ethnic minority, having low income, being from a non-English speaking family, and not having a medical home reduces the odds that youth with ASDs will receive comprehensive transition services. Even within medical homes, both parents and pediatricians have reported dissatisfaction with the time and resources dedicated to this transition.

Section 52.2

Federal Agency Activities Related to Transition for Autism

This section includes text excerpted from "Young Adults and
Transitioning Youth with Autism Spectrum Disorder," U.S.
Department of Health and Human Services (HHS), August 3, 2017.

It is important to note that many of these programs are not designed
specifically to serve or fund research focused on individuals with
ASD; however, as general population programs, or as efforts targeted
broadly to people with disabilities, these programs do inevitably serve
or include transition-age youth and young adults with ASD. Depending
on the fundamental goals of the program, they may or may not track
ASD status among those they serve or study. It is, thus, not possible
to know how many youth and young adults with ASD are receiving
services and supports from each specific agency. Information regarding
each of these programs follows.

U.S. Department of Health and Human Services

The majority of health-related federal research, programs, and services targeted to individuals with ASD are administered through the
United States. The U.S. Department of Health and Human Services
(HHS), which has as its mission enhancing and protecting the health
and well-being of all Americans. Youth and young adults with ASD
may, depending on eligibility requirements, benefit from, and/or participate in, supports and services provided by these programs, either
with their families or individuals. HHS includes 11 operating divisions,
nine of which administer programs relevant to this population:

Administration for Children and Families

This operating division promotes the social and economic health and
wellbeing of the nation's children and families. The Administration for
Children and Families (ACF) collects data through three mechanisms
about children/youth in the foster care system where child welfare
agencies are required through Title IV-E of the Social Security Act to
submit data. However, there are no ACF-source metrics that track the
number of children/youth in the United States foster care and/or the
larger child protection and welfare systems who have been diagnosed

431

with Autism/ASD. Nevertheless, valuable information about those involved in ACF programs is provided through ACF reports.

- **The Adoption and Foster Care Analysis and Reporting System (AFCARS)** collects case-level information from state and tribal IV-E (i.e., child protection and welfare) agencies on all children in foster care and those who have been adopted with Title IV-E agency involvement. Examples of data reported in AFCARS include demographic information on the child in care as well as the foster/adoptive parents, the number of removals the child may have experienced, and the current placement setting. ASD is included in a data element called "Other Medically Diagnosed Condition," and is not specifically identified in the collection of AFCARS data.

- **The National Child Abuse and Neglect Data System (NCANDS)** is a voluntary data collection system that gathers information from all 50 states, the District of Columbia and Puerto Rico about reports of child abuse and neglect. Key findings are published in the Child Welfare Outcomes Reports to Congress and in the annual Child Maltreatment reports. There are no data elements that specifically track whether clients have been diagnosed with Autism/ASD.

- **The National Youth in Transition Database (NYTD)** collects information on youth in foster care including demographic characteristics and the outcomes of youth that have aged out of the child welfare system. This tracking system began in 2010, and the first data were reported in May 2011. States are to collect information in a manner consistent with federal law on each youth who receives independent living services paid for or provided by the state agency that administers the John H. Chafee Foster Care Independence Program (CFCIP) of section 477 of the Social Security Act. States also collect demographic and outcome information on youth in foster care whom the state will follow overtime. This information allows ACF to track which independent living services states provide and to assess the outcomes of those participating youth. There is one data element that addresses whether or not a youth received a special education service; however, there is no particular information about a youth's specific diagnosis.

- Three Major Data Collection Projects have been funded in whole or in part by the ACF. The data can be accessed through the National Data Archive On Child Abuse and Neglect (NDACAN).

- **The Longitudinal Studies of Child Abuse and Neglect (LONGSCAN)** involved a consortium of research groups initiated in 1990 with grants from the ACF Children's Bureau and coordinated through the University of North Carolina Injury Prevention Research Center. LONGSCAN is a multisite longitudinal study of 1354 children identified in infancy or early childhood as being mistreated at risk of maltreatment. The children who were included in the study were culturally and ethnically diverse and from five distinct geographical areas. Maltreatment data were collected from multiple sources and yearly telephone interviews were conducted. This dataset did not specify whether a child had been diagnosed with Autism/ASD.

- **The National Incidence Study of Child Abuse And Neglect (NIS)** has been conducted approximately once each decade beginning in 1974 in response to requirements of the Child Abuse Prevention and Treatment Act. There Are four years of data available: 1980 (NIS-1), 1987 (NIS-2), 1996 (NIS-3), and 2006 (NIS-4). NIS studies are designed to estimate more broadly the incidence of child maltreatment nationally. A unique contribution of the NISHA's been the use of a common definitional framework for classifying children according to types and severity of maltreatment. Information Specifically about Autism/ASD is not collected.

- **The National Survey of Child and Adolescent Well-Being (NSCAW)** contains information about Autism/ASD. NSCAW is a nationally representative, longitudinal survey of children and families who have been the subjects of investigation by Child Protective Services. There have been two cohorts of children enrolled in the survey, which includes data from reports by children, parents, and caregivers; reports from caseworkers and teachers collected in a manner consistent with federal law; and reviews of administrative records. NSCAW also examines child and family well-being outcomes in detail and seeks to relate those outcomes to experience with the child welfare system and to family characteristics. This dataset represents the child welfare population in states that do not require first contact with agencies in order to participate in research studies. The prevalence rate of ASD was 3 percent, or approximately doubled what it is (1.47%) in the general child population according to the CDC's surveillance system. It should be noted that the NSCAW is a survey rather than a surveillance system, and as such uses parent self-report rather than diagnostic evaluation to determine the presence of ASD. However, using a similar self-report methodology, the 2011–2012 National Survey of Children's Health (NSCH, 2011–2012 vii) reported a national prevalence rate of currently diagnosed children with ASD of 1.8 percent, much closer to the official estimate of 1.47 percent derived from the CDC's epidemiological surveillance system. Thus, compared to a data source that also employs parent self-report of diagnosed ASD, the rate of ASD found among children tracked through the nation's child protective service system is still two-thirds higher than the rate reported in the general population.

Administration for Community Living (ACL)

The ACL works to increase access to community support systems for older Americans and for people with disabilities across the lifespan. Its main activities and statutory authorities include administration of disability programs that support community living from which young adults with ASD may benefit.

- The Administration on Intellectual and Developmental Disabilities (AIDD) administers programs under the Developmental Disabilities Assistance and Bill of Rights Act of 2000 (the DD Act). This Act was authorized to ensure that individuals with developmental disabilities and their families participate in the design of, and have access to, needed community services, individualized supports, and other forms of assistance that promote self-determination, independence, productivity, and integration and inclusion in all facets of community life through culturally competent programs authorized under the law. These programs include:

  - State Councils on Developmental Disabilities

  - Protection and Advocacy Systems

  - University Centers for Excellence in Developmental Disabilities Education (UCEDD) Research and Service Projects of National Significance

- The Rehabilitation Act of 1973, as amended in 2014 by the Workforce Innovation and Opportunities Act of 2014 (WIOA), authorizes the following programs:

  - The Independent Living Services (ILS) Program provides 63 formula grants, based on population, to states and territories to fund independent living services programs and activities for individuals with significant disabilities.

  - The Centers for Independent Living (CIL) Program provides 356 discretionary grants centers that are consumer-controlled, community-based, cross-disability, nonresidential, private nonprofit agencies to provide independent living services to individual with significant disabilities. One of the Core Services for these centers added under WIOA is the transition to adulthood among youth with significant disabilities aged 14 to 24, who were eligible for an Individualized Education Program (IEP), and who have completed their secondary education or otherwise left school.

  - The National Institute on Disability, Independent Living, and Rehabilitation Research (NIDILRR) funds research on disability and rehabilitation. NIDILRR mission includes: (a) generating and promoting the use of new knowledge in order to enable people with disabilities to perform activities of their choice in the community, and (b) expanding society's capacity to provide full opportunities and accommodations for its citizens with disabilities.

- The Assistive Technology Act of 1998, amended in 2004, helps make assistive technology available to people with disabilities so they can more fully participate in education, employment, and other daily activities as full members of their communities. The law covers people of all ages and types of disabilities, and in all environments, including in school and at work.

  - The State Grant for Assistive Technology Program supports state efforts to improve the provision of assistive technology to individuals with disabilities of all ages through comprehensive, statewide programs that are consumer responsive. The State Grant For Assistive Technology Program makes assistive technology devices and services more available and accessible to individuals with disabilities and their families. The program provides one grant to each of the states, the District of Columbia, Puerto Rico, and territories (American Samoa, the Commonwealth of the Northern Mariana Islands, Guam, and the U.S. Virgin Islands). The State Grant for Assistive Technology Program is a formula-based grant program, and thus there are no grant competitions. The amount of each state's annual award is based largely on state population.

- The State Protection and Advocacy for Assistive Technology (PAAT) Program Provides Protection and advocacy services to assist individuals of all ages with disabilities in the acquisition, utilization or maintenance of assistive technology services or devices. ACL provides formula grants to Protection and Advocacy agencies established under the Developmental Disabilities Assistance and Bill of Rights Act (DD Act).

Agency for Healthcare Research and Quality

Agency for Healthcare Research and Quality (AHRQ) produces evidence for the nation focused on healthcare safety and quality. This HHS operating division supports the following project with direct relevance to young adults and transitioning youth with ASD:

- **"A Deliberative Approach to Develop Autism Data Collection in Massachusetts"** is a health services research grant funded in 2016 that involves a deliberative citizen jury, the majority of which are individuals on the autism spectrum, to provide guidance to the Massachusetts Executive Office of Health and Human Services (EOHHS) regarding the creation of a statewide registry for ASD. A patient registry is a collection of standardized information about a group of patients who share a particular condition or experience. When complete, the registry will provide an integrated data system to track diagnosis, treatment, services, and outcomes for individuals with ASD, with the long-term goal of improving coordination of care and disseminating information on best practices. Although not specifically targeted to transition-age youth and young adults, it will, when completed, provide a way to track services and outcomes for this population in Massachusetts.

Centers for Disease Control and Prevention

The Centers for Disease Control and Prevention (CDC) protects the health of the U.S. population through surveillance activities and large-scale responses to significant disease threats. The Children's Health Act of 2000 mandated that the CDC establish autism surveillance and research programs to address the number, incidence, correlates, and causes of ASD and related developmental disabilities.

- **The Autism and Developmental Disabilities Monitoring Network (ADDM)** is overseen by the CDC's National Center on Birth Defects and Developmental Disabilities (NCBDDD). The purpose of ADDM is to estimate the prevalence of autism among children living in select communities. ADDM has conducted autism surveillance on 8-year-old children who were born in 1992, 1994, 1996, 1998, 2000, 2002, and 2004; children who were born in 1994, 1996, 1998, and 2000 are now between 16 and 24 years of age, and thus may provide a useful source of information for additional research efforts on transition age youth and young adults with ASD. ADDM continues to monitor and report, biannually, the estimated prevalence of autism in network sites throughout the United States.

- **The Study to Explore Early Development (SEED)** is a multi-site, case-control study designed to assess risk factors for children with ASD aged two to five years, and characterize behavioral, developmental, and medical features of ASD with the goal of defining potentially etiologically distinct ASD subtypes. In 2007, NCBDDD funded six sites to conduct the first phase of SEED. In 2017, the oldest children enrolled in the first phase of SEED will reach adolescence. The SEED Teen study, which is currently under development, seeks to investigate the health and functioning, healthcare utilization, and educational attainment, of children 12–15 years old with ASD, as compared to those without ASD, as well as family impacts of having a child with ASD.

- **The National Health Interview Survey (NHIS)** provides information on the health of the civilian noninstitutionalized population of the United States, and is one of the major data collection programs of the CDC's National Center for Health Statistics (NCHS). The NHIS was authorized through the National Health Survey Act of 1956, and its data are used to monitor trends in illness and disability; track progress toward achieving national health objectives; identify barriers to accessing and using appropriate healthcare services; and evaluate federal health programs.

Centers for Medicare and Medicaid Services

The Centers for Medicare and Medicaid Services (CMS) is committed to strengthening and modernizing the nation's healthcare system to enhance quality, accessibility and improved outcomes in the most cost-effective manner possible.

- The federal Medicaid program is a state-federal partnership in which Medicaid provides health coverage to millions of Americans, including eligible low-income adults, children, pregnant women, elderly adults and people with disabilities. Medicaid is administered by states, according to federal requirements. The program is funded jointly by states and the federal government. Each state has a Medicaid State Plan where the state sets forth its coverage of certain mandatory and optional eligibility groups and mandatory and optional services.

- Medicaid's Early and Periodic Screening, Diagnostic And Treatment (EPSDT) requires the states to provide medically necessary services authorized in section 1905(a) of the Social Security Act Medicaid beneficiaries under the age of 21. This benefit requires screening services as well as physical, mental, vision, hearing, and dental services for persons under age 21 that are needed in order to correct or ameliorate a physical or mental condition.

- Medicare Is the federal health insurance program for people who are 65 or older, certain young people with disabilities, and people with End-Stage Renal Disease (ESRD) (permanent kidney failure requiring dialysis or a transplant).

- The Children's Health Insurance Program (CHIP) provides health coverage to eligible children, through both Medicaid and separate CHIP programs. CHIP is administered by states, pursuant to federal requirements.

- The Medicaid Health Home State Plan Option, authorized under the Affordable Care Act (Section 2703), allows states to design Health Homes to provide comprehensive care coordination for Medicaid beneficiaries with chronic conditions. States will receive enhanced federal funding during the first eight quarters of implementation to support the roll out of this integrated model of care; thereafter they will receive their regular service match rate. Health Home services include:

1. Comprehensive Care Management;

2. Care Coordination And Health Promotion;

3. Comprehensive Transitional Care, including appropriate follow-up, from inpatient to other settings;

4. Patient and Family Support (including authorized representatives);

5. Referral to Community And Social Support Services, if relevant; and

6. Use of health information technology to link services, as feasible and appropriate.

CMS guidance indicates services must be persons and family-centered, include self-management support to individuals and their families, and provide access to individual and family support services. Individual and family supports could include providing caregiver counseling or skills to help the individual improve function, obtaining information about the individual's disability conditions, and navigating the service system. In addition, individual and family supports help families identify resources to assist individuals and caregivers in acquiring, retaining, and improving self-help, socialization, and adaptive skills and provide information and assistance in accessing services such as self-help services, peer support services, and respite services. These supports and services are available to those who meet the eligibility requirements, including youth and young adults with ASD.

- Additional autism-related policies have been published on the CMS website.

  - The Center for Medicaid and CHIP Services has published information on Medicaid home and community-based services (CBS) including guidance. States may provide CBS optionally to certain populations, and they manage their own waiting lists. CMS is available to provide technical assistance to states on the various coverage authorities for treatment of ASD, including state plan and HCBS waiver authorities.

  - CMS guidance on the implementation of the Community First Choice State Plan Option a home and community-based benefits package available to states to promote community integration, can be found online.

439

- CMS offers information about person-centered planning on its website.

- States may also offer Medicaid Health Homes as an optional benefit, to provide care coordination for beneficiaries with certain chronic conditions.

- Some Mental health services are available through Medicare.

Health Resources and Services Administration

Health Resources and Services Administration (HRSA) focuses on improving health equity among all Americans through access to care and a skilled health workforce, with special consideration for underserved populations. Through its Maternal and Child Health Bureau, HRSA supports the following programs and initiatives to address ASD through education, early detection, and intervention:

- Training

  - The Leadership Education in Neurodevelopmental and Other Related Disabilities (LEND) grant program provides medical, allied health professionals, family members, and self-advocates with interdisciplinary, graduate-level training that emphasizes family-centered care, the medical home, and lifespan issues. The primary goal of LEND is to train health professionals to improve the health of children who have, or are at risk of developing, neurodevelopmental disabilities including ASD. LEND programs may include activities focused on transition activities for youth with ASD and other developmental disabilities.

  - The Leadership Education in Developmental-Behavioral Pediatrics (DBP) program trains developmental-behavioral pediatricians (i.e., fellows), pediatricians and primary care providers, and other health and allied health professionals through its training and continuing education programs. DBP training programs provide didactic and clinical based training and continuing education events on all aspects of care for children and adolescents with ASD, including transition from pediatric to adult care and services. DBP grantees support activities related to transition for youth with ASD and other developmental and behavioral issues in a variety of ways, including providing training and technical assistance on transition to families, community

440

service providers, adolescent and adult medical providers, educational institutions; developing resources on transition, and conducting research on transition.

- The Interdisciplinary Technical Assistance Center (ITAC) supports LEND and DBP programs by providing technical assistance, disseminating information and resources, and promoting collaboration among Autism CARES grantees.

- Research

  - The Autism Research Networks (ATNs) Program funds five interdisciplinary research networks that serve to connect leaders in ASD research with healthcare providers, policymakers, and children and their families. The Networks form a common research platform for identifying autism research priorities, conducting ASD research, building capacity by mentoring junior researchers in the field, developing toolkits for parents and providers and guidelines for standards of care, increasing public awareness, and improving ASD service delivery. Of the five research networks receiving funds from 2014 through 2016, two have covered transition topics through their research studies and research-related activities.

  - The R40 Autism Research Program supports field-initiated empirical research through two funding mechanisms that together advance the evidence base on the health and wellbeing of children and adolescents with ASD with a special focus on underserved populations. The R40 Autism Field-Initiated Innovative Research Studies (Autism FIRST) Program supports research on interventions designed to improve health and healthcare service delivery systems. The R40 Autism Secondary Data Analysis Research (Autism-SDAR) Program funds secondary analysis studies using existing national databases. Among the 22 R40 Autism Research grantees first funded in 2013–2015, three projects focused on transition for youth with ASD.

  - Both the 2009–2010 National Survey of Children with Special Health Care Needs (NS-CSHCN) and the 2011–2012 National Survey of Children's Health (NSCH) include measures of the health and well-being, including transition planning, for adolescents with ASD. The national surveys identify households with one or more children under 18 years old.

441

The NS-CSHCN and the NSCH are being redesigned and will become a single survey that will be conducted annually. Both the content and methodology of this combined survey have been refined in 2016 to ensure that it meets the future needs of data users. The first public release of data is scheduled for summer 2017.

- State Services

  - The State Systems Grants Support efforts to build more comprehensive, coordinated State-based systems of care for individuals with ASD, with a special emphasis on medically underserved populations. Although The state grants focus primarily on early identification of ASD and placement in early intervention services, at least 5 of the 14state grantees active between 2014 and 2016 reported activities related to transition for youth with ASD.

  - The State Public Health Autism Resource Center (SPHARC) provides ongoing technical assistance to the state grantees funded under the 2014 Autism CARES Act and facilitates collaboration and coordination among the state grantees and other Autism CARES program areas.

  - The Title V Maternal and Child Health (MCH) Services Block Grant Program (Section 501(a) of Title V of the Social Security Act) intends"to improve the health of all mothers and children consistent with the applicable health status goals and national health objectives...."Administered through well-established federal/state partnerships, states have broad discretion in implementing programs that meet their specific priority needs. The MCH Block Grants are public health programs that are responsible for assessing needs in their state for the entire MCH population and prioritizing programs to meet those needs. States and jurisdictions use their Title V funds to design and implement a wide range of MCH and Children with Special Healthcare Needs (CSHCN) activities.

- The Got Transition/Center for Health Care Transition Improvement is a cooperative agreement between HRSA and the National Alliance to Advance Adolescent Health. Focused on special healthcare needs broadly, Got Transition has developed clinical resources on transition from pediatric to adult healthcare, including the Six Core Elements of Transition (6 core elements) that define the basic components of transition support. These core elements, available in English and Spanish, are consistent with 2011's "Clinical Report on Health Care Transition," which was jointly developed by the American Academy of Pediatrics (AAP), the American Academy of Family Physicians (AAFP), and the American College of Physicians (ACP). The six core elements have been shown to be an effective quality improvement intervention model.

Section 52.3

Legal and Financial Planning Related to Transition for Autism

This section includes text excerpted from "Young Adults and Transitioning Youth with Autism Spectrum Disorder," U.S. Department of Health and Human Services (HHS), August 3, 2017.

The U.S. Department of Justice (DOJ) ensures fair and impartial administration of justice for all Americans. Within DOJ, the Civil Rights Division (CRD) works to uphold the civil and constitutional rights of people with disabilities, including people with autism spectrum disorder and other developmental disabilities. The Division coordinates the activities of the various federal agencies that have obligations under Section 504 and Title II of the Americans with Disabilities Act (ADA). The Civil Rights Division collaborates with other federal agencies to promulgate guidance for schools, localities and state agencies to guarantee equal opportunity for all people, including people with disabilities.

Educational Opportunities Section

Educational Opportunities Section (EOS) enforces antidiscrimination statutes and court decisions in elementary and secondary schools and institutions of higher education, including the ADA, Section 504 of the Rehabilitation Act, the Equal Educational Opportunities Act (EEOA), Title VI of the Civil Rights Act, and upholds rights under the 14th Amendment to the U.S. Constitution in educational settings.

- The Supportive School Discipline Initiative (SSDI) (www. juvenilecouncil.gov/index.html) was created by DOJ and U.S. Department of Education (ED) to address the use of disciplinary policies and practices that push students out of school and into the justice system, which tend to disproportionately impact students with disabilities. The initiative supports school discipline practices that foster safe, inclusive and positive learning environments while keeping students in school.

- In 2014, DOJ and ED released a School Discipline Guidance Package (www.ed.gov/school-discipline) to assist states, districts, and schools in developing practices and strategies to enhance school climate, and ensure those policies and practices comply with federal law.

Disability Rights Section

Disability Rights Section (DRS) enforces Titles I, II and III of the ADA and administers the ADA. The Section uses the broad tools of the ADA to achieve equal opportunity for people with disabilities in the United States. The Section also coordinates the activities of the federal agencies under Section 504 of the Rehabilitation Act and Title II of the ADA. Key concepts that are common to the Department's section 504 and ADA regulations include: reasonable accommodations/ modifications; program accessibility; and effective communication.

- Guidance on the Application of the Integration Mandate of Title II of the Americans with Disabilities Act and *Olmstead v. L.C.* to State and Local Governments' Employment Service Systems for Individuals with Disabilities was released in 2016 and explains the requirements of the ADA integration mandate and Olmstead as applied to employment service systems for individuals with disabilities, which includes youth with autism spectrum disorders in transition from secondary school.

- Guidance on Testing Accommodations (www.ada.gov/regs2014/ testing_accommodations.pdf) was released in 2015 to ensure that people with disabilities who are taking standardized gateway examinations for the purpose of gaining entry to high school, college, or graduate programs, or for those attempting to obtain professional licensure or certification for a trade, have the opportunity to fairly compete for and pursue such opportunities by requiring testing entities to offer exams in a manner that is accessible to people with disabilities and does not measures a person's disability, but instead measures the individual's aptitude or achievement level.

- Guidance on Effective Communication (www.ada.gov/effective-comm.pdf) was released in 2014 to ensure that state and local governments and businesses and nonprofit organizations that serve the public communicate with people with vision, hearing, or speech disabilities in a manner that is equally as effective as their communication with people without disabilities.

- In collaboration with ED's Office for Civil Rights (OCR) and Office of Special Education and Rehabilitative Services (OSERS), DOJ's Civil Rights Division released Frequently Asked Questions on Effective Communication for Students with Hearing, Vision, or Speech Disabilities in Public Elementary and Secondary Schools (www.ada.gov/doe_doj_eff_comm/doe_doj_eff_comm_faqs. pdf) in 2014 to address the obligation of public schools to meet the communication needs of students with disabilities.

Special Litigation Section

SPL enforces Title II of the ADA, the Civil Rights of Institution-alized Persons Act (CRIPA), and Section 14141 of the Violent Crime Control and Law Enforcement Act of 1994. The Section's work has addressed conditions at healthcare facilities for individuals with disabilities, the rights of individuals with disabilities to live in their communities and not facilities, and the appropriate diversion of individuals with disabilities from the criminal justice system.

U.S. Department of Justice Office of Justice Programs

Office of Justice Programs (OJP) provides leadership to federal, state, local, and tribal justice systems through national dissemination of state-of-the-art knowledge and practices, and the provision of grants for the implementation of crime-fighting strategies.

Bureau of Justice Assistance

Bureau of Justice Assistance (BJA) provides leadership and assistance to local criminal justice programs that improve and reinforce the nation's criminal justice system. BJA works to reduce and prevent crime, violence, and drug abuse and to improve the way in which the criminal justice system functions. In 2013 BJA funded The Arc of the United States, Inc.'s project for the National Center on Justice and Disability, to build a national resource center to address challenges the justice system faces when it encounters people with disabilities in the areas of law enforcement, courts, and corrections. The Center's "Pathways to Justice" initiative works to increase the capacity of criminal justice professionals to respond to individuals with disabilities by providing training, technical assistance, and education. The Center brings together professionals from the disability and criminal justice fields to share expertise and provides training using a team approach, with the goal of becoming the go-to resource in their community or state on issues related to criminal justice and disability.

Chapter 53

Finding Appropriate and Affordable Housing

The U.S. Department of Housing and Urban Development (HUD) works to strengthen the housing market in order to bolster the economy and protect consumers; meet the need for quality affordable rental homes; utilize housing as a platform for improving quality of life; and build inclusive and sustainable communities free from discrimination.

The U.S. Department of Housing and Urban Development (HUD) administratively enforces several civil rights laws prohibiting housing discrimination, including the Fair Housing Act, Section 504 of the Rehabilitation Act, and the Americans with Disabilities Act (ADA). With few exceptions, the Fair Housing Act covers housing throughout the country.

Section 504

Section 504 provisions apply to recipients of HUD financial assistance, including the Community Development Block Grant, Public Housing, Multifamily, Housing Choice Voucher, and other programs. HUD's Section 504 regulations (at 24 CFR § 8.4c) permit exclusion of nondisabled persons from the benefits of a program if the program is limited by federal statute or executive order to individuals with

This chapter includes text excerpted from "Young Adults and Transitioning Youth with Autism Spectrum Disorder," U.S. Department of Health and Human Services (HHS), August 3, 2017.

disabilities, and also permits exclusion of a specific class of individuals with disabilities from a program if the program is limited by federal statute or executive order to a different class of individuals. However, HUD does not have disability-specific programs, such as housing specifically for persons with autism-spectrum disabilities.

Section 811 Supportive Housing for Persons with Disabilities

Section 811 program, HUD provides funding to develop and subsidized rental housing with the availability of supportive services for very low- and extremely low-income adults with disabilities.

Chapter 54

Adult Autism and Employment

Chapter Contents

Section 54.1

Employment Training for Adolescents with Autism Spectrum Disorder

This section includes excerpted from "Protecting
Students with Disabilities," U.S. Department of
Education (ED), September 25, 2018.

Placement

Once a student is identified as being eligible for regular or special
education and related aids or services, a decision must be made regarding
the type of services the student needs.

If a Student Is Eligible for Services under Both the Individuals with Disabilities Education Act (IDEA) and Section 504, Must a School District Develop Both an Individualized Education Program (IEP) under the IDEA and a Section 504 Plan under Section 504?

No. If a student is eligible under Individuals with Disabilities Education Act (IDEA), she or he must have an individualized education
program (IEP). Under the Section 504 regulations, one way to meet
Section 504 requirements for a free appropriate public education is to
implement an IEP.

Must a School District Develop a Section 504 Plan for a Student Who Either "Has a Record of Disability" or Is "Regarded as Disabled"?

No. In public elementary and secondary schools, unless a student
actually has an impairment that substantially limits a major life activity, the mere fact that a student has a "record of" or is "regarded as"
disabled is insufficient, in itself, to trigger those Section 504 protections that require the provision of a free appropriate public education
(FAPE). This is consistent with the Amendments Act, in which Congress clarified that an individual who meets the definition of disability solely by virtue of being "regarded as" disabled is not entitled to
reasonable accommodations or the reasonable modification of policies,
practices or procedures. The phrases "has a record of disability" and
"is regarded as disabled" are meant to reach the situation in which a

student either does not have or never had a disability, but is treated by others as such.

In the Amendments Act, Congress clarified that an individual is not "regarded as" an individual with a disability if the impairment is transitory and minor. A transitory impairment is an impairment with an actual or expected duration of six months or less.

What Is the Receiving School District's Responsibility under Section 504 toward a Student with a Section 504 Plan Who Transfers from Another District?

If a student with a disability transfers to a district from another school district with a Section 504 plan, the receiving district should review the plan and supporting documentation. If a group of persons at the receiving school district, including persons knowledgeable about the meaning of the evaluation data and knowledgeable about the placement options determines that the plan is appropriate, the district is required to implement the plan. If the district determines that the plan is inappropriate, the district is to evaluate the student consistent with the Section 504 procedures at 34 C.F.R. 104.35 and determine which educational program is appropriate for the student. There is no Section 504 bar to the receiving school district honoring the previous IEP during the interim period.

What Are the Responsibilities of Regular Education Teachers with Respect to Implementation of Section 504 Plans? What Are the Consequences If the District Fails to Implement the Plans?

Regular education teachers must implement the provisions of Section 504 plans when those plans govern the teachers' treatment of students for whom they are responsible. If the teachers fail to implement the plans, such failure can cause the school district to be in noncompliance with Section 504.

What Is the Difference between a Regular Education Intervention Plan and a Section 504 Plan?

A regular education intervention plan is appropriate for a student who does not have a disability or is not suspected of having a disability but may be facing challenges in school. School districts vary in how they address performance problems of regular education students. Some districts employ teams at individual schools, commonly referred to as "building teams." These teams are designed to provide regular education classroom teachers with instructional support and strategies for helping students in need of assistance. These teams are typically composed of regular and special education teachers who provide ideas to classroom teachers on methods for helping students experiencing academic or behavioral problems. The team usually records its ideas in a written regular education intervention plan. The team meets with an affected student's classroom teacher(s) and recommends strategies to address the student's problems within the regular education environment. The team then follows the responsible teacher(s) to determine whether the student's performance or behavior has improved. In addition to building teams, districts may utilize other regular education intervention methods, including before-school and after-school programs, tutoring programs, and mentoring programs.

Procedural Safeguards

Public elementary and secondary schools must employ procedural safeguards regarding the identification, evaluation, or educational placement of persons who, because of disability, need or are believed to need special instruction or related services.

Must a Recipient School District Obtain Parental Consent Prior to Conducting an Initial Evaluation?

Yes. Office for Civil Rights (OCR) has interpreted Section 504 to require districts to obtain parental permission for initial evaluations. If a district suspects a student needs or is believed to need special instruction or related services and parental consent is withheld, the IDEA and Section 504 provide that districts may use due process hearing procedures to seek to override the parents' denial of consent for an initial evaluation.

If So, in What Form Is Consent Required?

Section 504 is silent on the form of parental consent required. OCR has accepted written consent as compliance. IDEA, as well as many state laws, also require written consent prior to initiating an evaluation.

What Can a Recipient School District Do If a Parent Withholds Consent for a Student to Secure Services under Section 504 after a Student Is Determined Eligible for Services?

Section 504 neither prohibits nor requires a school district to initiate a due process hearing to override a parental refusal to consent with respect to the initial provision of special education and related services. Nonetheless, school districts should consider that IDEA no longer permits school districts to initiate a due process hearing to override a parental refusal to consent to the initial provision of services.

What Procedural Safeguards Are Required under Section 504?

Recipient school districts are required to establish and implement procedural safeguards that include notice, an opportunity for parents to review relevant records, an impartial hearing with opportunity for participation by the student's parents or guardian, representation by counsel and a review procedure.

What Is a Recipient School District's Responsibility under Section 504 to Provide Information to Parents and Students about Its Evaluation and Placement Process?

Section 504 requires districts to provide notice to parents explaining any evaluation and placement decisions affecting their children and explaining the parents' right to review educational records and appeal any decision regarding evaluation and placement through an impartial hearing.

Is There a Mediation Requirement under Section 504?

No.

Section 54.2

Disability Employment

This section contains text excerpted from the following sources:
Text beginning with the heading "Job Seekers" is excerpted from
"Disability Employment," U.S. Office of Personnel Management
(OPM), November 14, 2010. Reviewed October 2018; Text beginning
with the heading "U.S. Department of Labor (DOL)" is excerpted
from "Young Adults and Transitioning Youth with Autism
Spectrum Disorder," U.S. Department of Health and
Human Services (HHS), August 3, 2017.

Job Seekers

The federal government is actively recruiting and hiring persons with disabilities. It offers a variety of exciting jobs, competitive salaries, excellent benefits, and opportunities for career advancement.

Hiring people with disabilities into federal jobs is fast and easy. People with disabilities can be appointed to federal jobs noncompetitively through a process called Schedule A. Learn how to be considered for federal jobs under the noncompetitive process. People with disabilities may also apply for jobs through the traditional or competitive process.

Getting a Job

Learn the difference between the competitive and noncompetitive hiring processes, how to use the Schedule A Authority, and how to conduct a job search in the federal government.

Find a Selective Placement Program Coordinator

Most federal agencies have a Selective Placement Program Coordinator, a Special Emphasis Program Manager (SEPM) for Employment of Adults with Disabilities, or equivalent, who helps to recruit, hire and accommodate people with disabilities at that agency.

Reasonable Accommodations

The federal government may provide you reasonable accommodation in appropriate cases. Requests are considered on a case-by-case basis.

Federal Agencies

As the Nation's largest employer, the federal government has a special responsibility to lead by example in including people with disabilities in the workforce. This website contains important information for federal agencies to use in recruiting, hiring, and retaining individuals with disabilities and targeted disabilities.

Background

On July 26, 2010, President Obama issued Executive Order 13548, which provides that the federal government, as the Nation's largest employer, must become a model for the employment of individuals with disabilities. The order directs Executive departments and agencies (agencies) to improve their efforts to employ federal workers with disabilities and targeted disabilities through increased recruitment, hiring, and retention of these individuals. This is not only the right thing to do, but it is also good for the government, as it increases the potential pool of highly qualified people from which the federal government draws its talent. Importantly, the Executive Order adopts the goal set forth in Executive Order 13163 of hiring 100,000 people with disabilities into the federal government over 5 years, including individuals with targeted disabilities.

The Executive Order also instructed the Director of the Office of Personnel Management (OPM), in consultation with the Secretary of Labor, the Chair of the Equal Employment Opportunity Commission (EEOC), and the Director of the Office of Management and Budget (OMB), to design model recruitment and hiring strategies for agencies to facilitate their employment of people with disabilities.

In addition to the Executive Order, federal agencies are obligated under the Rehabilitation Act of 1973, as amended to affirmatively employ people with disabilities. The specific requirements of this obligation are spelled out in the Equal Employment Opportunity Commission Management Directive (MD) 715.

Recruiting

This section contains recruiting information and resources for selective placement program coordinators, human resources professionals, managers and hiring officials.

Hiring

There are two types of hiring processes. In the noncompetitive hiring process, agencies use a special authority to hire persons with disabilities without requiring them to compete for the job. In the competitive process, applicants compete with each other through a structured process.

Retention

Retention is essential to making the investment of identifying and hiring people pay off. Learn helpful practices for retaining people with disabilities.

Providing Accommodation

In order to meet their accommodation obligations, agencies should think creatively about ways to make their workplace more accessible and create an environment where their employees who have disabilities can thrive. Here are some suggestions that relate specifically to reasonable accommodation issues.

U.S. Department of Labor

The U.S. Department of Labor (DOL) works to improve full access to gainful employment opportunities for all Americans, including Americans with disabilities. DOL also supports career pathways for youth and adults through its support for workforce development and job training programs.

Office of Disability Employment Policy

- Office of Disability Employment Policy (ODEP) in DOL developed the Guideposts for Success in conjunction with its grantee, the National Collaborative on Workforce and Disability for Youth. The Guideposts for Success is an evidence-based policy and practice framework for serving all youth, including youth with disabilities. The Guideposts indicate that all youth, including those with significant disabilities, should receive high quality supports and services in the areas of: career exploration and development, school-based preparation, family involvement, youth leadership and development, and connecting activities.

- The Pathways to Careers Demonstration Grants support researching, developing, testing and evaluating innovative approaches to providing comprehensive, coordinated, and integrated inclusive education and career development services to youth and young adults with disabilities ages 14–24, including youth and young adults with significant disabilities. The grants are also intended to increase institutional capacity within the community college system by building an evidence base of policies and practices that are most effective in helping youth and young adults with disabilities to thrive in community college settings.

- Employment First is a policy framework for systems change that is centered on the premise that all citizens, including those with significant disabilities, are capable of fully participating in competitive integrated employment (CIE) and community life. ODEP manages the Employment First State Leadership Mentoring Program (EFSLMP) with 14 participating states. Through EFSLMP, ODEP provides training and technical assistance to these states to assist with their development and implementation of holistic systems change. EFSLMP also assists states in sharing information, resources, and recommendations for implementing Employment First policies and practices. The objectives of the EFSLMP are to provide mentoring, intensive technical assistance and training from a national pool of subject matter experts and peer mentors to core states as they transform existing policies, service delivery systems, and reimbursement structures to reflect an Employment First approach. EFSLMP also facilitates virtual training and knowledge translation on effective practices, facilitates dialogue on shared experiences related to effectuating Employment First policies and practice, links participating states with federal initiatives that are focused on promoting state-level systems-change conducive to Employment First objectives, and evaluates the impacts of the investments in state Employment First systems change efforts over time to identify common challenges faced by state governments and validate innovative strategies and effective practices that lead to the successful implementation of Employment First objectives.

Disability Employment Initiative

The Disability Employment Initiative (DEI) is a collaborative of ODEP and DOL's Employment and Training Administration (ETA) to increase the capacity of the national American Job Center network to provide services to job seekers with disabilities. Since 2010, DOL has awarded grants totaling $126 million to 49 DEI projects in 28 states in order to improve workforce development services for job seekers with disabilities, including those with significant disabilities. The most DEI projects have incorporated a focus on career pathways and alignment with the Workforce Innovation and Opportunity Act of 2014 (WIOA).

Advisory Committee on Increasing Competitive Integrated Employment for Individuals with Disabilities

The Advisory Committee on Increasing Competitive Integrated Employment for Individuals with Disabilities was established under the Rehabilitation Act of 1973, as amended by the WIOA, to advise in three areas:

- Ways to increase competitive integrated employment (CIE) opportunities for individuals with intellectual or developmental disabilities (I/DD) or other individuals with significant disabilities;

- The use of a certificate program carried out under Section 14(c) of the Fair Labor Standards Act (FLSA) for the employment of individuals with I/DD or other individuals with significant disabilities; and

- Ways to improve oversight of the use of such certificates.

The Committee was established in September 2014 according to the provisions of the Federal Advisory Committee Act (FACA), which helps ensure the independent nature of the Committee in providing advice and recommendations to the Administration. The primary purpose of the work of the Committee was to address issues and make recommendations to improve the employment participation of people with I/DD and others with significant disabilities by ensuring opportunities for CIE.

Section 54.3

Self-Employment for People with Disabilities

This section includes text excerpted from "Self-Employment
for People with Disabilities," U.S. Department of Labor (DOL),
December 15, 2013. Reviewed October 2018.

Many Americans are the descendants of people who came to the
United States from across the globe to realize opportunity and exercise
freedom. Steeped in the spirit of independence, the earliest Americans
were self-employed, primarily in agriculture. However, as the nation's
economic base shifted from farming to manufacturing and then on to
the "Information Age," the nature of employment in America did as
well, with wage employment replacing self-employment as the primary
means of livelihood.

Yet, America continues to be associated the world over with the
spirit of self-determination that embodies its roots as an entrepreneurial, self-reliant society. Furthermore, in economic downturns, job
loss and lack of employment opportunities may produce additional
incentive to pursue self-employment for people in a variety of situations and circumstances.

People with disabilities demonstrate the same passion, independence, and self-direction as all Americans, and given certain characteristics—including being on average older and less educated—it is
not surprising that the rate of self-employment for people with disabilities in the labor force in 2011 was about 50 percent higher than
the corresponding rate for people without disabilities. In 2011, among
employed individuals, a higher proportion of those with disabilities
were unincorporated self-employed (11.8%) than individuals without
disabilities (6.6%).

Self-Employment among People with Disabilities

Self-employment allows people to customize their work experiences
specifically to their needs and to design a work environment that opti-
mizes flexibility and accommodation. Several public programs support
employment preparation and work incentives to achieve self-sufficiency. Although limited, available statistics indicate that there has
been little engagement by public programs to help people with disabilities explore self-employment as a viable work option. Prior to
Start-Up, several federal programs acknowledged self-employment

as an outcome for people both with and without disabilities, but with few exceptions, it is fair to say that not many programs specifically promoted self-employment.

The Workforce Investment Act (WIA), which authorizes DOL's American Job Centers (AJCs) (formerly known as One-Stop Career Centers), makes numerous references to self-employment. In fact, self-employment, entrepreneurship and small businesses are mentioned in WIA, as amended, in several titles and sections: definitions; migrant and seasonal farmworkers programs; demonstration, pilot, multi-service research, and multistate projects; employment statistics; people with significant disabilities; vocational rehabilitation (VR) services for individuals and groups; research; special projects and demonstrations; and provider and individual training. Furthermore, self-employment is an allowed exit outcome for individuals receiving services authorized by WIA. In 2010, the Employment and Training Administration (ETA) issued guidance on self-employment to state and local workforce agencies and rapid response coordinators. But the proportion of AJC exciters who entered self-employment is unknown. AJCs report outcomes as employment of any type, with no distinction between self-employment and wage employment.

In 2011, ETA reported that 4.3 percent of all 2010 WIA exiters disclosed disabilities, and 3 percent who exited for employment reported disabilities. ETA reported that less than 1 percent of WIA exiters in 2010 received entrepreneurial training, suggesting that a very small percentage of all exiters (with and without disclosed disabilities) prepared for self-employment. The U.S. Social Security Administration (SSA) sponsors work incentive programs to encourage employment of people with disabilities who receive Social Security Disability Insurance (SSDI) and Supplemental Security Income (SSI) due to disability. SSI's Plan to Achieve Self-Support (PASS) and Ticket to Work incentive programs include self-employment as an outcome for people with disabilities, but available data suggest self-employment is an infrequent outcome for program exiters. ETA sponsored a study that matched AJC clients in four states (Colorado, Iowa, Maryland, and Oregon) with SSI and SSDI records to find out what proportion received SSA disability benefits (information not routinely recorded by AJCs). In Program Years 2002–2007, in all four states, only 2 to 4 percent of AJC users were SSA beneficiaries when they registered for services; slightly higher percentages (3–6%) had once been SSA beneficiaries. Despite these low percentages, AJCs served a substantial percentage of all SSA beneficiaries actively seeking employment (26% in Iowa and Colorado). These percentages are similar to, or much greater than, the percentage of SSA beneficiaries receiving employment services from vocational rehabilitation (VR) agencies in the same states.

People with disabilities may prepare for employment through their state VR programs, funded by the Rehabilitation Services Administration (RSA) in the Department of Education. RSA collects data on self-employment outcomes for people with disabilities who receive VR services. The Rehabilitation Act of 1973, Sections 7(11) (C) and 103(a) (13), supports state VR agencies in offering a self-employment outcome as follows:

> *(C) Satisfying any other vocational outcome the Secretary may determine to be appropriate (including satisfying the vocational outcome of self-employment, telecommuting or business ownership), in a manner consistent with the Act.*

> *(13) Technical assistance and other consultation services to conduct market analyses, develop business plans, and otherwise provide resources, to the extent such resources are authorized to be provided through the statewide workforce investment system, to eligible individuals who are pursuing self-employment or telecommuting or establishing a small business operation as an employment outcome.*

Despite this authority, an analysis of RSA case closure statistics for VR clients indicated that self-employment remains a small percentage of overall VR status 26 closures in employment, ranging from 1.97 percent in 2003 to 1.66 percent in 2007 and 1.99 percent in 2009, although there has been a small increase to 2.40 percent in 2012.

VR agencies with the highest percentage of self-employment outcomes were in states generally considered to have more disbursed populations and generally more rural communities.

Average hourly and weekly earnings for individuals closed in self-employment were consistently higher than the average wages for all Status 26 (successfully employed) closures. The average hourly wage for persons closed in self-employment in FY 2012 was $14.46, compared to $11.33 for all Status 26 closures. Average weekly wage in self-employment in FY 2012 was $445, compared to $365 for all Status 26 closures.

The mean average case service expenditure by VR agencies for persons closed in self-employment in FY 2012 was approximately $7,910. In comparison, the average expenditure for all Status 26 closures in FY 2012 was approximately $5,436.

The mean average time period from the point that the Individual Plan for Employment was initiated to closure in self-employment in FY 2012 was 663 days. The comparative time period for all Status 26 closures in employment was 630 days.

VR State agency involvement in facilitating self-employment outcomes does vary substantially from state to state, particularly for persons with a primary intellectual disability. There are states, such as Florida and Ohio, whose VR agencies are involved in initiatives to implement policies and practices that expand participation in self-employment. These agencies are implementing a step-by-step vocational rehabilitation process that provides a variety of resources to the individual with a disability potentially interested in self-employment. This process focuses on individual support needs and emphasizes the development of a business design team to assist and support the self-employment initiative. It also focuses on the ongoing support needed for the development of a viable business plan and the successful implementation and maintenance of the self-employment venture.

Chapter 55

The Affordable Care Act and Autism and Related Conditions

What Is the Affordable Care Act?

The Affordable Care Act (ACA) is a historic healthcare reform law to improve healthcare coverage and access while putting in place new protections for people who already have health insurance. Under the law, health insurance coverage will become affordable and accessible for millions of people, a factor that will help reduce health disparities. By 2019, it is estimated that 32 million individuals will obtain health insurance coverage as a result of the ACA. The ACA affects everyone in the United States, so it is important to understand what the law means for community members that you will interact with during your education and outreach activities. This chapter is designed to help you understand what the law is and how it will benefit individuals and families in your target communities.

This chapter contains text excerpted from the following sources: Text beginning with the heading "What Is the Affordable Care Act?" is excerpted from "The Affordable Care Act Resource Kit," Office of Minority Health (OMH), U.S. Department of Health and Human Services (HHS), February 18, 2014. Reviewed October 2018; Text under the heading "Affordable Care Act and Autism" is excerpted from "The Affordable Care Act and Autism and Related Conditions," U.S. Department of Health and Human Services (HHS), April 9, 2015. Reviewed October 2018.

Why Is the Affordable Care Act Important?

Prior to the ACA, insurance companies could turn away the 129 million Americans with preexisting conditions. Premiums had more than doubled over the last decade. Tens of millions were underinsured, many had coverage but were afraid of losing it, and 50 million individuals had no insurance at all. Racial and ethnic minorities continued to lag behind in many health indicators, including prevalence of chronic illness and access to quality care.

Rising health insurance costs previously meant that fewer people could afford or access healthcare. From 2003–2010, the average health insurance premium for a worker with a family was approximately $14,000 per year. The high cost of health insurance forced many individuals and families to choose between paying for coverage or other basic needs.

In addition to the problem of rising healthcare costs, many people did not have the security that health insurance is suppose to provide. Prior to the Affordable Care Act, individuals could be denied coverage because of a preexisting condition; health insurance companies could raise costs if people were sick, making coverage unaffordable for many small businesses and individuals; and insurance companies could place lifetime limits on benefits.

The Affordable Care Act offers solutions to the problems outlined above. Essentially, the ACA ends many insurance company abuses, makes health insurance more affordable, strengthens the Medicare program, and provides better options for getting health coverage. Together, the law takes a big step forward towards eliminating health disparities.

Improvements in coverage have already been documented:

- 3.1 million young adults have gained insurance through their parents' plans

- 6.1 million people with Medicare through 2012 received $5.7 billion in prescription drug discounts

- An estimated 34 million people with Medicare received a free preventive service in 2012

- 71 million privately insured people gained improved coverage for preventive services

- 105 million individuals have had lifetime limits removed from their insurance

What Are the Major Themes of the Affordable Care Act?

The Affordable Care Act:

1. Strengthens insurance coverage by generally ending discrimination based on preexisting conditions or gender and doing away with lifetime limits on essential health benefits.

2. Makes healthcare more affordable by offering eligible individuals new tax credits to lower premiums, reduced cost-sharing, and better access to Medicaid and the Children's Health Insurance Program (CHIP).

3. Strengthens the Medicare program by eliminating cost-sharing for most preventive services, adding an Annual Wellness Visit, and lowering beneficiaries' prescription drug costs when they hit the prescription drug coverage gap known as the "donut hole."

4. Expands access to coverage and care for uninsured and underinsured individuals, including people with low or no incomes, people who live in medically underserved areas, people in rural communities, and youth.

Affordable Care Act and Autism

The ACA contains important provisions for individuals with autism and related conditions and their families:

- Most health insurance plans are no longer allowed to deny, limit, exclude, or charge more for coverage to anyone based on a preexisting condition, including autism and related conditions.

- All Marketplace health plans and most other private insurance plans must cover preventive services for children without charging a copayment or coinsurance. This includes autism screening for children at 18 and 24 months.

- Health plans cannot put a lifetime dollar limit on most benefits you receive. The law also does away with annual dollar limits a health plan can place on most of your benefits. Prior to the ACA, many plans set a dollar limit on what they would spend for covered benefits during the time individuals were enrolled in the plan, leaving individuals on the autism spectrum and their families to pay the cost of all care exceeding that limit.

- Young adults can remain covered under their parents' insurance up to the age of 26. For a young adult with autism or related conditions and their family, that means more flexibility, more options, and greater peace of mind.

- Individuals on the autism spectrum and families of children on the autism spectrum now have expanded access to affordable insurance options through the new Health Insurance Marketplace and expansion in Medicaid.

- New health plans sold in the individual and small group markets, including the Marketplace, must cover "essential health benefits," including hospitalizations, preventive services, and prescription drugs, to help ensure you have the coverage you need to stay healthy. Health insurers will also have annual out-of-pocket limits to protect families' incomes against the high cost of healthcare services.

Part Eight

Additional Help and Information

Chapter 56

Acronyms and Glossary of Autism Spectrum Disorder Terms

Autism Spectrum Disorder-Related Acronyms

ABA: applied behavior analysis

ADA: Americans with Disabilities Act

ADD: attention deficit disorder

ADHD: attention deficit hyperactivity disorder

ADI: Autism Diagnostic Interview—a diagnostic tool developed in London by the Medical Research Council

ADOS: Autism Diagnostic Observation Schedule

AS: Asperger syndrome

ASA: Autism Society of America

ASD: autism spectrum disorder

CARS: Childhood Autism Rating Scale

CHAT: Checklist for Autism in Toddlers—a diagnostic tool

DD: developmental disabilities

This glossary contains terms excerpted from documents produced by several sources deemed reliable.

EEG: electroencephalogram

FC: facilitated communication

GARS: Gilliam Autism Rating Scale

HFA: high-functioning autism

IDEA: Individuals with Disabilities Education Act

IEP: individualized education plan

LRE: least restrictive environment

NOS: not otherwise specified

OCD: obsessive-compulsive disorder

OT: Occupational therapist

PDD: pervasive developmental disorder

PDD-NOS: pervasive developmental disorder not otherwise specified

PECS: picture exchange communication system

PRT: pivotal response training

PT: physical therapy

SI: sensory integration

SIB: self-injurious behavior

SIT: sensory integration therapy

TEACCH: Treatment and Education of Autistic and Related Communication Handicapped Children

Autism Spectrum Disorder-Related Terms

Affordable Care Act (ACA): The comprehensive healthcare reform law enacted in March 2010.

Angelman syndrome: Microdeletion of 15q-13, of maternal origin, resulting in mental retardation, ataxia, paroxysms of laughter, seizures, characteristic facies, and minimal speech.

aphasia: Total or partial loss of the ability to use or understand language; usually caused by stroke, brain disease, or injury.

apraxia of speech: A speech disorder, also known as verbal apraxia or dyspraxia, in which a person has trouble speaking because of inability to execute a voluntary movement despite normal muscle function.

Asperger disorder: A pervasive developmental disorder character-ized by severe and enduring impairment in social skills and restrictive and repetitive behaviors and interests, leading to impaired social and occupational functioning but without significant delays in language development.

assistive devices: Technical tools and devices such as alphabet boards, text telephones, or text-to-speech conversion software used to aid individuals who have communication disorders perform actions, tasks, and activities.

assistive technologies: Products, devices, or equipment that help maintain, increase, or improve the functional capabilities of people with disabilities.

audiologist: Healthcare professional who is trained to evaluate hear-ing loss and related disorders, including balance (vestibular) disorders and tinnitus, and to rehabilitate individuals with hearing loss and related disorders. An audiologist uses a variety of tests and procedures to assess hearing and balance function and to fit and dispense hearing aids and other assistive devices for hearing.

auditory nerve: Eighth cranial nerve that connects the inner ear to the brainstem and is responsible for hearing and balance.

autism spectrum disorders (ASDs): A spectrum of developmen-tal disorders that begin in early childhood and persists throughout adulthood; autism spectrum disorders affect three crucial areas of development: communication, social interaction, and creative or imag-inative play.

autistic disorder (also called classic autism): This is what most people think of when hearing the word autism. People with autistic disorder usually have significant language delays, social and commu-nication challenges, and unusual behaviors and interests. Many people with autistic disorder also have intellectual disability.

biomarker: A specific physical trait or a measurable biologically pro-duced change in the body connected with a disease or health condition.

childhood disintegrative disorder (CDD): Loss of such skills as vocabulary are more dramatic in CDD than they are in classical autism. The diagnosis requires extensive and pronounced losses involv-ing motor language, and social skills. CDD is also accompanied by loss of bowel and bladder control and oftentimes seizures and a very low intelligence quotient (IQ).

clonic seizures: Seizures that cause repeated jerking movements of muscles on both sides of the body.

cochlear implant: A medical device that bypasses damaged structures in the inner ear and directly stimulates the auditory nerve, allowing some people who are deaf or hard of hearing (HoH) to learn to hear and interpret sounds and speech.

cognition: Thinking skills that include perception, memory, awareness, reasoning, judgment, intellect, and imagination.

community first choice option: The Community First Choice Option lets states provide home and community-based attendant services to Medicaid enrollees with disabilities, under their State Plan.

community provider: A community provider is a medical or educational professional who works with children with developmental disabilities (including psychologist, physician, teacher, learning specialist, speech/language pathologist, occupational therapist, physical therapist, nurse, social worker, etc.) within the ADDM Network communities.

comorbid: The existence of one or more co-occurring disorders in addition to a primary disorder.

compulsion: Uncontrollable thoughts or impulses to perform an act, often repetitively, as an unconscious mechanism to avoid unacceptable ideas and desires which, by themselves, arouse anxiety; the anxiety becomes fully manifest if performance of the compulsive act is prevented; may be associated with obsessive thoughts.

convulsions: Sudden severe contractions of the muscles that may be caused by seizures.

corpus callosotomy (CC): Surgery that severs the corpus callosum, or network of neural connections between the right and left hemispheres.

cost-sharing: The share of costs covered by your insurance that you pay out of your own pocket. This term generally includes deductible, coinsurance and copayments, or similar charges, but it doesn't include premiums, balance-billing amounts for nonnetwork providers, or the cost of noncovered services.

developmental delay: A developmental delay is a persistent delay experienced by a child in reaching one or more developmental milestones—how children grow, move, communicate, interact, learn, and play.

*de novo***:** New, for the first time.

developmental disability: Loss of function brought on by prenatal and postnatal events in which the predominant disturbance is in the acquisition of cognitive, language, motor, or social skills; for example, mental retardation, autistic disorder, learning disorder, and attention deficit hyperactivity disorder.

donut hole: Most plans with Medicare prescription drug coverage (Part D) have a coverage gap (called a "donut hole"). This means that after you and your drug plan have spent a certain amount of money for covered drugs, you have to pay most costs out-of-pocket for your prescriptions up to a yearly limit.

dravet syndrome: A type of intractable epilepsy that begins in infancy.

drop attacks: Seizures that cause sudden falls; another term for atonic seizures.

echolalia: Involuntary parrot-like repetition of a word or sentence just spoken by another person.

encephalitis: Inflammation of the brain caused by a virus. Encephalitis can result in permanent brain damage or death.

epilepsy syndromes: Disorders with a specific set of symptoms that include epilepsy.

etiology: The cause of.

focal seizures: Seizures that occur in just one part of the brain.

fragile X syndrome (FXS): This disorder is the most common inherited form of mental retardation. It was so named because one part of the X chromosome has a defective piece that appears pinched and fragile when under a microscope.

gene expression: The process by which the information encoded in a gene is used to direct the assembly of a protein molecule; different subsets of genes are expressed in different cell types or under different conditions.

generalized seizures: Seizures that result from abnormal neuronal activity in many parts of the brain.

genetics: The study of particular genes, DNA, and heredity.

genomics: The study of the genome (the entire genetic makeup) of an organism.

grand mal seizures: An older term for tonic-clonic seizures.

health disparities: A health disparity is a particular type of health difference that is closely linked with social, economic, and/or environmental disadvantage.

Health Insurance Marketplaces: Health Insurance Marketplaces are designed to make buying health coverage easier and more affordable.

hearing aid: An electronic device that brings amplified sound to the ear; it usually consists of a microphone, amplifier, and receiver.

hemispherectomy: Surgery involving the removal or disabling of one hemisphere of the brain.

hemispheres: The right and left halves of the brain.

hemispherotomy: Removing half of the brain's outer layer (cortex).

idiopathic: Relating to a disease or disorder that arises spontaneously or without a known cause.

immunization: The process by which a person or animal becomes protected against a disease. This term is often used interchangeably with vaccination or inoculation.

infantile spasms: Clusters of seizures that usually begin before the age of 6 months. During these seizures the infant may bend and cry out.

intellectual disability: Intellectual disability means that a person has difficulty learning at an expected level and functioning in daily life. In this report, intellectual disability is measured by intelligence quotient (IQ) test scores of less than or equal to 70.

intractable: Hard to treat; about 30 to 40 percent of people with epilepsy will continue to experience seizures even with the best available treatment.

ketogenic diet: A strict diet rich in fats and low in carbohydrates that causes the body to break down fats instead of carbohydrates to survive.

Landau-Kleffner syndrome: Childhood disorder of unknown origin which often extends into adulthood and can be identified by gradual or sudden loss of the ability to understand and use spoken language.

language disorders: Any of a number of problems with verbal communication and the ability to use or understand a symbol system for communication.

language: System for communicating ideas and feelings using sounds, gestures, signs, or marks.

learning disabilities (LD): Childhood disorders characterized by difficulty with certain skills such as reading or writing in individuals with normal intelligence.

lesion: Damaged or dysfunctional part of the brain or other parts of the body.

lesionectomy: Surgical removal of a specific brain lesion.

lobectomy: Surgical removal of a lobe of the brain.

Medicaid: Each state operates a Medicaid program that provides health coverage for some lower-income people, families and children, the elderly, and people with disabilities.

Medicare: Medicare is health insurance for people age 65 or older, people under 65 with certain disabilities, and people of all ages with end-stage renal disease.

monotherapy: Treatment with only one antiepileptic drug.

multiple subpial transection (MST): A type of operation in which surgeons make a series of cuts in the brain that are designed to prevent seizures from spreading into other parts of the brain while leaving the person's normal abilities intact.

mutation: A change in a DNA sequence that can result from DNA copying mistakes made during cell division, exposure to ionizing radiation, exposure to chemical mutagens, or infection by viruses.

nonepileptic seizures: Any phenomena that look like seizures but do not result from abnormal brain activity.

nonverbal: Denoting communication without words, for example, by signs, symbols, facial expressions, gestures, posture.

obsession: A recurrent and persistent idea, thought, or impulse to carry out an act that is ego-dystonic, that is experienced as senseless or repugnant, and that the individual cannot voluntarily suppress.

pervasive developmental disorder (PDD): A group of mental disorders of infancy, childhood, or adolescence characterized by distortions in the acquisition of the multiple basic psychologic functions necessary for the elaboration of social skills, language skills, and imagination; also characterized by restricted or stereotypical activities and interests.

pervasive developmental disorder-not otherwise specified (PDD-NOS): People who meet some of the criteria for autistic disorder or Asperger syndrome, but not all, may be diagnosed with PDD-NOS. People with PDD-NOS usually have fewer and milder symptoms than those with autistic disorder. The symptoms might cause only social and communication challenges.

phenotype: An individual's physical and behavioral characteristics.

placebo: A substance or treatment that has no effect on human beings.

prevalence: The number of people in a population that have a condition relative to all of the people in the population.

Rasmussen encephalitis (RE): A progressive type of epilepsy in which half of the brain shows continual inflammation.

responsive stimulation: A form of treatment that uses an implanted device to detect a forthcoming seizure and administer intervention such as electrical stimulation or a fast-acting drug to prevent the seizure from occurring.

Rett syndrome (RTT): A pervasive developmental disorder characterized by the development of several specific deficits after an apparently normal prenatal and perinatal period, including deceleration in head growth, loss of purposeful hand skills with deterioration into stereotypical hand movements, impairment in expressive and receptive language, and significant psychomotor retardation.

screening: Examination of a group of usually asymptomatic individuals to detect those with a high probability of having a given disease, typically by means of an inexpensive diagnostic test. Also, in the mental health professions, initial patient evaluation that includes medical and psychiatric history, mental status evaluation, and diagnostic formulation to determine the patients suitability for a particular treatment modality.

seizure focus: An area of the brain where seizures originate.

seizure triggers: Phenomena that trigger seizures in some people.

sign language: Method of communication for people who are deaf or hard of hearing in which hand movements, gestures, and facial expressions convey grammatical structure and meaning.

The Small Business Health Options Program (SHOP): The SHOP marketplace makes it possible for small businesses to provide qualified health plans to their employees.

specific language impairment (SLI): Difficulty with language or the organized-symbol system used for communication in the absence of problems such as mental retardation, hearing loss, or emotional disorders.

speech disorder: Any defect or abnormality that prevents an individual from communicating by means of spoken words. Speech disorders may develop from nerve injury to the brain, muscular paralysis, structural defects, hysteria, or mental retardation.

speech-language pathologist (SLP): Health professional trained to evaluate and treat people who have voice, speech, language, or swallowing disorders (including hearing impairment) that affect their ability to communicate.

status epilepticus: A potentially life-threatening condition in which a seizure is abnormally prolonged.

stuttering: A speech disorder in which sounds, syllables, or words are repeated or prolonged, disrupting the normal flow of speech.

Surveillance (also known as 'tracking'): In public health, surveillance is defined as the continuous, systematic collection, analysis, and interpretation of health-related data.

temporal lobe epilepsy: The most common epilepsy syndrome with focal seizures.

temporal lobe resection: A type of surgery for temporal lobe epilepsy in which all or part of the affected temporal lobe of the brain is removed.

tonic-clonic seizures: Seizures that cause a mixture of symptoms, including loss of consciousness, stiffening of the body, and repeated jerks of the arms and legs.

Tourette syndrome (TS): Neurological disorder characterized by recurring movements and sounds (called tics).

tuberous sclerosis: Tuberous sclerosis is a rare genetic disorder that causes benign tumors to grow in the brain as well as in other vital organs. It has a consistently strong association with ASD.

vagus nerve stimulator (VNS): A surgically implanted device that sends short bursts of electrical energy to the brain via the vagus nerve and helps some individuals reduce their seizure activity.

Chapter 57

Directory of Additional ASD Resources

Government Organizations

Agency for Healthcare Research and Quality (AHRQ)
5600 Fishers Ln.
Seventh Fl.
Rockville, MD 20857
Phone: 301-427-1104
Website: www.ahrq.gov

Brain Resources and Information Network (BRAIN)
P.O. Box 5801
Bethesda, MD 20824
Toll-Free: 800-352-9424
Fax: 301-402-2186
Website: www.ninds.nih.gov/
Disorders/Support-Resources/
Gov-Organizations
E-mail: braininfo@ninds.nih.gov

CDC Act Early
Centers for Disease Control and Prevention (CDC)
1600 Clifton Rd.
Atlanta, GA 30329-4027
Toll-Free: 800-CDC-INFO (800-232-4636)
Toll-Free TTY: 888-232-6348
Website: www.cdc.gov/ncbddd/
actearly/index.html

Resources in this chapter were compiled from several sources deemed reliable; all contact information was verified and updated in October 2018.

479

CDC Autism Information Center

Centers for Disease Control and
Prevention (CDC)
1600 Clifton Rd.
Atlanta, GA 30329-4027
Toll-Free: 800-CDC-INFO
(800-232-4636)
Toll-Free TTY: 888-232-6348
Website: www.cdc.gov/ncbddd/
autism/index.html

Centers for Autism and Developmental Disabilities Research and Epidemiology (CADDRE)

National Center on Birth
Defects and Developmental
Disabilities (NCBDDD)
1600 Clifton Rd.
Atlanta, GA 30329-4027
Toll-Free: 800-CDC-INFO
(800-232-4636)
Toll-Free TTY: 888-232-6348
Website: www.cdc.gov/ncbddd/
autism/caddre.html

Centers for Disease Control and Prevention (CDC)

1600 Clifton Rd.
Atlanta, GA 30329-4027
Toll-Free: 800-CDC-INFO
(800-232-4636)
Toll-Free TTY: 888-232-6348
Website: www.cdc.gov

Office of Disability Employment Policy (ODEP)

U.S. Department of Labor (DOL)
200 Constitution Ave. N.W.
Washington, DC 20210
Toll-Free: 866-487-2365
Website: www.dol.gov/odep

ED Pubs

U.S. Department of Education
(ED)
400 Maryland Ave. S.W.
Washington, DC 20202
Toll-Free: 877-4-ED-PUBS
(877-433-7827)
Toll-Free TTY: 800-877-8339
Website: www.ed.gov/edpubs

Eunice Kennedy Shriver National Institute of Child Health and Human Development (NICHD)

P.O. Box 3006
Rockville, MD 20847
Toll-Free: 800-370-2943
Toll-Free TTY: 888-320-6942
Toll-Free Fax: 866-760-5947
Website: www.nichd.nih.gov
E-mail: NICHDInformation
ResourceCenter@mail.nih.gov

Genetic and Rare Diseases Information Center (GARD)

P.O. Box 8126
Gaithersburg, MD 20898-8126
Toll-Free: 888-205-2311
Phone: 301-251-4925
Toll-Free TTY: 888-205-3223
Fax: 301-251-4911
Website: rarediseases.info.nih.
gov/about-gard/contact-gard

Lister Hill National Center for Biomedical Communications (LHNCBC)
U.S. National Library of Medicine (NLM)
8600 Rockville Pike
Bethesda, MD 20894
Toll-Free: 888-346-3656
Phone: 301-496-4441
Fax: 301-402-0118
Website: lhncbc.nlm.nih.gov

National Institute of Environmental Health Sciences (NIEHS)
P.O. Box 12233
MD K3-16
Research Triangle Park, NC 27709-2233
Phone: 919-541-3345
Fax: 301-480-2978
Website: www.niehs.nih.gov/about/od/ocpl/contact
E-mail: webcenter@niehs.nih.gov

National Institute of Mental Health (NIMH)
6001 Executive Blvd.
Rm. 6200 MSC 9663
Bethesda, MD 20892-9663
Toll-Free: 866-615-6464
Toll-Free TTY: 866-415-8051
TTY: 301-443-8431
Fax: 301-443-4279
Website: www.nimh.nih.gov/index.shtml
E-mail: nimhinfo@nih.gov

National Institute of Neurological Disorders and Stroke (NINDS)
P.O. Box 5801
Bethesda, MD 20824
Toll-Free: 800-352-9424
Phone: 301-496-5751
Website: www.ninds.nih.gov

National Institute on Deafness and Other Communication Disorders (NIDCD)
31 Center Dr.
MSC 2320
Bethesda, MD 20892-2320
Fax: 301-402-0018
Website: www.nidcd.nih.gov
E-mail: nidcdinfo@nidcd.nih.gov

National Database for Autism Research (NDAR)
6001 Executive Blvd.
Rm. 7162 MSC 9640
Bethesda, MD 20892-9645
Phone: 301-443-3265
Website: ndar.nih.gov

Office for Civil Rights (OCR)
U.S. Department of Education (ED)
400 Maryland Ave. S.W.
Washington, DC 20202
Toll-Free: 800-872-5327
Toll-Free TTY: 800-730-8913
Website: www2.ed.gov/about/offices/list/ocr/aboutocr.html

U.S. Department of Education (ED)
400 Maryland Ave. S.W.
Washington, DC 20202
Toll-Free: 800-872-5327
Toll-Free TTY: 800-877-8339
Website: www.ed.gov

U.S. Department of Health and Human Services (HHS)
200 Independence Ave. S.W.
Washington, DC 20201
Toll-Free: 877-696-6775
Website: www.hhs.gov

U.S. Department of Labor (DOL)
200 Constitution Ave. N.W.
Washington, DC 20210
Toll-Free: 866-487-2365
Website: www.dol.gov; www.
disability.gov

U.S. Food and Drug Administration (FDA)
10903 New Hampshire Ave.
Silver Spring, MD 20993
Toll-Free: 888-INFO-FDA
(888-463-6332)
Website: www.fda.gov

U.S. National Library of Medicine (NLM)
8600 Rockville Pike
Bethesda, MD 20894
Toll-Free: 888-346-3656
Phone: 301-496-4441
Fax: 301-402-1384
Website: www.nlm.nih.gov
E-mail: custserv@nlm.nih.gov

U.S. Office of Personnel Management (OPM)
1900 E. St. N.W.
Washington, DC 20415-1000
Phone: 202-606-1800
Toll-Free TTY: 800-877-8339
Website: www.opm.gov

Private Organizations

American Speech-Language-Hearing Association (ASHA)
2200 Research Blvd.
Rockville, MD 20850-3289
Phone: 301-296-5700
TTY: 301-296-5650
Fax: 301-296-8580
Website: www.asha.org

Asperger Syndrome
Autism Spectrum Coalition
P.O. Box 524
Crown Point, IN 46308
Website: www.
aspergersyndrome.org

Asperger Syndrome Education Network (ASPEN)
9 Aspen Cir.
Edison, NJ 08820
Phone: 732-321-0880
Website: www.aspennj.org

Association for Behavior Analysis International (ABAI)
550 W. Centre Ave.
Portage, MI 49024
Phone: 269-492-9310
Website: www.abainternational.
org/welcome.aspx

Association for Science in Autism Treatment (ASAT)
P.O. Box 1447
Hoboken, NJ 07030
Website: www.asatonline.org
E-mail: info@asatonline.org

Autism National Committee (AUTCOM)
Website: www.autcom.org

Autism Network International (ANI)
P.O. Box 35448
Syracuse, NY 13235-5448
Website: www.
autismnetworkinternational.org

Autism Research Institute (ARI)
Website: www.autism.com/index.
asp

Autism Science Foundation (ASF)
106 W. 32nd St.
Ste. 182
New York, NY 10001
Phone: 914-810-9100
Website: www.
autismsciencefoundation.org
E-mail: contactus@
autismsciencefoundation.org

Autism Society of America (ASA)
4340 East-West Hwy
Ste. 350
Bethesda, MD 20814
Toll-Free: 800-328-8476
Website: www.autism-society.
org

Autism Speaks
1 E. 33rd St.
Fourth Fl.
New York, NY 10016
Phone: 646-385-8500
Fax: 212-252-8676
Website: www.autismspeaks.org/
index2.php

Autism Support Network (ASN)
P.O. Box 1525
Fairfield, CT 06824
Phone: 203-404-4929
Fax: 203-404-4969
Website: www.
autismsupportnetwork.com
E-mail: info@
AutismSupportNetwork.com

Autism Today
244 Fifth Ave.
New York, NY 10001
Toll-Free: 866-9AUTISM
(866-928-8476)
Phone: 780-416-4448
Fax: 780-416-4330
Website: www.autismtoday.com
E-mail: sales@autismtoday.com

AutismCares
Website: autismcares.org

AWAARE Collaboration
Website: awaare.
nationalautismassociation.org

483

Birth Defect Research for Children, Inc. (BDRC)
976 Lake Baldwin Ln.
Ste. 104
Orlando, FL 32814
Phone: 407-895-0802
Website: www.birthdefects.org
E-mail: staff@birthdefects.org

Center for Autism and Related Disorders Inc. (CARD)
21600 Oxnard St.
Ste. 1800
Woodland Hills, CA 91367
Toll-Free: 855-345-2273
Phone: 818-345-2345
Fax: 818-758-8015
Website: www.centerforautism.com

Center on Technology and Disability (FCTD)
Website: www.ctdinstitute.org
E-mail: ctd@fhi360.org

Children's Craniofacial Association (CCA)
13140 Coit Rd.
Ste. 517
Dallas, TX 75240
Toll-Free: 800-535-3643
Phone: 214-570-9099
Fax: 214-570-8811
Website: www.ccakids.com
E-mail: contactCCA@ccakids.com

Easterseals
141 W. Jackson Blvd.
Ste. 1400A
Chicago, IL 60604
Toll-Free: 800-221-6827
Website: www.easterseals.com

FHI 360
359 Blackwell St.
Ste. 200
Durham, NC 27701
Phone: 919-544-7040
Website: www.fhi360.org

First Signs, Inc.
P.O. Box 358
Merrimac, MA 01860
Website: disabilityinfo.org/records/first-signs-inc
E-mail: FirstSigns1@gmail.com

Guiding Eyes for the Blind
611 Granite Springs Rd.
Yorktown Heights, NY 10598
Toll-Free: 800-942-0149
Phone: 914-245-4024
Fax: 914-245-1609
Website: www.guidingeyes.org

Indiana Resource Center for Autism (IRCA)
Indiana Institute on Disability and Community (IIDC)
1905 N. Range Rd.
Bloomington, IN 47408-9801
Toll-Free: 800-825-4733
Phone: 812-855-6508
Fax: 812-855-9630
Website: www.iidc.indiana.edu/pages/irca

Interactive Autism Network (IAN)
Kennedy Krieger Institute (KKI)
707 N. Bdwy.
Baltimore, MD 21205
Website: www.ianresearch.org
E-mail: ian@kennedykrieger.org

International Rett Syndrome Foundation
4600 Devitt Dr.
Cincinnati, OH 45246
Toll-Free: 800-818-7388
Phone: 513-874-3020
Fax: 513-874-2520
Website: www.rettsyndrome.org
E-mail: admin@rettsyndrome.
org

March of Dimes
1275 Mamaroneck Ave.
White Plains, NY 10605
Toll-Free: 888-MODIMES
(888-663-4637)
Website: www.marchofdimes.org

Medical Home Implementation
c/o American Academy of
Pediatrics (AAP)
345 Park Blvd.
Itasca, IL 60143
Toll-Free: 800-433-9016
Phone: 630-626-6605
Website: medicalhomeinfo.aap.
org/Pages/Contact.aspx
E-mail: medical_home@aap.org

Moebius Syndrome Foundation
P.O. Box 147
Pilot Grove, MO 65276
Toll-Free: 844-MOEBIUS
(844-663-2487)
Website: www.
moebiussyndrome.org
E-mail: info@moebiussyndrome.
org

National Center on Accessible Instructional Materials at Cast, Inc.
40 Harvard Mills Sq.
Ste. 3
Wakefield, MA 01880-3233
Phone: 781-245-2212
Website: aem.cast.org
E-mail: aem@cast.org

National Organization for Rare Disorders (NORD)
55 Kenosia Ave.
Danbury, CT 06810
Phone: 203-744-0100
Fax: 203-263-9938
Website: www.rarediseases.org

Operation Autism
2000 N. 14th St.
Ste. 240
Arlington, VA 22201
Toll-Free: 866-366-9710
Website: www.
operationautismonline.org

PACER Center
8161 Normandale Blvd.
Bloomington, MN 55437
Toll-Free: 800-537-2237
Phone: 952-838-9000
Fax: 952-838-0199
Website: www.pacer.org

Parent Center Hub
Center for Parent Information
and Resources (CPIR)
35 Halsey St.
Fourth Fl.
Newark, NJ 07102
Phone: 973-642-8100
Website: www.parentcenterhub.
org

Resource Guide for Military Families

Center for Autism & Related Disabilities (CARD)
University of South Florida (USF)
13301 Bruce B. Downs Blvd.
MHC 2113A
Tampa, FL 33612-3899
Toll-Free: 800-333-4530
Phone: 813- 974-2532
Fax: 813-905-9812
Website: card-usf.fmhi.usf.edu
E-mail: card-usf@usf.edu

Organization for Autism Research (OAR)
2000 N. 14th St.
Ste. 300
Arlington, VA 22201
Toll-Free: 866-366-9710
Website: researchautism.org
E-mail: info@researchautism.org

PEDSTest
1013 Austin Ct.
Nolensville, TN 37135
Toll-Free: 877-296-9972
Phone: 615-776-4121
Fax: 615-776-4119
Website: www.pedstest.com
E-mail: evpress@pedstest.com

Rehabilitation Engineering and Assistive Technology Society of North America (RESNA)
1560 Wilson Blvd.
Ste. 850
Arlington, VA 22209
Phone: 703-524-6686
Fax: 703-524-6630
Website: www.resna.org
E-mail: info@resna.org

Rett Syndrome Research Trust (RSRT)
67 Under Cliff Rd.
Trumbull, CT 06611
Phone: 203-445-0041
Website: www.reverserett.org
E-mail: info@rsrt.org

Tourette Association of America (TAA)
42-40 Bell Blvd.
Ste. 205
Bayside, NY 11361
Toll-Free: 888-4-TOURET
(888-486-8738)
Website: tourette.org
E-mail: support@tourette.org

Index

Index

N